DATE DUE

FEB - 3 1997	
NOV 2 4 1998	
APR 1 7 1999	
SEP 2 9 1999	
FEB 3 0 2001	
OCT 5 2001	

BRODART   Cat. No. 23-221

IMPROVING QUALITY AND PERFORMANCE

Concepts, Programs, and Techniques

IMPROVING QUALITY AND PERFORMANCE

Concepts, Programs, and Techniques

Patricia Schroeder, RN, MSN

Nursing Quality Consultant
Quality Care Concepts, Inc.
Thiensville, Wisconsin

with 94 illustrations

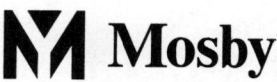 Mosby

St. Louis Baltimore Boston Chicago London Madrid Philadelphia Sydney Toronto

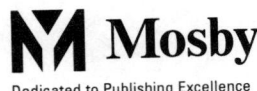

Mosby

Dedicated to Publishing Excellence

Executive Editor: N. Darlene Como
Associate Developmental Editor: Brigitte Pocta
Project Manager: Barbara Bowes Merritt
Editing and Production: Carlisle Publishers Services
Designer: Betty Schulz

Printed in the United States of America
Composition by Carlisle Communications, Ltd.
Printing/binding by Maple Vail–Binghamton

Mosby–Year Book, Inc.
11830 Westline Industrial Drive
St. Louis, Missouri 63146

Library of Congress Cataloging in Publication Data

Improving quality and performance : concepts, programs, and techniques
/ [edited by] Patricia Schroeder. — 1st ed.
    p.   cm.
    Includes bibliographical references and index.
    ISBN 0-8016-7003-9
    1. Total quality management.   2. Nursing—Quality control.
3. Medical care—Quality control.   I. Schroeder, Patricia S.
    [DNLM: 1. Quality Assurance, Health Care.   2. Nursing Services—
standards.   3. Nursing Care—standards.   WY 100 T348 1994]
RT85.5.I55   1994
610.73'068'5 — dc20
DNLM/DLC
for Library of Congress   93-2547
                                                                  CIP

93 94 95 96 97 / 9 8 7 6 5 4 3 2 1

CONTRIBUTORS

P. Mardeen Atkins, BSN, RN

Manager, Nursing Quality Management
Cleveland Clinic Foundation
Cleveland, Ohio

Dawn Bailey, BSN, RN

Nurse Manager
Cleveland Clinic Foundation
Cleveland, Ohio

Lori Blashford, BSN, RN

Staff Nurse
Cleveland Clinic Foundation
Cleveland, Ohio

Mary Ellen Blatt, BSN, RN, CNN

Nurse Manager
Cleveland Clinic Foundation
Cleveland, Ohio

Lisa A. Bonadonna, RN, MS

Director, Staff Support
Medical University of South Carolina Medical Center
Charleston, South Carolina

Catherine J. Buck, MS, RN

Patient Care Director—Dialysis Unit
Froedert Memorial Lutheran Hospital
Milwaukee, Wisconsin

Sharon J. Coulter, MN, MBA, RN

Chairman, Division of Nursing
Cleveland Clinic Foundation
Cleveland, Ohio

Cheryl Czech, RN, C

Cardiac Floor Section Leader
Bellin Hospital
Green Bay, Wisconsin

Geri Day, MS, RN, CPHQ

Quality, Standards, and Research Specialist
Bon Secours Hospital
Grosse Pointe, Michigan

Barbara Dianda-Martin

Manager, Cardiac Surgical Intensive Care
St. Vincent Medical Center
Toledo, Ohio

Rita S. Fogel, MS, RN, CNA

Associate Administrator for Nursing Education
Quality Improvement and Research
Long Island Jewish Medical Center
New Hyde Park, New York

Mary E. Geary, MN, RN, ARNP

Clinical Nurse Specialist
Lakeland Regional Medical Center
Lakeland, Florida

Beatrice Hessen, RN, C

Staff Nurse
Bon Secours Hospital
Grosse Pointe, Michigan

Mimi Jenko, MN, RN

Clinical Nurse Specialist
formerly, Lakeland Regional Medical Center
Lakeland, Florida

Pete Knox, BS, MS

Quality Education Manager
Bellin Hospital
Green Bay, Wisconsin

Judy Malinowski, BSN, RN, C

Nurse Manager
Bon Secours Hospital
Grosse Pointe, Michigan

Nancy E. Miller, RN, MS

Nurse Specialist—QA and Special Projects
Beth Israel Hospital
Boston, Massachusetts

G. John Pandl, MSW, MBA

Director of Continuous Quality Improvement
Froedert Memorial Lutheran Hospital
Milwaukee, Wisconsin

Lenard L. Parisi, MS, RN

QA Coordinator—Critical Care
The New York Hospital
New York, New York

Patricia Schroeder, MSN, RN

Nursing Quality Consultant
Quality Care Concepts, Inc.
Thiensville, Wisconsin

Sandra Shumway, MSN, RN

Assistant to the Chairman, Division of Nursing
Cleveland Clinic Foundation
Cleveland, Ohio

Elaine L. Smith, MS, RN, CNA

Assistant Director of Nursing Education
Long Island Jewish Medical Center
New Hyde Park, New York

Toni C. Smith, EdD, RN

Program Director, Nursing Methods, Procedures,
and Quality
Assistant Professor
University of Rochester Medical Center
Strong Memorial Hospital
Rochester, New York

Rhonda R. Stockard, RN, MS

Assistant Vice President for Nursing Quality Assurance, Education, and Research
St. Vincent Medical Center
Toledo, Ohio

Pamela A. Triolo, PhD, RN

formerly, Director, Quality Management Training and
Development
University of Iowa Hospitals and Clinics
Iowa City, Iowa
currently, Chief Nursing Officer, University Hospital
and Assistant Dean, College of Nursing
University of Nebraska Medical Center
Omaha, Nebraska

Jo Marie Walrath, RN, MS

Director of Nursing
The Johns Hopkins Hospital
Baltimore, Maryland

Jean Walters, MS, RN

Vice President
Patient Care Services
Froedert Memorial Lutheran Hospital
Milwaukee, Wisconsin

Cathleen Krueger Wilson, PhD, RN

Senior Partner
Specialty Applications
Scottsdale, Arizona

Janet E. Yskes, BSN, RN

Staff Nurse
Critical Care Unit
Bellin Hospital
Green Bay, Wisconsin

To my family

Steve and *Amy*
Walter and *Irene*
Jeanne, Chuck, Mike, Liz, and *Tim*—

A very high quality group—
With much love and gratitude

PREFACE

Improving quality and performance has become the commitment of the 1990s for health care organizations. Society, enamored of industrial models for quality improvement and outraged at spiraling health care costs, is calling for the use of new approaches to quality. Governmental, regulatory, and accrediting agencies have labeled quality improvement as the key to many of the overwhelming problems in the U.S. health care system. Health care professionals and organizations have begun to commit to the philosophies of quality improvement with unprecedented energy and resources. Quality improvement holds the potential for creating a new paradigm for health care delivery.

Beyond the passion and enthusiasm, however, lies a mandate. The Joint Commission on Accreditation of Healthcare Organizations has incorporated expectations for quality and performance improvement in its standards for accreditation. This mandate has created more than a little concern. Those agencies that have been the forerunners in adopting quality improvement principles and programs have no more than five years of experience, a time span considered by industry to be minimal and premature in disclosing program benefits. Can multiple health care agencies across the United States reasonably adopt approaches that are relatively untested in health care settings, with evidence of success that is only now being demonstrated?

This book describes the concepts, programs, and tools and techniques used in quality improvement. It is intended to provide real-world perspectives on this evolving science. It demonstrates that quality improvement is a powerful tool to positively change care and service, yet it is not fast, not foolproof, and not without a need for major investment in people and other resources.

Commitment to quality improvement may be the most significant action we can take to move forward into the 21st century, but it cannot be considered a religion or be undertaken with blind obedience. Quality improvement must be considered a science and a process that require personal and organizational commitment, continuous critical thinking, and a willingness to create change to meet the needs of patients, families, and other customers.

Improving Quality and Performance: Concepts, Programs and Techniques is a book rich with insight and examples. Section I addresses the building blocks of improving quality in organizations. Chapters describe QI concepts, programs, techniques, and roles. They blend theory, literature, and practical experience, and can serve as an ongoing reference for clinical settings.

Section II provides examples of quality improvement activities carried out in health care settings. These chapters reflect hospital-based activities, because hospitals generally have been the first settings of care delivery to adopt QI approaches. As you will see, however, the experiences can be applied to other health care settings. The chapters reflect organizations at various stages in QI implementation, from those that began a total QI commitment several years ago, to those that have made early steps into the process. Readers will be able to relate to the examples, irrespective of the current state of their own agency.

The examples provided share important lessons about the impact of QI on professionals, organizations, and patients. Authors have graciously shared both their successes and failures in early QI efforts. They show that there is much to learn from industrial examples, but the unique features of health care settings must always be acknowledged. They reinforce the message that QI is not a "magic bullet" and that it requires constant support and nurturing in order to flourish. These authors and organizations are leaders and trailblazers, and we own them a debt for helping us to learn from their experience.

Quality improvement is an exciting opportunity in health care today, one that I believe will be energizing and supportive to nurses in particular. It is a science based on getting to know the *customer* (patients and families), constant attention to better meeting the customer's needs, careful analysis of processes of care and service, empowerment of front-line providers, and collaboration with others. These are all issues that nurses have long sought to achieve. The time has come to create organizationwide approaches to move forward in synchrony. Through strategic efforts and the sharing of our lessons, perhaps the best is yet to be.

ACKNOWLEDGMENTS

Whenever a project requires a prolonged and coordinated effort to complete, there are always those whose participation and support must be acknowledged.

First, and foremost, my thanks to contributing authors, who were generous in sharing their work, but also courageous in their willingness to put forward early experiences and allow others to learn from their examples.

Sincere thanks also goes to Darlene Como, an exceptional woman, friend, and editor, who has taught me much over our 12 years of collaboration; Jackie Katz and Jay Katz, treasured colleagues and friends, who have catalyzed outstanding efforts to improve health care quality, expanded my horizons, made the world a better place, but, most significantly, enriched my life; Madeline Wake and Judith Fitzgerald Miller, leaders whose wisdom, creativity, and mentoring have always served as a beacon to me; and Rhonda Stockard, Len Parisi, Ellie Green, Nancy Gorham, and Cheryl Anderson, valued colleagues whose ideas never cease to inspire me and whose friendship provides invaluable support.

CONTENTS

IMPROVING QUALITY AND PERFORMANCE

Concepts, Programs, and Techniques

SECTION I

IMPROVING QUALITY AND PERFORMANCE

Concepts and Strategies

Section I contains the nuts and bolts for improving quality and performance in health care. It begins with the concepts of quality improvement (QI) and the principles that form the basis of today's continuous quality improvement initiatives. These concepts are then integrated into discussions of programs and models for QI implementation in Chapter 2. While no two models are alike, this chapter describes core components and real-world experiences to plan and effectively implement a QI initiative.

Chapter 3 provides a how-to overview of common QI tools and techniques, and adds examples to help in their application. Chapters 4, 5, and 6 describe functions and roles that are essential to and are significantly affected by QI and its impact. These chapters address the roles of the team facilitator, manager, and staff developers. The examples add depth and perspective to the discussions.

These building blocks will provide readers with the necessary tools to get started on the never-ending journey. They should be considered not so much as a mandatory step-by-step procedure but rather as a map to guide early efforts.

IMPROVING QUALITY AND PERFORMANCE: THE CONCEPTS

Patricia Schroeder

Today's approaches to managing and improving quality in health care are moving in a new and positive direction. While strategies in this movement may vary somewhat among applications in different settings, in general, the new efforts in quality improvement can be characterized as organization-wide, collaborative, enthusiastic, and focused on refining processes of care rather than assigning blame to people. Expectations have been redefined. The goal for quality initiatives in many health care organizations has shifted from achieving accreditation to improving care and service. Philosophically, quality has shifted from mandate to opportunity. Many organizations can accurately claim improvements in both effectiveness and efficiency as a result of this new commitment and approach to quality.

Quality improvement has taken health care by storm. Current concepts about quality and how to achieve it, most notably as applied in manufacturing industries, have been the subject of much discussion, literature, education, and debate. The concepts are being addressed by professional associations, consumer groups, payers, regulators, and accreditors, as well as by the providers and organizations themselves. They are considered the key to survival in the 1990s and beyond.

But what exactly is quality improvement (QI), and how does it relate to health care? This chapter will answer that question and will provide perspectives on the fit of QI initiatives in U.S. health care organizations.

UNDERSTANDING THE TERMS

The field of quality assurance always had a language of its own. Terms were complex, subject to change, and frequently redefined within different settings.

QI also carries a complex changing vocabulary. Even the very term *quality improvement* is not consistently used as the primary label for quality-related concepts. Other labels include the following:

- Continuous quality improvement (CQI)
- Total quality management (TQM)
- Total quality systems (TQS)
- Quality systems improvement (QSI)
- Total quality (TQ)

The list could continue. Most confusingly, while some terms dealing with quality do have unique meanings, many people use the terms interchangeably.

This ongoing problem of vocabulary requires all to look carefully beneath the terms and labels themselves, and to clarify the definitions before making assumptions about an author's ideas. For the purpose of this book, *quality improvement* will be used generically as the label for the new approach described by these terms.

A glossary of QI-related terms is provided. Its terms and definitions may vary slightly from those used in other settings. It is unlikely that terms will be universally defined and used consistently any time soon. It is, therefore, most helpful to seek consistent use of terms within one's own organization or setting.

WHAT IS QUALITY IMPROVEMENT?

Quality improvement is the commitment and approach used to continuously improve every process in every part of an organization, with the intent of meeting and exceeding customer expectations and outcomes. It stimulates individuals and teams to look at the way they deliver care and service, to identify the root causes of problems in systems, and then to innovate to make improvements. QI integrates strategic leadership, an empowered workforce, and a data-driven effort to refine one's product and service constantly. It is a long-term approach, established through incremental steps: it is an approach that must be tailored to the setting, service, people, and consumers of an organization.

Some consider QI a management approach. Others see it as an attitude or mindset. All concur that QI goes far beyond a set of techniques or a circumscribed "program," and instead is a way of "being" for organizations. QI is a way of doing business that pervades every aspect of the organization.

Discussions of QI in the United States frequently identify it as a paradigm shift in American organizations (with *paradigm* defined as one's fundamental beliefs about something, the model on which thought and action is based). QI has wrought a significant

Twelve Paradigm Shifts to World-Class Quality	
Former Paradigm	**New Paradigm**
Control management	Commitment management
Task-focused	Process- and customer-focused
Command decisions	Consensus decisions
Individual work	Teamwork
Experts and labor	Experts all
Control through punishment and fear	Control through positive reinforcement
One right way	Continuous improvement
Record-keeping	Scorekeeping
Tall and rigid structure	Flat and flexible structure
Unstated values and vision	Shared values and vision
Tough on people	Tough on competition
Wealth-exploiting	Wealth-creating

change in thinking about quality and its pursuit in the workplace generally and in health care specifically. This change is summarized in the "Twelve Paradigm Shifts to World Class Quality" (Miller and Howard, 1991, p. 228), shown in the box above. These shifts describe different approaches to organizational structure, management, work design, and attitudes. They speak to a new organization, one that is refocused on its mission.

It is essential to note, however, that the move to quality improvement is not the first time that health care in general and nursing in particular have identified a need for new approaches. In fact, aspects of these paradigm shifts have been identified over the years in discussions of decentralization, work redesign, shared governance, and general team building. Nurse leaders have long sought to implement many of these changes under other labels or titles.

A crucial aspect of quality improvement, one often cited as a major strength, is its organizational focus. That is, it emphasizes that all facets and members of the organization will move with identified principles, thereby providing a synergy to efforts. This synergy extends beyond the organization because QI also is strongly understood and supported by many external customers of health care, including patients and families, payers, business, and government. External customers may also include health care services, settings, and providers involved before or after the time of health care delivery. The global nature of quality improvement is a strength that may serve to increase the likelihood that the goals of QI can be achieved in organizations.

THE LEADERS AND THEIR CONCEPTS

The concepts of quality improvement have been attributed to work that stems from at least as far back as the 1920s. Shewhart, Deming, Juran, Ishikawa, Fiegenbaum, and Crosby are some of the names most commonly acknowledged as forerunners.

The three gurus of quality most frequently cited in the United States today are W. Edwards Deming, Joseph Juran, and Philip Crosby. Fig. 1-1 spells out the major tenets of their work (Cambridge Research Institute Management Consultants, 1992).

Deming, an American engineer and statistician, is perhaps the most well known of the three. His early efforts, in a post–World War II society, launched Japan on its internationally renowned quest for quality (Walton, 1986). Deming's frequently cited 14 points have been described as "changing the philosophy of the organization, empowering the worker to be more productive, and leadership and teambuilding" (Dieneman, 1992, p. 25). Deming's principles have been applied in a variety of manufacturing and service settings, and are considered the most commonly used framework for QI efforts.

Juran, also a participant in the Japanese quality transition of the 1940s and 50s, developed a trilogy to guide quality improvement, which includes quality planning, quality control, and quality improvement. He is also attributed with addressing the costs of poor quality, which include wasted efforts, extra expenses, and defects.

Crosby came to international prominence in 1979 with the book *Quality Is Free*. His 14 steps emphasize quality as "conformance to requirements" and prevention systems to assure zero defects.

The approaches proposed by Deming, Juran, and Crosby contain key conceptual differences. Some of these have been summarized by the Cambridge Research Institute Management Consultants (see the box on p. 6). Beyond these distinctions, however, are many more common tenets. All three, as well as the other aforementioned leaders, believe QI to be an unceasing, organization-wide effort that focuses on improving processes of work rather than blaming people for errors. Customers of the service or industry must be identified, and their needs must be met. Teamwork and innovation must guide the organization to greater effectiveness and efficiency.

MAJOR PREMISES OF QUALITY IMPROVEMENT

Certain major premises or concepts underlie quality improvement, irrespective of the model, and will be discussed here. They are focus on organizational mission, continuous improvement, customer orienta-

Deming's 14 Points	Crosby's 14 Steps	Juran Trilogy
1. Create constancy of purpose	1. Management commitment	*I. Quality Planning*
2. Adopt the new philosophy	2. Quality improvement team	1. Determine customers
3. Cease dependence on inspection	3. Quality measurement	2. Determine customers' needs
4. End the practice of awarding business on the basis of price	4. Cost-of-quality evaluation	3. Develop products for customers
5. Improve constantly	5. Quality awareness	4. Develop processes to produce products
6. Institute training on the job	6. Correction action	*II. Quality Control*
7. Institute leadership	7. Ad hoc committee for zero defects	1. Evaluate performance
8. Drive out fear	8. Supervise training	2. Compare performance to goals
9. Break down barriers between departments	9. Zero defects day	3. Act on differences
10. Eliminate slogans, exhortations	10. Goal setting	*III. Quality Improvement*
11. Eliminate work standards (quotas). Eliminate management by objectives	11. Error-cause removal	1. Establish infrastructure
12. Remove barriers to employees	12. Recognition	2. Identify needs for improvement/projects
13. Institute education	13. Quality councils	3. Establish project teams
14. Transform everyone's job	14. Do it over again	4. Provide teams with: • Resources • Motivation • Training

Four Quality Absolutes

1. Quality defined as conformance to requirements, not "goodness"
2. The system for causing quality is prevention, not appraisal
3. The performance standard must be zero defects, not "that's close enough"
4. The measurement of quality is the price of nonconformance, not indexes

Fig. 1-1 Guru overview. *Modified with permission of Cambridge Research Institute Management Consultants, Cambridge, Mass.*

tion, leadership commitment, empowerment, collaboration/crossing boundaries, focus on processes, and focus on data and statistical thinking.

Focus on Organizational Mission

Quality requires consistent efforts toward achievement of the organization's mission. The mission of any organization is its basic purpose and reason for being. If the mission is to be achieved, it must be:

• Articulated in a mission statement
• Understood by all members of the organization
• Valued
• Visible
• Used consistently to guide all plans, goals and actions

The organization's mission must guide both short- and long-range efforts.

McCabe (1992) suggests that the process of vertical alignment will assist individuals and departments in understanding and working toward the organization's mission. Vertical alignment threads mission-focused goals, plans, and efforts through all organizational levels, from the individual employee to the governing board. Measurable quality goals, linked to the mission, must be identified in job descriptions, performance plans, and department expectations. This alignment of people and efforts will move the organization in a consistent and positive direction. As decentralization proceeds or key processes change, it is the mission that keeps the organization moving in a planned and consistent direction.

Continuous Improvement

Quality improvement (or continuous quality improvement) is grounded in the premise that every plan, every effort, every process, can always be made better. Rather than striving to achieve an arbitrary endpoint or threshold, or attempting to only solve a problem, organizations must make efforts to get better constantly.

Continuous improvement requires deep valuing of the consumer (both internal and external) and a commitment to critical thinking and innovation. It also creates a different organization, replacing the tradi-

---

Some Conceptual Differences

- Crosby believes in slogans. Deming insists on eliminating slogans.
- Deming says drive out fear. Juran states, "Fear can bring out the best in people."
- Juran focuses on the "vital few versus the trivial many." For Crosby, no problem is too small to address.
- For training, Deming stresses statistical techniques. Juran emphasizes quality management processes and problem-solving techniques. Crosby's training is targeted toward developing a new quality culture.
- Juran and Crosby focus on the cost of quality as the main quality measurement tool and use it to select quality improvement projects. Deming opposes the use of cost of quality as a measurement tool, because, he says, the largest factor—customer satisfaction—is left out.
- Deming emphasizes quality as being "a predictable degree of uniformity and dependability," Juran as "fitness of use" or correspondence to customers' needs, and Crosby as "zero defects" or conformance to requirements.
- Deming's thrust is to identify systemic quality problems and PDCA; Juran's is to identify customers and their needs and to start the QI process in a project-by-project or "breakthrough sequence" way; and Crosby's main thrust rests in his ability to launch an improvement process, removing the causes of error, changing the culture.

Modified with permission of Cambridge Research Institute Management Consultants, Cambridge, Mass.

---

tional protection of the status quo with a willingness, even eagerness, to change. Flexibility is coupled with an eternal quest for improvement.

Zuckerman and Hatala (1992, pp. 66-69) believe, however, that this premise may present a significant problem in American society. Their research suggests that workers in the American culture do not innately embrace the concepts of diligent pursuit of continuous improvement toward a goal of perfection. Whereas the Japanese can be totally dedicated to incremental improvement and getting closer and closer to market expectations, Americans as a culture often find this constrictive and boring. Americans, Zuckerman and Hatala suggest, may actually need crises to occur before they provide all-out efforts to improve. Periodic crises are likewise necessary to maintain excitement, energy, and interest in quality.

Organizational cultures as well as societal cultures must hear and live the message that improving quality is a dynamic process necessary for all. Organizations that survive will be those that constantly seek to get better at meeting customer needs. Quality cannot be considered a destination. It must be considered an ongoing journey.

Customer Orientation

Quality is increasingly defined as meeting and exceeding customer expectations. This idea involves a dramatic shift for health care, which previously defined quality solely from professional perspectives. All quality improvement initiatives emphasize an identification of one's customers as well as the unique needs those customers seek to meet. One can provide products and services of quality only if one has a clear understanding of the needs of the customer.

Customers can be specified as internal and external customers. Internal customers are persons within the organization who depend on our performance in order to perform well themselves. This might be a colleague covering one's caseload on the next shift, a housekeeper cleaning a unit prior to a patient's admission, or a pharmacist requiring patient-data follow-up. External customers are those from outside the organization who depend on our performance to meet their needs. External customers include patients and families, payer groups, physicians not employed by the organization, and the government.

The terms *customer* and *consumer* have been difficult for many health care providers to accept, despite their generic use in QI discussions. Some observers anecdotally report that it demeans the professional relationship or suggests a more trivial commitment to service. As terms, however, *customer* and *consumer* are used frequently in other industries, including service industries. While they may be difficult words to use, they are part of a consistent language for quality improvement that transcends peculiarities of specific businesses and industries.

Leadership Commitment

Theory and experience show unequivocally that quality improvement efforts will not succeed in an organization unless senior managers commit to personal, long-term involvement. Such involvement is necessary to achieve the following:

- Emphasize the value and importance of quality
- Establish a pervasive commitment to quality that runs through all levels of an organization
- Allocate resources and support for quality

Improving quality is not fast or easy. To move forward requires consensus building and strategy. It is imperative, then, that the quality initiative be established from a position of strength. The involvement of senior managers, providing day-to-day attention to improving the organization's product or service, is a serious message of the importance of quality. "Quality improvement can sprout from the middle, but only leaders can help it take root as a companywide organizational strategy," write Berwick, Godfrey, and Roessner (1990, p. 157). Leaders must plan changes, deploy methods, and integrate quality throughout the corporate strategy.

Empowerment

Quality improvement is grounded in the concept that the people on the front line of production or service delivery know their product and customers better than anyone else. From the QI perspective, employees are not seen as perpetrators of problems, but as the organization's greatest resource. Empowerment may be viewed as placing decision making as close as possible to the front line of service, or as helping others to use the personal, professional, or situational power that they already possess. The key to improvement is to empower these people through infrastructures that promote increased participation and shared authority. Wilson (1992, p. 132) suggests that participation falls into four broad categories: goal setting, decision making, problem solving, and participating in the change process. This degree of involvement not only increases the quality of the product, but it also increases productivity and job satisfaction and decreases overall costs.

To be effective, empowerment must move beyond a statement and into a planning and action mode. Employees must be prepared for their new, participative role. Knowledge and skills as well as experience and support are needed to make this extensive workplace change. A long-term commitment is needed, along with a willingness to support the model, even when the decisions reached may not have been the same as those of senior managers. Shanon (1991, p. 63) writes: "There are no magical ways for leaders to empower themselves and others. It all boils down to simple behavioral changes."

Collaboration/Crossing Boundaries

Despite the vertical, hierarchical structures of most organizations, the majority of functions and processes cross the boundaries of disciplines and departments. Completing even the most simple act often depends on the actions of other people, on the availability of space and supplies, and on issues of time (what happened before a patient arrived for a test, or what follows today's situation). Changing and improving these functions and processes, therefore, also requires the input of all involved, with everyone working as a collaborative team to achieve a quality goal.

A hallmark of quality improvement is the use of collaborative teams to analyze and improve functions and processes. These teams, representing diverse disciplines, functions, and viewpoints, are able to identify different and at times simultaneous strategies necessary to improve. Team members are selected, based on being a stakeholder in the process. Through the use of group-process techniques, group members seek to identify their viewpoints and perspectives, analyze the process, seek the root causes of problems or defects, and initiate changes across the organization to create process improvements.

The effectiveness of multidisciplinary teams is based on many factors, including the selection and training of key team members, the use of group-process skills by leaders and members of groups, effective collection and use of data, and efforts toward integrative decision making. Teams are most successful when members cross traditional lines of authority and adopt a shared decision-making approach (Fargason and Haddock, 1992).

Focus on Processes

Failures in quality most commonly are the result not of faulty people but of faulty processes. Quality improvement concepts emphasize that improvement will happen when we stop assigning blame and instead study and change the way the system works.

All activities carried out in an organization can be described in terms of processes. *Processes* are a series or set of actions carried out to achieve a certain result. In health care, the kinds of processes carried out can be clinical (e.g., postoperative wound care), managerial (e.g., feedback on performance), or systems-oriented (e.g., ordering supplies) (Katz and Green 1992).

Processes are usually complex, and they are linked to what preceded and what follows specific actions. That is, actions are rarely isolated; they first are related to input, or what preceded the current state of being. For example: Are the needed supplies present? Are people appropriately trained? Is time available? Is the equipment useful and effective? Attention to improving inputs is the essence of "building quality" into a product or service.

Actions are also linked to outputs or those things that follow them. For example: Were the actions effective? Did they meet presenting needs? In what ways did the end results change the situation? Inputs, actions, and outputs/outcomes are interrelated, and effective improvements must take all three into consideration.

Most processes are carried out in a variable way. That is, they may be done differently by different people, at different times of the day, or in different departments. Some of the greatest opportunities to create improved care and service, as well as to increase efficiency and cost savings, is to understand and control (and ultimately decrease) process variation. Variation may be minor or significant, and may be related to predictable causes or unique situations. Most of the tools of quality improvement measure or study process variation, and assist in identifying more effective ways to decrease variation when processes are carried out (see chapter 3). Reducing variation in processes has been found to enhance performance and to promote predictable and positive outcomes.

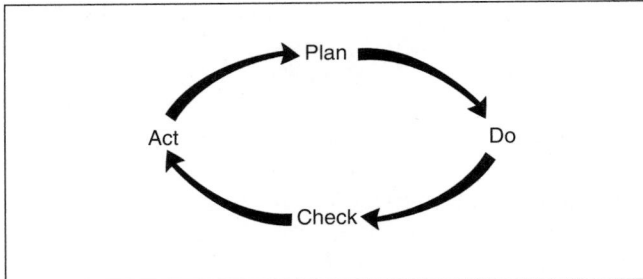

Fig. 1-2 PDCA cycle.

Focus on Data and Statistical Thinking

Traditional QA approaches have provided some basic principles by which health care providers are to use data and statistics in planning change. Imprecise measures and punitive approaches were the common practice and were too often linked with the QA process. These misguided or unproductive approaches were the result of a sparsely stocked bank of solid measures of quality. We too long believed that health care quality was unmeasurable, leaving us hesitant or unwilling to identify or measure it. At other times, data collection was done as an inspection, attempting only to identify those who performed poorly or committed errors rather than to better understand the care/service delivered and how it could be improved. This approach was considered "state of the art," and reflected prevailing thought on authority and organizational culture.

Deming is a strong advocate of the need for data to improve quality. Three key points underlie his beliefs (Walton, 1986, p. 96). First, data are essential to identify and describe process variation. Until one is able to clearly understand the processes and make them consistent, there is little hope for improvement. Second, data must be accurate and put into proper context in order to be useful. Third, one must take care not to depend on statistical methods alone to address quality.

The use of measurement and statistical thinking speaks to the application of scientific methods to the field of quality. Some define this scientific method in terms of the PDCA cycle: that is, Plan, Do, Check, Act (see Fig. 1-2). This process specifies that one should:
Plan
- Identify one's customer groups
- Define their unique needs and the characteristics of quality they hold most dear
- Develop your product or service to meet these needs

Do
- Deliver your product or service

Check
- Continuously measure and analyze key aspects of quality
- Contrast these data to customer needs and expectations (Some suggest this step should be renamed "Study," yielding the PDSA approach.)

Act
- Refine/improve the system and product/service

This scientific method, easily comparable to the nursing process or the Joint Commission on Accreditation's Ten Step Process for Monitoring and Evaluation, can guide the approach to quality. See Fig. 1-3. In all approaches, one uses a logical thinking process that requires careful assessment and planning, the delivery of care/service, measurement, and actions.

Further variations on this scientific method are being coined in today's quality arena. Acronyms being used to describe these improvement processes include FOCUS-PDCA (Hospital Corporation of America); the FADE Method (Organizational Dynamics, Inc.); and the IMPROVE Process (Ernst & Young). While articulated in different ways, there is great similarity in the steps of the approaches.

Quality improvement concepts emphasize continuous measurement of the most significant aspects of processes in an effort to gauge and improve each per-

PDCA Cycle	Ten Step Process	Nursing Process
Plan	1. Responsibility	Assess
	2. Scope of care	Diagnose
	3. Important aspects of care	Plan
	4. Indicators	
	5. Thresholds	
Do	6. Collect data	Intervene
Check	7. Evaluate	Evaluate
Act	8. Take actions	
	9. Reassess	
	10. Communicate findings	

Fig. 1-3 Problem-solving methods.

son's performance, and find ways to improve results. As Berwick, Godfrey, and Roessner (1990, p. 41) put it, "Measurement is used so that everyone can control and improve processes, not so that some people can control other people."

More and better measures of characteristics of quality in health care are needed. But measurement cannot be considered an end in itself. It is in the analysis and in the use of critical and statistical thinking that opportunities for improvement will result. Extreme care must be taken to consider data and statistical tools as a strategy to tailor actions, rather than as the desired outcome.

APPLYING QI TO HEALTH CARE

Though the major concepts of quality improvement hold true from one QI model to another, it is clear that they can be implemented in a variety of ways to tap the strengths or meet the unique needs of various organizations. There is no single right way to address QI, no single approach that is guaranteed to achieve results. Rather, a QI initiative must be carefully tailored to the organization in order to be effective.

The concepts and premises of QI are difficult to dispute, for they are supported by theory, experience, and common sense. Health care management has struggled over the years to integrate its conflicting demands and move toward more effective and efficient care-delivery systems. Quality improvement may be just the vehicle needed in these chaotic times. Some might even suggest that QI is the last opportunity for health care to "repair itself" from within, rather than continuing to court further external regulation. In order to use QI effectively, however, one must clearly understand how it fits into health care organizations.

From QA to QI

While quality improvement brings new perspectives and approaches, it must still be viewed as an evolution of past efforts. The box above summarizes the contrasts between QA and QI. The differences are distinct, but readers must be careful not to interpret these evolutionary contrasts as bad to good, or as ineffective to effective.

Despite the contrasts, traditional QA is grounded in many of the cornerstones of QI. Both QA and QI:
- Are organized approaches intended to improve care/service
- Are linked to structure, process, and outcome
- Include standards, measurement, and actions
- Yield greater impact when many are involved
- Require leadership commitment
- Were mandatory or are strongly encouraged by the Joint Commission on the Accreditation of Health Care Organizations (Schroeder, 1992, pp. 1, 3)

Contrasts between QA and QI	
QA	**QI**
Externally driven	Internally driven
Follows organizational structure	Follows patient care
Delegated to a few	Embraced by all
Focuses on individuals	Focuses on processes
Works toward endpoints	Has no endpoints
"Assures" quality	"Improves" quality
Divided analysis of effectiveness and efficiency, cost and quality	Integrated analysis

Adapted from **William Jessee (1991), presentation at the Eighth Annual Conference of the International Society for Quality Assurance in Health Care, Washington, DC.**

QA has provided many lessons about both health care and quality, and that experience will help with the progression to the next step.

There has been great confusion across the country determining specifically which parts of the quality process will remain through this evolution and which ones will change. Should quality only be addressed in a multidisciplinary fashion? Do standards fit in today's QI approaches? Should the unit-based, discipline-specific QA program be disbanded? As the early flurry around QI begins to settle, the picture becomes more clear. Certain components within the quality function must be present in order to be comprehensive. These include:
- Standards and guidelines
- Individual performance appraisal
- Intradisciplinary assessment and improvement
- Interdisciplinary assessment and improvement
- Organizational culture
- Interorganizational benchmarking

Standards and Guidelines

Standards and guidelines will always be necessary in health care settings. They are tools that reflect the vision, values, and context for care and service. Standards are needed to:
- Establish consistent expectations and patterns for practice (i.e., decrease process variability)
- Articulate what we do, both when we are talking with colleagues and when we are talking with consumers
- Serve as a framework against which we measure, with intent to constantly improve

There is no hope of improving quality if we cannot clearly describe practice. Further, despite the prolific development of standards and guidelines by many groups across the country, these tools must be tailored in health care organizations to reflect the unique setting, practitioners, and patients/families served. While multidisciplinary standards and guidelines (such as case management critical pathways) are a direction for the future, individual disciplines require these tools if each profession is to clearly understand and articulate what it brings to the care arena.

Individual Performance Appraisal

Quality programs are moving away from the approach of looking for "bad apples." There will, however, always be a need for people to receive feedback on their performance. Strategies must be further refined to:

- Assess competence at employment and periodically thereafter
- Provide routine, nonpunitive feedback
- Conduct ongoing personal/professional development

Performance appraisal methods must include self-assessment, peer and leader feedback, some data reflecting quality performance, and an action plan for further development.

The shift away from using performance appraisal as a controlling and often punitive strategy does not, however, eliminate the need to assure professional accountability. Patient safety can never be sacrificed for staff accommodation. Rather, a balance must be achieved between systems accountability and professional accountability, with multiple opportunities taken both to improve the system and to further develop professional capacity.

Intradisciplinary Assessment and Improvement

There will always be a need for groups to assess, analyze, and improve their own performance. There are many unit- and department-specific systems that greatly influence care and service. Examples might include postoperative skin care on the orthopedic unit, promotion of self-care/grooming behaviors on the rehab unit, or accurate ECG interpretation on the telemetry unit. Practice issues like these will not be efficiently addressed if no forum is available, or if the available forum is focused on a broader scope of issues.

Every department has quality issues that can be most efficiently addressed internally. Mechanisms or groups must remain in place to allow that to happen. It is critical that unit-based or department-based quality committees not be disbanded, and instead be focused to:

- Coordinate the department's quality efforts
- Use the best measures, tools, and techniques to analyze and improve care/service

Interdisciplinary Assessment and Improvement

A hallmark of QI initiatives has been the interdisciplinary quality improvement project teams. They are based on the premise that much of health care is interdependent, and requires collaboration across departmental boundaries to analyze and improve. Interdisciplinary groups have been formed to share perspectives and viewpoints, analyze crossfunctional processes of care and service, and innovate to find better approaches to meet customer needs.

The size and number of interdisciplinary project teams may vary from organization to organization. What remains central is:

- The representation in the group of those who own or are affected by the process
- The linking of the input aspect of care/service and output stages of the process to better understand and refine it
- The use of group-process techniques to reach the goal, rather than traditional hierarchical authority or decision making
- Use of measurement and data-driven decisions to create planned change

Organizational Culture

Quality is not the result of a task, regulation, or committee. It is the result of a synergy of people, values, behaviors, and structures that are integrated and focused toward the common goal. While it is relatively easy to establish quality-specific committees or project teams, it is both difficult and time-consuming to take the essential step of reorienting an entire organization toward new values, mindsets, and behaviors.

The establishment of a pervasive quality culture will differentiate the winning organizations from the mediocre ones. Quality improvement, in its truest sense, requires a culture that links quality-related tasks, functions and structures, with all people, elements, and strategies of the organization.

Interorganizational Benchmarking

Striving toward excellence requires an organization to do more than look within itself to improve. It requires it to look beyond its walls, to other organizations that have created excellence in care/service. Benchmarking, according to the Xerox Corporation, is "the continuous process of measuring products, services, and practices against the company's toughest competitors and against companies recognized as industry leaders" (Fenwick, 1991, p. 65).

Benchmarking combines insights of cutting-edge practice with real-world experience. It allows one to gain realistic views of the highest achievements in service or care. As a result, it has been found to be an approach most effective in high-performing organizations. It also shifts the approach to improvement and away from asking the question "How can we make this approach better?" Instead, it allows the organization to say, "This particular example of best practice is achieveable and will be our goal by (a certain deadline)." Then we ask: "What resources will it take? What do we need to do to make it happen?"

Benchmarking is necessary to keep organizations on the cutting edge of best practice, especially in today's rapidly changing environment.

FUTURE DIRECTIONS FOR QUALITY

There are many uncertainties about the future in health care, but one thing remains clear. Quality and its continuous improvement will play a major role. The issue of quality will move far beyond regulation and accreditation, and instead will relate to organizational survival. Those organizations that hold quality as a major value and that aggressively manage for quality will survive and even thrive in the future. Those that maintain focus on short-term financial gains will struggle and fail (Garvin, 1988).

Many American health care organizations are heeding this message and are changing their structures and methods according to QI concepts. This trend is clearly demonstrated in the results of the International Quality Study (IQS) conducted by the American Quality Foundation and Ernst & Young (1992). The IQS as a whole encompassed four nations (United States, Japan, Canada, and Germany) and four specific industries in each country (health care, automotive, banking, and computers). This study is unrivaled in its scope and implications for tracking where we have been and where we are going in the name of quality.

In the study leaders of health care organizations responded to a lengthy set of questions regarding the pursuit of quality in the past (three years previous), the present, and the future (three years hence). The study results provide an advance view of anticipated directions for quality programs for the near future. Key findings regarding the future expectations for U.S. hospitals herald anticipated increases in the following areas:

- Expectations for quality performance and teamwork
- Employee involvement in quality-related meetings
- Employee education regarding quality
- Use of crossfunctional teams to assess and improve quality
- Implementation of process-improvement approaches
- Use of flowcharts and other tools and techniques of quality improvement
- Restructuring of the work of nursing departments to eliminate departmental barriers influencing patient care
- Use of quality measures as a determinant of suppliers (Ernst & Young, American Quality Foundation, 1992)

The IQS validates the expectation that implementation of quality improvement is very much a part of our future in U.S. health care organizations.

CONCLUSION

Quality improvement concepts hold important promise and opportunity for health care organizations. They are not, however, a magical tool that will produce a quick-fix solution to all organizational ills. It is as much a mistake to look at QI concepts as oracles as it is to ignore their obvious potential.

We must continue to study the concepts of QI and their early application in health care settings. We must identify ways to adapt QI concepts to the unique characteristics of health care and settings for care delivery. We must identify other variables, resources, and issues that must be coupled with QI concepts in order to achieve effective end results. Above all, we must maintain the vision for quality improvement not as a committee project or a discrete program, but as a strategic commitment of individuals, departments, and the organization as a whole to better meet patient needs.

REFERENCES

Berwick DM, AB Godfrey, JR Blanton (1990): *Curing health care: new strategies for quality improvement*, San Francisco, Jossey Bass Publishers.

Crosby P (1979): *Quality is free*, New York, McGraw-Hill.

Dieneman J, editor (1992): *Continuous quality improvement in nursing*, Washington, DC, American Nurses Association.

Ernst & Young, American Quality Foundation (1992): *International quality study SM: health care industry report*, Cleveland, American Quality Foundation and Ernst & Young.

Fargason CA, CC Haddock (1992): Cross functional integrative team decision making: essentials for effective QI in health care, *Quality Review Bulletin* 18:157-163, May 1992.

Fenwick AC (1991): Five easy lessons, *Quality Progress* 24(12):63-66, 1991.

Garvin D (1988): *Managing quality: the strategic and competitive edge*, New York, The Free Press.

Jessee W (1991): Presentation at the Eighth Annual Conference of the International Society for Quality Assurance in Health Care, Washington, DC, May 1991.

Katz J, E Green (1992): *Managing quality: a guide to monitoring and evaluating nursing services*, St Louis, Mosby.

McCabe WJ (1992): Total quality management in a hospital, *Quality Review Bulletin* 18(4):134-140, 1992.

Miller M, J Howard (1991): *Managing quality through teams: a workbook for team leaders and members*, Atlanta, Miller Consulting Group Inc.

Oberle J (1990): Quality gurus: the men and their message, *Training*: 47-52, January 1990.

Schroeder P (1992): Quality improvement: evolution or revolution, *Nursing Quality Connection* 1(4):1-3.

Shannon WC: Empowerment: the catchword of the 90s, *Quality Progress* 24(7):62-63, 1991.

Walton M (1986): *The Deming management method*, New York, Dodd, Mead, & Co.

Wilson CK (1992): *Building new nursing organizations: vision and realities*, Gaithersburg, Md, Aspen Publishers Inc.

Zuckerman MK, LJ Hatala (1992): *Incredibly American: releasing the heart of quality*, Milwaukee, ASQC Press.

IMPROVING QUALITY AND PERFORMANCE: THE PROGRAMS

Patricia Schroeder

"Most quality programs fail for one of two reasons. They have system without passion, or passion without system. You must have both," Tom Peters (1987, p. 90) has written. The concepts of quality improvement (QI) often generate a passionate response. That is, the ideas are seen as freeing, logical, and energizing. Yet these concepts will not succeed in establishing a synchronized and effective approach unless they are embodied into an organized program. This chapter will describe such approaches, and strategies for QI program implementation.

It is difficult to discuss the new QI approaches in health care without contrasting them to traditional quality assurance (QA)—a dangerous task for several reasons. First, not all QA programs were the same. While stemming from similar regulations and statutes, there were wide variations in actual QA programs and their degree of success. Some programs labeled "QA" implemented quality improvement concepts without calling them such. Approaches such as decentralization of quality to the level of service, multidisciplinary collaboration, and leadership commitment may have been a part of these programs.

Second, contrasting QA with QI programs often sounds like a comparison of bad and good, old and new, and wrong and right. Evolving approaches to quality improvement cannot be seen in such black-and-white terms. Some aspects of QA programs are the very building blocks of today's QI. For example, clinician involvement, critical thinking skills, quantitative measurements, and the use of standards are all rooted in the science of QA.

Third, the link of quality programs to Joint Commission regulation certainly has affected their structure and function. Programs for QA and QI have been and will be influenced by health care regulation. At times, the differences between the conceptual bases for these two programs may be hard to differentiate from what regulation mandates.

CONTRASTS BETWEEN QA AND QI PROGRAMS

Despite these concerns, it is essential to contrast QA and QI to understand the evolving approach to health care quality improvement and clarify the distinctions. QI programs differ conceptually from traditional QA programs in several ways.

A Larger Scope

Quality improvement programs are more broadly encompassing than traditional QA. They span issues of governance, management, and clinical and support-system performance. They integrate efficiency and effectiveness. They include planning, action, evaluation, and change.

Relative to QA, QI programs, then:
- Are broader in scope
- Require decisions to determine boundaries
- Require involvement of more people
- Require planned integration of information and functions

Coordination at a Higher Organizational Level

Personal involvement of upper managers is essential to the successful implementation of quality improvement philosophies. The quality guru Joseph Juran (1991, p. 82) states, "Upper managers must personally lead the effort. Having observed a great many companies in action, I am unable to point to a single instance in which stunning results were achieved without the active and personal leadership of upper managers. . . . They decided it was not delegatable, it required their personal leadership."

The need for leadership involvement in QI is so great that the first part of the Joint Commission's adapted "Quality Assessment and Improvement" standards address leadership. The leadership expectations remain a part of the Joint Commission's draft standards for "Assessment and Improvement of Organizational Performance," anticipated for 1994.

Quality improvement requires hands-on and visible commitment from those who have power to change the course of the organization and to allocate resources to the efforts.

QI programs, then, tend to:
- Be initiated and coordinated at a higher organizational level
- Require visible commitment from leaders
- Require more day-to-day efforts of upper managers

Collaboration across Boundaries

Traditional QA programs were focused on the role of one discipline. Successful conduct of those quality activities did not require perspective of how the entire organization worked nor did it mandate relationships with other disciplines. Efforts to improve quality stopped at the boundaries of the unit, discipline, turf, and budget.

QI concepts place the internal or external customer, rather than the discipline, as the central focus. Improvement in meeting customer needs can only be achieved through synchronized and consistent efforts of all people, departments, and systems involved.

While departments and disciplines will always have cause to assess and improve some aspects of their own performance, the QI program as a whole must organize the most complex component: those efforts and activities that are collaborative.

QI programs, then:
- Involve all disciplines and roles
- Require a common understanding of and commitment to quality
- Require coordination

Increased Data and Automation Needs

The science of quality improvement, created by engineers, is dependent on data for informed decision making. These data must then be manipulated through the use of statistical and problem-solving tests to create information about the product or service.

The flurry of data demands in health care today has spotlighted many problems in our current data systems. We often collect data that cannot tell us what we need to know. Data are often housed in different data banks and different departments, both of which might make it difficult to gain access or interrelate in a meaningful way. Data demands from outside the organization or departments frequently drain resources from the job of meeting internal data demands.

QI programs, then, require:
- Careful selection of the needed data
- Ongoing data collection
- Supportive automation to integrate data

A Personal Commitment

Commitment to quality requires more than committee participation. Those who participated in past QA programs too often looked at QA as a task or a tool. Phrases such as "I have to do my QAs" or "I'm not involved because I'm not a member this year" or "I've been QA'd" reflect a task-oriented and objectified view.

QI requires not only participation in definitive tasks, but also an extension of that critical thinking

and personal accountability into everyday performance. Ongoing education, decision-making capacity, and rewards must accompany such efforts.

QI, then, requires:
- A new organizational philosophy about quality
- Ongoing education
- Staff empowerment
- Rewards for quality
- Awareness that all roles relate to quality

CREATING A QUALITY IMPROVEMENT PROGRAM

While certain quality concepts are essential and integral to any quality improvement initiative, there is wide divergence in the structures and functions of programs. There is no single correct approach. The following approaches are more commonly used, but none is by any means the only (or necessarily the most effective) approach for each unique organization.

Quality Council

Establishment of a quality council is a common first step in creating a quality improvement program. This council typically is made up of upper managers, department directors, and, usually, a designated QI director or coach, or a consultant. It is commonly chaired by the chief executive officer.

The quality council has many important responsibilities. These include:
- Establishing a personal and organizational commitment to continuous improvement
- Articulating the vision, values, and mission of the organization
- Assessing readiness and preparing the organization for action
- Making decisions about the QA/QI relationship
- Designing the program policies and structure
- Initiating education on QI
- Establishing initial QI project teams
- Creating a plan for QI program extension
- Precipitating change in organizational conduct

The quality council may choose to carry out these responsibilities itself, or it may establish the overall policy and direction for the program and initiate task forces to complete parts of it. For example, the University of Michigan Hospitals used task forces to explore vision and values, management commitment, work reorganization, rewards and recognition, communication and materials, training and education, diversity, and other issues (Marszalek-Gaucher and Coffey, 1990, pp. 99, 102).

In other models used to initiate the QI program, upper managers join with staff members to plan the program implementation and carry out a process-improvement project. A common and necessary theme of all models, however, is the personal and ongoing involvement of upper managers in quality efforts.

Establishing a Personal and Organizational Commitment to Quality

The organizational commitment to improve quality begins an all-encompassing, unwavering, and an initially expensive journey. It holds the promise of uncharted changes, shifted priorities, and unknown results. Further, there are few empirical examples of long-term implications of health care quality improvement programs. These factors make the process a difficult one to start.

Yet, the potentials demonstrated in industry, as well as early success stories in health care, make it clear that the journey is required. If an organization has any possibility of achieving positive results, the QI program must begin with leaders who are prepared for its challenges and are convinced of its merit.

The quality council and organizational leaders must have education in the concepts and techniques of quality improvement. This information will guide future planning, establish a language for quality, be helpful in teaching others, and be useful in day-to-day process improvement. A sound knowledge base in QI will demonstrate a leader's commitment to the approach and the program as a whole.

Furthermore, leaders must begin to share the information and approaches in their day-to-day activities. They must begin to challenge the status quo, and send the message that change is necessary for survival. They must begin to market the concepts and pique the curiosity of others to know more about quality improvement. Raising the general level of awareness and interest will do much to encourage early participation. Early lessons learned about QI implementation at North Florida Regional Medical Center in Gainesville included increasing the staff and manager's awareness of the need to change and constantly reinforcing the premise that all processes can be improved (Duncan et al, 1991, p. 111).

Unless there is a visible, unanimous, and genuine commitment to quality on the part of upper managers and program leaders, coupled with a personal willingness to change, the program will flounder.

Articulating the Mission, Vision, and Values

The first of Deming's 14 points for quality is to "create constancy of purpose for the improvement of product and service" (Walton, 1986, p. 55). This point suggests that organizations can only survive and thrive if they have committed themselves to a long-range purpose and have oriented all functions toward its achievement. In addition, the organization must seek new ways to constantly improve the functions used to gain success.

Creating constancy of purpose requires statements that articulate a consensus view. Three types of statements are commonly used: a mission statement, a vision statement, and core-value statements. Marszalek-Gaucher and Coffey (1990, p. 66) define these statements in the following ways.

- *Mission:* The basic purpose of your organization—often names, types of products and services, customers, market areas, and other basic characteristics of the business.
- *Vision:* The guide to where your organization is going. Particularly important if leaders see the need for a substantial change in direction.
- *Values:* The basic beliefs that are most important to your organization and its workers.

These statements may already be developed in your organization. Attention and revision will be necessary if they are complex and difficult for all to understand, if they are not visible, available, and familiar to all staff, or if their intent is not commonly followed in all aspects of organizational conduct.

Writing or revising the mission and vision statements require input from and careful attention to internal and external customer groups. What do customers need, and how can we meet and exceed their expectations?

Statements of core values guide the way an organization works. They must frame the way we work together in pursuit of the mission and vision. They must come alive in day-to-day interactions, far beyond their visibility as a written document.

Values that are commonly identified in today's programs include customer satisfaction, involvement of all staff, measurement, systematic support, and constant improvement of processes (Doherty, 1990, p. 35). The Air Force Logistics Command summarizes its values as:

Quality = People + Process + Performance
$$+ \text{Product}$$

or "QP4" (Doherty, 1990, p. 34). The University of Michigan, Ann Arbor, defines its values as respect, compassion, integrity, efficiency, and excellence (Marszalek-Gaucher and Coffey, 1990, p. 69).

Attending to the mission, vision, and values of an organization must not be considered an academic exercise. It is the way to chart a direction of where we are going and how we will get there. It underlies the organizational conduct as well as the formal quality improvement program. It must guide the business we do and the way we do it.

Assessing Readiness and Preparing for Action

Preparing for an organizational change requires careful preliminary assessment and planning. Obviously, the point at which we begin this journey will influence how we should proceed.

Some organizations carry out an assessment of their culture, addressing communications, decision making, roles, relationships, effectiveness, efficiency, and employee or internal-customer satisfaction. Patient and external-customer satisfaction is also measured. Such assessments could be comprehensive (more complete, yet time-consuming and expensive) or could focus on select or high-risk (or high-cost) variables. Proprietary agencies and consulting firms are two sources of organizational assessment tools. Many agencies choose to develop their own assessment plan based on available tools in the literature, or tools that they create themselves. The ability to measure future improvement and success might be based on having data available that reflect preprogram status.

In a service industry such as health care, quality comes from people. Establishing an organizational commitment to quality (and a quality improvement program) will be successful only to the extent that people are prepared for it.

Accountability for quality cannot be conveyed by dictate. Bergman (1981) identifies three preconditions to accountability, conditions that must be met before one can expect performance or results. They include (1) knowledge, skills, and values, (2) responsibility, and (3) authority to carry out the charge. To ready the environment for continuous quality improvement, people must learn about the concepts. They must understand and commit themselves to the values held, and see the same in the behavior of others.

A formal quality program will articulate responsibility for quality. If, however, the concepts are to be carried out in all functions of the organization and by all people, commitment to quality should be reflected in other documents, programs, and activities. Quality must be included in job descriptions, performance appraisals, standards, measures, and plans. Consistent vision and values should thread through all parts of the organization.

Finally, authority to carry out the charge will be the visible result of true empowerment of staff and the new role of manager. Staff members must use this authority to create improvements to better meet consumer needs. Such actions must be recognized and rewarded. Accountability must be placed at the level closest to the care or service.

These approaches will require long-term efforts that go far beyond the scope of the quality council and program. As the quality council and upper managers begin the formal quality improvement initiatives, they must simultaneously address other parts of the organization to create a consistent and pervasive approach.

Making Decisions about the QA/QI Relationship

While quality improvement programs have captured the spotlight, quality assurance programs have re-

Models of Relationships between QA and QI
Parallel structures: separate programs QI integrated into non-QA program QA and QI integrated Matrix approach: Core quality program with crossfunctional responsibilities and reporting
General Health Inc., cited by D Barry, editor: Integrating QA and QI: marriage or mayhem? *Quality Exchange* 1(2): 1-3, 9, 1991.

mained a part of the reality of health care settings. Evolving regulatory expectations for quality assurance are most likely the main reason for their presence, yet QA continues to suit a valuable purpose: namely, ongoing review of performance within clinical departments.

Questions such as "Does QI replace QA?" have long stalled the planning and implementation of quality programs. General Health Inc., a health care system in southern Louisiana, has identified four models that alter the QA/QI relationship (see the box above). The most common model is the parallel structure, by which QA and QI are distinctly separate programs, frequently with separate participants, goals, and directions. A second model is to integrate QI into a non-QA program, such as a guest relations program or a human resource or education department. A third model is to restructure the QA to integrate QI. Finally, a matrix approach could be used, with activities carried out by a crossfunctional quality resource group (Barry, 1991, p. 3).

Whatever model is selected for the QA/QI relationship, several key premises should be followed.

1. Be sure that the program plan(s) clearly describe the program(s) focus and boundaries. It should be clear to the potentially uninvolved reader how this program works, what it does, who is involved, and how it differs from other programs.

2. Build a common language for quality. Quality-related vocabulary has been noted for its complexity and ever-changing nature. Employees of the organization must be able to understand and use a given set of terms, or they could be quickly disengaged from the value of the program.

3. Keep the programs as closely aligned as possible (if not integrated). Employees will find it difficult to differentiate the "quality program" from the "quality program," preventing it from being used and valued to its greatest extent. Furthermore, employees may feel overloaded and grow resentful if they perceive a duplication of quality efforts for an illogical purpose.

4. Involve those who previously participated in QA as early members of QI project teams. Those who

have supported previous quality efforts may be eager and ready to try the new approach. The attention and resources being provided to QI, in contrast to limitations accorded with QA, may be misinterpreted personally, and disengage our quality champions.

Regulatory standards are moving in the direction of quality improvement, but there will always be a need for standards, and discipline-specific, departmentally based quality assessment and improvement activities—which collectively some may refer to as quality assurance. It is essential that QI program planning address this level of activity, as well as the organizational and multidisciplinary team approach.

Designing the Program Structure

The structure of the QI program will be based on decisions made in the previously described responsibilities. Some agencies elect to adopt a QI program structure based on the recommendations of a consultant or consulting group. Such program models reflect experiences and successes achieved in other agencies (within and outside health care). The assistance of external consultants and trainers may provide a jump-start to settings that lack the internal expertise of available resources to plan and implement independently.

Some agencies can benefit from assistance and models established at the corporate level. Multiagency health care corporations of all types are building quality-related support structures and teams to assist member organizations in their QI program planning. The availability of expert assistance from within the corporation may influence the program model ultimately selected.

Other organizations look to literature and reports of successful QI programs to make structural decisions. Questions asked during the planning stages often include:

1. What is the role of the quality council?
2. Who are its members? Do they have terms? How are the members to function?
3. How will project teams be established?
4. What will be the reporting structure?
5. Are teams permanent and ongoing, or time-limited and process-specific?
6. How will quality projects be prioritized?
7. How will resource allocation for quality be planned?

The role of the quality council at North Florida Regional Medical Center changed over phases of implementation. In early program planning, the council's role was to identify educational needs and develop programs. In later stages of development, the council was needed to monitor and facilitate program growth and expansion (Duncan et al, 1991).

Initiating Education in QI

Education about quality improvement and its tools and techniques is perhaps the most time-consuming and costly issue in bringing a program to life. It moves the concepts off the paper and into action.

Early education for QI often targets team leaders or facilitators for training, as well as top and middle managers. Clinical leaders must be included as well. In addition to learning about the new imperatives for quality and the concepts of quality improvement, participants are taught tools and techniques in group process as well as process assessment and improvement. (Additional information about the role of the team leader and education will be found in later chapters.)

Deming suggests that extensive education is necessary for all employees, citing the critical-mass approach. That is, if a knowledgeable critical mass is formed, significant results will occur. Walton (1986, p. 88) writes: "Just as workers cannot act alone, neither can top management. Enough people must understand the 14 points [of Deming's QI approach] to know what to do and how to do it."

The experience of the hospitals that first implemented QI programs has suggested that overeducation might be as great a concern as undereducation. According to Michael Pugh, president and chief executive officer of Parkview Episcopal Medical Center in Pueblo, Colorado, the critical-mass theory doesn't work. "It's the same thing as dressing everybody up for the dance with no dance to take them to," he says (Kennedy et al, 1992, p. 84).

Revised approaches have supported the effectiveness of "just in time" (JIT) training. The employees involved in QI projects are given education at times when they can immediately apply it. For example, a project team discussing a work-flow issue may be initially coached in the use of flowcharts by the involved team facilitator. The immediate application of this skill helps group members better understand and value its use. Often, education is provided in a cascade approach, with early groups taught by external sources. These group members then teach the next in line, who subsequently teach the next, and so on. This approach both provides the needed education and demonstrates the commitment and knowledge base of those leading the charge.

Education for quality improvement is often considered one of the most expensive parts of program implementation, yet it can yield great return. Organizations that have won the Malcolm Baldrige National Quality Award, the United States' most prestigious quality award, report that for every dollar they spend

TABLE 2-1 Characteristics of Successful QI Project Teams

Number of members	Could be from 2 to 20
Representation	Those with experience in process and with a vested interest in the outcome
	Team leader or coach
	Facilitator
Frequency of meetings	Weekly
	Every other week
	Monthly, with members or teams carrying out activities in between
Knowledge/skills needed	QI concepts
	Process to be reviewed
	Mission, vision, values
	Group-process skills
	Problem-analysis techniques
	Data-collection strategies and basic statistical process control tools

on employee training in quality measurement techniques, they can account for a 30 to 40 times return on the investment.

Establishing Initial QI Project Teams

Early QI project teams are often selected on the basis of processes and issues that are visible, interesting, and worthwhile and that have a high potential for achieving success. It may also help to target an issue that would likely yield willing and effective team members, and one that could be resolved relatively quickly. To enhance commitment, early successes could then be used to market the benefits of QI.

In most QI models, a process is selected for review, and a team is established to assess and improve it (see Table 2-1). After achievement of the goals the team is then disbanded. (Some models have preestablished teams that remain intact, moving from work on one process to the next.) Team members are selected on the basis of their experience and involvement with the process, as well as a vested interest in the outcome. Ford Motor Company and IBM Corporation, both noted for their experience in quality improvement, report that multifunctional groups are essential because most opportunities to improve quality lie outside the natural departmental work group (Peters, 1987, p. 93).

Team members must be provided with quality improvement education. At the minimum, the curriculum must include or cover:

- Basic concepts of quality improvement
- The mission, vision, and values of the organization
- Basic team skills and group-process techniques
- Basic data-collection methods
- Basic analysis techniques
- Basic use of statistical process-control tools

Once the group begins work on the actual projects, members must be supported in use of this knowledge and skills with trained facilitators or coaches.

Michael Pugh of Parkview Episcopal Medical Center in Colorado reports that based on his experience education must be frequent and must take a variety of forms. Adults learn in different ways. Not everyone sits down and reads a book. Some prefer video; some learn by doing. Educational programs need to allow for different learning styles, and must repeat key principles over and over again. "Learning doesn't happen in one shot," note Kennedy et al (1992, p. 87).

Basic concepts for effective group process apply to QI project teams. In reality, no absolute number of group members is ideal for effective functioning. Tackett (1991) recommends five members in addition to the team leader and facilitator. Reported work of the National Demonstration Project (NDP), a large-scale, grant-supported, collaborative project to assess the outcomes and implications of using QI in various health care settings, describes successful project teams involving anywhere from two to twenty members, with a median of nine (Berwick et al, 1990, p. 70).

Anecdotal reports of the QI project teams in the NDP also stated that simply having a project team meet would often move the group toward improvement, even without the use of other tools or techniques. Project directors believed that crossfunctional teams served to provide members with previously unseen information about how organizations worked, and how each person and action influences the other, and the way processes are carried out (Berwick et al, 1990, p. 70).

Frequency of meetings of QI project teams varies within and across organizations, yet regularity is essential. Weekly meetings, every-other-week meetings, or monthly meetings with work completed in between have been reported as successful. Management support for sending employees to meetings is essential.

Creating a Plan for QI Program Expansion

When the commitment is set, the education begun, and the pilot teams under way, it is important to project how you want quality efforts to proceed when they are fully implemented. The following questions might help identify issues to be considered in your program expansion.

1. Should the structure or function of the quality council change?

- Who should be standing members?
- Should the council have some rotating members or participants who are included based on the issues being reviewed?
- How often does the council need to meet?
- Should the council have ongoing task forces to address specific issues or functions?
- Who should lead the council?
- Will the council have authority to initiate or reject QI projects?
- If so, how will projects be prioritized?

2. Should the coordination of quality assessment and quality improvement change?
   - Are specific functions being duplicated?
   - Can QA/QI programs be streamlined, integrated, or extended?
   - Can regulatory requirements be met in more efficient and effective ways?

3. How can quality issues be best communicated and coordinated?
   - Is information about the quality of care or service being communicated to all parties affected by it?
   - Do employees have the information they need to innovate and improve?
   - Do employees know about the quality commitment and efforts currently under way?
   - Is there duplication of efforts on similar quality projects, or, conversely, are there major gaps in areas that need improvement but are not being addressed?

4. What can be done to support QI project teams?
   - Are education and training available to everyone?
   - Are team members prepared to participate?
   - Does the education provided meet the needs of participants?
   - Are team leaders capable of successfully leading project teams?
   - Do we have enough prepared team leaders to meet the current and future needs of groups?
   - Are QI project teams given enough time and resources to function effectively?

5. Are data and information-systems needs being met?
   - Is needed data available to project teams and the council?
   - Are information-systems services available?
   - Is technical support available for assistance in data analysis and management?
   - Does the council (and all affected parties) have an ongoing perspective and data on the quality of care and service provided in the organization?

6. Is quality recognized and rewarded throughout the organization?
   - Has quality been integrated into all functions, departments, and services?
   - Is quality a major component of reward systems?
   - Are there mechanisms in place to recognize exceptional quality efforts?

Despite good planning and extra effort in implementation, quality programs often lose their energy within 12 to 18 months after implementation (Peters, 1987, p. 88). The intrigue of a "new thing," the rush of great expectations, and the improvement in the easily solved problems give way to slower progress and sometimes stale expectations. Times like these call for new approaches, creative efforts, and changed rewards. True commitment requires ongoing persistence. Periodic review of the quality program will allow its leaders to make changes that maintain its vigor and strengthen its impact.

Precipitating Change in Organizational Conduct

Successful implementation of QI implies the creation of a new organization. With the consumer as the focus, and an enlightened and empowered staff, the organization must function entirely differently than before. There are new ways to make decisions, to communicate, to create change, and to innovate. "Improvements" and "quality" are not confined within the operational boundaries of the quality program.

Implementation and integration of these concepts requires many years and many champions. The message that must be sent and heard is that the organization cannot remain status quo. It must change, and a focus on quality will be the direction of the change.

The quality council must work to elevate quality issues both within and outside of its own program. This level of influence can only be achieved through the ongoing personal involvement of upper managers. Experience of those in the National Demonstration Project demonstrated that "there appears to be no effective substitute for the time of top leaders, at least in early stages of the QI effort" (Berwick et al, 1990, p. 70).

Strategies promoted by the quality council must also be carefully monitored to assure that progress is resulting. Reports of the International Quality Study (Ernst & Young, American Quality Foundation, 1992) note that not all QI approaches are effective in all settings. One part of the study categorized hospitals into high performers, medium performers, and low performers, based on data about productivity, profitability, and self-assessment on quality. Responses rating the effectiveness of various QI strategies varied, according to the respondent's performance category (see Table 2-2). Quality teams, already common in high-performing organizations, were not seen by these participants as an approach that increased effectiveness. Low-performing organizations, however, believed they made a great difference. Quality-related meetings were considered of mixed benefit by high performers, while medium performers found

TABLE 2-2 Effectiveness of QI Techniques Reported by Organizations in the International Quality Study (1992)

	Organizational Performance Ranking		
	High	Medium	Low
Quality Teams	−	+/−	+
Quality Meetings	+/−	+	−
Quality Training	+/−	+/−	+
Benchmarking	+	+/−	−

+ Highly beneficial
+/− Of mixed benefit
− Not beneficial

them highly beneficial. Low performers reported that these meetings were not helpful, perhaps because there was insufficient direction or resources available. Education for quality, once heralded as being universally positive, received mixed reviews from high and medium performers, but was most effective in low-performing organizations. Benchmarking, while effective for high-performing organizations already on the cutting edge, had mixed effectiveness in medium organizations and was ineffective in low-performing organizations. Low performers were apparently likely to be so far from the identified best practice that comparison served to demotivate rather than encourage performance. The IQS report reinforces the need for critical thinking and close ongoing assessment of the effectiveness of QI approaches. Organizations can learn from the experiences of others, but they must tailor their efforts to their people, their culture, their unique situations, and the resources available to them.

IMPLEMENTING THE QUALITY IMPROVEMENT PROGRAM

Implementation of an initiative with the magnitude of quality improvement requires a planned-change approach to achieve success. Lewin (1947) has described one commonly used approach which includes unfreezing of the current approach, implementing the change or transition, and then refreezing, or creating an acceptance and consistent use of the new approach or concept. Fluctuations between phases may occur; that is, progress may not always occur as a one-way, linear motion.

The *unfreezing* phase occurs when there is recognition that the status quo is no longer acceptable. For health care quality, this includes societal dissatisfaction with aspects of the health care system and increasing expectations from savvy patients and families. The increased competition in the health care marketplace, as well as the dramatic issues of health

care costs, have intensified the need for new approaches to quality. Staff dissatisfaction with ineffective, paper approaches to quality has also created a state of readiness for implementing quality improvement concepts and programs. The final component needed for unfreezing the current state of being is the commitment of upper managers and leaders, and a strong and persistent message that quality improvement will be the direction in which to move.

The change or transition phase involves initial implementation, with the formation of a quality council, the implementation of education and training, and the establishment of QI project teams. This phase could go on for several years, through stages of change to achieve full implementation of the program.

"Striving Toward Improvement: Six Hospitals in Search of Quality" (Joint Commission, 1992, p. 221) details the initial QI efforts of six hospitals. The report finds that after 3 years of intensive efforts, these hospitals are 10 to 15 percent along the way to full transition.

Refreezing occurs with visible acceptance of this new way of doing business. The culture of the organization has been changed to support participative decision making, accountability, information sharing, and boundary crossing, all with the purpose of better meeting the needs of internal and external customers. The refreezing phase is supported within the organization by the commitment of leaders, written statements of mission, vision, and values, the conduct of relevant programs, and the assignment of resources to carry out the charge. Further, the internal structure of the organization will have changed to support the new culture.

Forces outside the organization will also influence the refreezing process, creating quality improvement concepts as the new way of being. These include new regulations for quality, new payor mandates, and revised expectations of consumer groups. Other health care agencies will likewise be implementing these changes, making QI the community standard and almost the basis for competition within society. Finally, the availability of functional helpers, such as consultants, educational offerings, and literature will make the change easier and will validate the journey for participants (Prevost, 1991).

For each of these phases, it will be helpful to identify those factors that move the process forward (driving forces) and those that hold it back (restraining forces). Obviously, the goal is to ignite and sustain the driving forces, to use them to move as far as possible. Restraining forces must be identified so that one can eliminate them, or at least decrease their impact, so as to continue to progress (Lewin, 1951). "It may be tempting to focus efforts solely on enhancing driving forces. It is easier to add new accelerators than to confront the process and managerial and social paradigms that inhibit change. However, thinking in terms of Lewin's force field analysis is the only way to achieve progress; we are well aware that the removal of inhibitors and barriers [restraining forces] is the only effective method to leverage accelerators [driving forces]. In other words, we found that in the absence of effective resolution of inhibitors, increasing the number of accelerators by itself will not achieve a paradigm transition," said Chip Caldwell, president and CEO of West Paces Medical Center in Atlanta (1993, p. 43).

SUCCESSFUL QUALITY PROGRAMS

There is no single correct program model to achieve success in quality improvement. Though various consultants and experts might have us think that their approach is the only "guaranteed" method, in fact many program models have yielded some success in today's organizations.

Tom Peters, in *Thriving on Chaos* (1987, pp. 85-98), identifies what he believes to be consistent traits shared by successful quality programs:

1. *Management is obsessed with quality.* This commitment requires personal involvement, consistent attention, and emotion.
2. *There is a guiding system or ideology.* An organized program must be established and followed faithfully.
3. *Quality is measured.* The program and all participants must consistently collect and use data to create improvements.
4. *Quality is rewarded.* Quality rewards and incentives must be built into every role in the organization.
5. *Everyone is trained in technologies for assessing quality.* Quality programs cannot be elitist or exclusive. Everyone in the organization must be trained in the use of basic problem solving, statistical process-control tools, and group techniques.
6. *Teams involving multiple functions/systems are used.* QI project teams must include members from various departments and roles who have experience with the process and hold a stake in the outcome.
7. *Small is very beautiful.* Improvements need not be grand to be valued.
8. *There is constant stimulation.* The program must be attended to with new approaches, themes, and ideas in order to stay vital.
9. *There is a parallel organizational structure devoted to quality improvement.* Special-event programs, recognition programs, and steering committees can create energizing forces and new champions for quality. These time-limited groups can support the ongoing work of the quality program.
10. *Everyone plays.* Quality must involve suppliers, employees, leaders, and consumers.
11. *When quality goes up, costs go down.* The quality program must integrate cost perspectives, and will ultimately be the predominant strategy for decreasing costs.
12. *Quality improvement is a never-ending journey.* A fully integrated program strives daily, in many ways, to do things better. It can never be considered "finished business" because each situation presents new ways to improve.

CONCLUSION

The creation of a quality-oriented, consumer-focused organization requires a vision, an approach, and champions. Quality programs are central to all three. The program established will be the approach used to embody the vision and to guide the champions. It must reflect the best of research and experience, as well as the unique character of the organization itself.

While there is no single correct approach to program structure, and ambiguity exists in defined strategies for implementation and integration, one truth remains. Quality improvement programs are the unavoidable reality for today's health care settings. The greatest danger lies not in creating an imperfect program but in not getting started.

REFERENCES

Barry D, editor (1991): Integrating QA and QI: marriage or mayhem? *Quality Exchange* 1(2):1-3, 9.

Bergman R (1981): Accountability: definitions and dimensions, *International Nursing Review* 28:53-59.

Caldwell C (1993): Accelerators and inhibitors to organizational change in a hospital, *Quality Review Bulletin* (19)2:42-46.

Doherty SD (1990, Oct): Developing a blueprint for quality, *Journal of Quality Assurance*: 34-37.

Duncan RP, E Fleming, T Gallant (1991, April): Implementing a continuous quality improvement program in a community hospital, *Quality Review Bulletin*: 106-112.

Ernst & Young, American Quality Foundation (1992): International quality study SM: health care industry report. Cleveland, American Quality Foundation and Ernst & Young.

Joint Commission (1992): *Accreditation manual for hospitals,* 1992, Oakbrook Terrace, Ill, Joint Commission on Accreditation of Healthcare Organizations.

Joint Commission (1991, June 24): Draft, *Quality improvement standards for the accreditation manual for hospitals,* 1994 edition, unpublished document.

Joint Commission (1992): *Striving toward improvement: six hospitals in search of quality,* Oakbrook Terrace, Ill, Joint Commission on Accreditation of Healthcare Organizations.

Juran J (1991, March): Strategies for world class quality, *Quality Progress:* 81-85.

Kennedy M, J Prevost, MP Carr, JW Dilley (1992, March): A roundtable discussion: hospital leaders discuss QI implementation issues, *Quality Review Bulletin* 18(3):78-96.

Lewin K (1947): Frontiers in group dynamics: concept, method, and reality in social science: social equilibria and social change, *Human Relations* 1:5-41.

Lewin K (1951): *Field theory in social science,* New York, Harper & Row.

Marszalek-Gaucher E, RJ Coffey (1990): *Transforming health-care organizations: how to achieve and sustain organizational excellence,* San Francisco, Jossey-Bass Publishers.

Peters T (1987): *Thriving on chaos: handbook for management revolution,* New York, Harper & Row.

Prevost J (1991, March 7): Presentation. Creating change in the organization, San Antonio, Meetings of the Robert Wood Johnson Foundation, Improving the quality of hospital care grant recipients.

Tackett SA (1991, Oct): The quality council: a catalyst for improvement, *Journal of Quality Assurance* 13(5):30-36.

Walton, M (1986): *The Deming management method,* New York, Dodd, Mead, and Company.

CHAPTER THREE

IMPROVING QUALITY AND PERFORMANCE: TOOLS AND TECHNIQUES

Patricia Schroeder

Quality assurance in health care has long been equated with retrospective chart audits. This approach was relatively easy to accomplish, inexpensive, and could be carried out at any given time with little advance planning. Resulting data were collated, put into percentages, and reported to staffs. Analysis often focused on whether staff members had done a good job or bad job. At times, individuals with the greatest "noncompliance" were identified and counseled.

The use of this single approach to quality assessment had many limitations.

- It limited the availability and accuracy of data, especially data regarding outcomes.
- It fit with an inspection-oriented perspective on quality assessment.
- It ignored the multiplicity of other data sources.
- Its findings were easy to discount as "We did it but didn't document it."
- It worked by rote, was isolated, and often lacked the "real world" feel of practice.

Quality improvement opens new doors to data and allows the translation of data into information. Furthermore, it helps individuals and groups use information to create changes in care and systems.

QI tools clarify trends, patterns, relationships, and inefficiencies and can be used to find ways to improve. Rather than seeking to "expose the noncompliant," QI tools help individuals and groups identify opportunities to improve, root causes of problems, and the multiple approaches people can use to make things better. It constantly addresses these questions:

- What is happening?
- Why?
- How can we improve it?

Yet not all QI tools and techniques are brand new to health care. Many of the QI techniques cited are basic approaches used to promote effective group process. These include brainstorming and nominal group process. Teambuilding approaches may be included in this list as well.

Some of the QI tools used in data collection are also familiar. For example, "check sheets" are the label given to traditional data-collection forms on which the data collector uses hatch marks (tally marks) to identify whether a patient outcome, situation, or action met or did not meet the indicator statement. Logs are also familiar tools, used to identify patients, events, or concerns for later follow-up.

A crucial difference between then and now is how the tools are used. Too often, QA approaches stopped immediately after the point of data collection. Little analysis was done, because we focused more on the question of who rather than why. Actions were also limited, often because there was too little information to provide clear direction for improvements.

The use of QI tools and techniques requires a willingness to seek new perspectives and to gain new knowledge and skill; in addition, it frequently requires the involvement of a group of individuals who participate in (or are affected by) the process being studied. QI tools and techniques also require resources, including team facilitators and coaches, reference materials, and time to work through the process. This chapter helps in this pursuit, providing a reference in the use of basic QI tools and techniques.

FROM DATA TO INFORMATION

A key to creating improvements is to understand the current state or processes of care/service, and their relationship to where one wants to be. Processes are a series or set of activities carried out to achieve a certain end result. Processes are always linked to what precedes them—inputs—as well as what follows them—outputs/outcomes. Variations in the conduct of processes of care/service are typical and may be the result of common causes (i.e., minor differences that consistently appear because of such things

Note: As the needs of individuals and groups advance, other references will be helpful. Two excellent and frequently cited references are Brassard's *The memory jogger plus +* and Leebov and Ersoz's *The health care manager's guide to continuous quality improvement.*

as person-to-person nuances, time of day, etc.) or of special causes (i.e., aberrations that occasionally arise, such as missing supplies, errors, etc.).

QI theory states that understanding processes and their variations, and then decreasing those variations, is a prerequisite for effective improvement. Tools and techniques for QI were developed to help people clarify processes, understand their variations, and identify and implement more effective approaches to care and service.

Understanding the current state requires data or facts regarding processes of care and their outcomes: for example, How many IV sites become infected? When? What IV catheters are most commonly involved?

Collecting Data

Collecting data first requires a clear identification of the data source. One must ask, "Where can I get the facts that I need to know?" Data sources include records and documentation, but also direct observation, staff feedback, and patient/family feedback—a vast, underused data source. Frequently, a person needs more than one source to understand the situation or to gain a clearer perspective on the facts. Selection of the data source is based on issues of time, access, skills, and resources; one should always attempt to obtain as direct a source as possible.

Once the data source(s) is/are identified, the data-collection method must be selected. The approach selected should be determined by assessing its fit with the following statements:

- It has potential to generate/produce the necessary data.
- It respects issues of confidentiality and rights.
- It fits with traits of the group.
- It is efficient in terms of time, sample size, population, and staff availability.
- It creates the least possible disruption in the settings.
- Knowledge and skill in its construction and use are available.

Table 3-1 describes the data-collection methods possible for each data source. It is essential, however, that data collection be considered the beginning rather than the end of the improvement process.

Using Data

The intent of quality improvement is not to document data, nor is it to demonstrate one's strengths. It is to find ways to improve. QI tools and techniques were created to help in various stages of the improvement and problem-solving process. The box on p. 25 categorizes the tools that are effective at different points in the improvement process. Fig. 3-1 outlines the problem-solving steps differently and with more detail, and highlights commonly used tools for each step (Berwick, Godfrey, Roessner, 1990, p. 179).

TABLE 3-1 Collection Methods Available for Data

Data Source	Data-Collection Method
Patient/family	Interview
	In person
	Telephone
	Focus group
	Written survey/questionnaire
Observed event	Check sheet
	Log
Staff	Interviews
	Focus groups
	Written survey/questionnaire
	Brainstorming
	Nominal group process
Documentation (medical record or unit/department records)	Record review, using:
	Check sheet
	Log
	Questionnaire

With the array of tools available, it may be difficult at first to determine which tool to use at any given time. Keep in mind that there are no absolute right or wrong selections. There are only choices that produce greater or lesser insight into the aspects of the process that can be improved. Practice and experience will provide users with a greater feel for the use of different tools at different times, in different conditions, and with different groups.

QI TOOLS AND TECHNIQUES

The following section provides a simple overview of common QI tools and techniques. Each description highlights the tool's most common use and provides a step-by-step approach to creating and applying these tools in health care settings. Despite the relative simplicity of this discussion, some of these tools and techniques require substantial knowledge and skill for accurate, effective use. Readers are encouraged to seek out in-depth literature and expert assistance.

Logs

A log is a simple and basic tool used to identify or track events or problems (generally ones that are relatively uncommon or infrequent). It requires the periodic entry of data as events or situations occur, such as patients leaving the hospital against medical advice, specific patient complaints, or incidents of unavailable equipment. The resulting data allow the reviewer to follow up on specific situations or can be summarized periodically to identify trends.

To create a log:
1. Clarify the focus and intended purpose of the log.
2. Identify the information that will be necessary to adequately cover the focus and purpose.

Steps in Problem Solving		Flow Diagrams	Brainstorming	Cause-Effect Diagrams	Data Collection	Graphs and Charts	Stratification	Pareto Analysis	Histograms	Scatter Diagrams	Control Charts
Quality Improvement Tools											
Defining the Problem	1. List and prioritize problems	○	○	●	○	○	●				
	2. Define project and team	○				○	○				
The Diagnostic Journey	3. Analyze symptoms	●		●	○	○	●	○		○	
	4. Formulate theories of causes	○	●	●			○				
	5. Test theories	●			●	●	●	●	●	●	
	6. Identify root causes	●			●	●	●	●	●	●	
The Remedial Journey	7. Consider alternative solutions	●	●	○			○				
	8. Design solutions and controls	●			●	●	○		○	●	●
	9. Address resistance to change	○	●	○							
	10. Implement solutions and controls	●				○		○	○	○	
Holding the Gains	11. Check performance	○			●	●	●	●	●	○	●
	12. Monitor control system	○			●	●	●		○		●

● Primary or frequent application of tool   ○ Secondary, infrequent, or circumstantial   ☐ None or very rare

Fig. 3-1 Applications for quality improvement tools. *From Berwick et al (1990): Curing health care: new strategies for quality improvement, San Francisco, Jossey Bass.*

3. Create vertical columns on the page, labeled with each requested piece of information.
4. Keep the log in a place convenient to those intended to use it.
5. Analyze or use the log on a routine basis to keep others aware of its value and to promote its continued use.
6. Summarize the data periodically, to identify trends or patterns.

Fig. 3-2 provides examples of two logs.

Check Sheets

Check sheets are tools used to tally the frequency of events. They are common, easy-to-use data-collection

---

Tools Available to Assist in the Improvement Process

Tools to Identify Opportunities for Improvement

Brainstorming	Interviews
Nominal group process	Focus groups
Checksheets	Pareto charts
Logs	Flowcharts
Surveys/questionnaires	Run charts

Tools to Analyze Processes

Commonly Used

Cause-and-effect diagrams	Scatter diagrams
Flowcharts	Run charts
Brainstorming	Control charts
Nominal group process	Is/Is Not diagrams
Pareto charts	Deployment charts
Histograms	Other charts and graphs

Less Commonly Used

Affinity diagrams	Tree diagrams
Force field analysis	

Tools to Plan and Implement the Change

Commonly Used

Brainstorming	Tree diagrams
Nominal group process	Force field analysis
Flowcharts	

Less Commonly Used

Cause and effect diagrams	Scatter diagrams
Pareto charts	Affinity diagrams
Histograms	

Tools to Follow Up/Hold the Gains Achieved

Commonly Used

Checksheets	Histograms
Logs	Pareto charts
Surveys/questionnaires	Run charts
Interviews	Control charts
Focus groups	

Less Commonly Used

Flowcharts	Scatter diagrams

---

forms that can be adapted to a variety of situations. Check sheets are often a starting point in data collection. Traditional QA data-collection forms are a variation of check sheets.

To create a check sheet:

1. Identify the event or occurrence to be studied and the variable or items to be counted.
2. Specify variables or items under study in the left-hand column.
3. Provide vertical columns to specify the category in which the counting will occur, such as dates, locations, groups, records. Allow enough room in columns to use tally marks or check marks for recording.
4. Add a column on the right-hand side for total of data in each variable or item. A total line may be added at the bottom as well, to provide a total for each category, if relevant.

Clarify the sample or time frame for the check sheet to be used.

Fig. 3-3 provides examples of check sheets.

Surveys/Questionnaires

Surveys and questionnaires are preplanned, written tools used to elicit responses to selected questions from key people. Some use the terms *survey* and *questionnaire* interchangeably. Some classify surveys as briefer tools, and questionnaires as more detailed.

Surveys and questionnaires have the advantage of being easy to use and efficient to distribute to large numbers of people. These tools can collect quantitative or qualitative data, and they can allow for anonymous responses. They can be distributed by mail or in person or, at times, are circulated in a convenient place, such as a waiting area. The method of distribution may affect the response rate.

Considerable knowledge and skill are necessary for developing surveys/questionnaires that will provoke valid and reliable responses, or even any responses at all. Much literature is available to guide tool development. Keep in mind that some groups of individuals are unlikely to complete surveys or questionnaires at all (for example, those who are feeling very sick, those who are depressed, the elderly). In those instances, obtaining written feedback is not the data-collection method of choice.

Vocabulary and a respondent's reading level must also play a role in strategic tool development. In general, eliminate any health care jargon and write at no higher than a sixth-grade reading level. If the respondent group is non–English speaking, the text should be translated, or other data-collection methods considered.

To create a survey/questionnaire:

1. Carefully define both the survey/questionnaire focus and the respondent group. Both elements should be kept uppermost in mind during tool construction.
2. Write clear, simple, and brief directions at the top.
3. Keep the survey/questionnaire as brief as possible while ensuring that it is complete enough to elicit the necessary feedback.
4. Be sure to state where to send or return the survey/questionnaire when completed. If it is mailed, enclose a self-addressed stamped envelope.
5. Allow respondents to remain anonymous if they so choose.
6. Pilot-test the tool with sample members of the intended respondent group. Get feedback regarding:
   - Appropriateness of the vocabulary
   - Clarity of questions

PATIENTS WHO LEAVE AGAINST MEDICAL ADVICE (AMA)

Date	Time	Patient Number	Admission Date	Patient Stated Reason for Leaving

UNAVAILABLE EQUIPMENT

Date	Time	Type of Equipment	Date/Time of Availability

Fig. 3-2 Examples of logs.

- Time it takes to complete the tool
- Any other feedback about the approach

Use this insight in revising the tool and approach to its use.

7. Reevaluate the tool, its content responses, the response rate, and the distribution process on a periodic basis.

Fig. 3-4 provides an example of a survey.

Interviews

Interviews are a guided approach to eliciting verbal responses to preestablished questions from an individual or small group. They can be conducted in person or by phone.

Interviews have several advantages. They:
- Are relatively easy to conduct
- Are often therapeutic
- Provide the opportunity to follow up on responses

Disadvantages to interviews include their potential to be time-consuming if much feedback is requested, and the inherent preclusion of anonymous responses. As with questionnaires, careful develop-

ment of this tool is essential for the collection of valid, reliable, and useful information. Assistance from literature or experts is encouraged.

Interviews must be planned in advance and responses must be documented, either during or immediately after the process.

To interview:

1. Carefully clarify both the interview focus and the respondent group. Both elements should be kept uppermost in mind during the planning stage as well as the interview itself.

2. Plan the interview for a time convenient to the respondent.

3. Develop a clear, simple, and brief introduction of yourself and the interview that can be used on first contact with prospective respondents. Always request permission to conduct the interview.

4. Keep the interview as brief as possible, particularly with respondents who are ill.

5. Encourage clarification of responses whenever necessary.

SUPPLIES UNAVAILABLE ON THE UNIT SUPPLY CART

	7 am-3:30 pm	3:30 pm-11:30 pm	11:30 pm-7 am
IV start kits	ℍℍ I	II	I
Urinary catheter kits		I	
Catheter care kits	III	II	I
Nasogastric tubes			I
IV Solution: • D5W	II	I	
• D5W/.45NS		II	
• D5W/.9NS	I		
Other (Specify):			

REASONS FOR GREATER THAN 15-MINUTE DELAY IN STARTING SURGERY

Reasons	Week 1	Week 2	Week 3	Week 4
Previous surgery still in progress	III	I	II	I
Room not ready		I		
Equipment not available	I		I	
Surgeon delay		I		II
Nurse delay	I	I	I	
Patient delay		I		I
Other (Specify):				

Fig. 3-3 Examples of check sheets.   *Continued.*

6. Avoid questions that place respondents in a vulnerable position. For example: "Who is your favorite care provider and why? Who is your least favorite care provider and why?"
7. Pilot-test the interview guide with sample members of the proposed respondent group. Get feedback on:
   • Appropriateness of vocabulary
   • Clarification of questions
   • Time it takes to complete the interview
   • Any other feedback about the approach
8. Record responses to the interview as soon as possible.
   Fig. 3-5 provides a sample interview guide.

Focus Groups

Focus groups are meetings of individuals (usually a representative sample of consumers) brought together to provide feedback on a predetermined topic. These groups are lead by a facilitator, who is trained to elicit responses from group members about their preferences, experiences, perceptions, or concerns. These data can then be used to adapt care and service to better meet consumer needs. Focus groups are carefully planned in advance, and they promote free flow of information among participants.

To conduct a focus group:
1. Prepare a room conducive to the size of your group. Groups of 5 to 12 are effective, typically

DATA COLLECTION FORM

1 DATES: Beginning of study: _____
     End of study: _____

2 DATA COLLECTOR: _____
    (name & title)

3 FOCUS OF STUDY: ☐ Patient ☐ Staff ☐ System: _____

6 OBJECTIVE OF MONITORING: _____

4 ASPECT OF CARE
BEING REVIEWED: _____

☐ High-volume ☐ High-risk ☐ Problem-prone ☐ High-cost

5 SAMPLE SIZE: _____ Number

KEY

+ met criteria
– did not meet
e exception

7 Indicators	8 Exceptions	9 Data-Retrieval Method	10 ID #'s	11 Demographic Data	12 Totals (+ / – / e)	13 Threshold for Eval. (projected / actual (A_1))	14 Remarks
1							
2							
3							
4							
5							
6							

Fig. 3-3, cont'd.

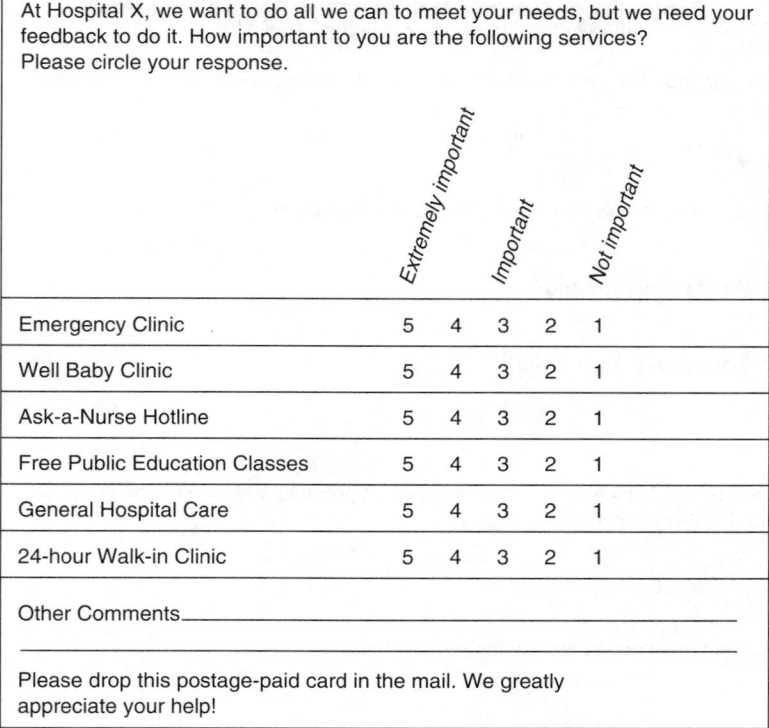

At Hospital X, we want to do all we can to meet your needs, but we need your feedback to do it. How important to you are the following services? Please circle your response.

	Extremely important	Important	Not important
Emergency Clinic	5 4	3 2	1
Well Baby Clinic	5 4	3 2	1
Ask-a-Nurse Hotline	5 4	3 2	1
Free Public Education Classes	5 4	3 2	1
General Hospital Care	5 4	3 2	1
24-hour Walk-in Clinic	5 4	3 2	1
Other Comments_____			

Please drop this postage-paid card in the mail. We greatly appreciate your help!

Fig. 3-4 Example of a survey.

working for a 60 to 90 minute session (Leebov, Ersoz 1991, p. 106).

2. The group facilitator should be prepared for the role. Traits of effective facilitators include an ability to convey an accepting attitude, and sophisticated group-process and communication skills. A guide of open-ended questions that address the group's focus or topic should be developed in advance.

3. At the beginning of the meeting, the facilitator introduces herself or himself and the topic at hand. Participants introduce themselves.

4. The facilitator initiates discussion, clarifies responses, and encourages interaction among group members. The goal is to get a clear picture of the preferences, experiences, perceptions and concerns of participants—all of which are useful in planning customer-focused improvements.

5. At the conclusion of the session, convey sincere thanks to group members for their participation.

6. Record responses of group members as soon as possible.

Brainstorming

Brainstorming is a group activity used to identify the range or scope of:
- Problems or situations
- Options or possibilities
- Strategies
- Reasons underlying a situation
- Ideas

It is an effective approach that promotes creativity and encourages the involvement of all group members.

Successful brainstorming requires group members to generate lists without feedback or discussion. That is, as points are identified by successive group members, no feedback or critique is allowed by others. This approach encourages those who are hesitant to respond for fear of being challenged or looking foolish, and increases potential for the identification of new ideas.

To brainstorm:

1. Identify the group leader/recorder if not already established.

2. Clarify the question under discussion. Be as specific as possible.

3. Review the ground rules of brainstorming for all participants:
   - Ideas will be called out without discussion or rationale. (If preferred, go around the room and let each person take a turn.)
   - All ideas are of value; none are too abstract.
   - All ideas will be recorded.
   - The goal is to exhaust the list of possibilities.

4. Provide a brief time (1 or 2 minutes) for participants to generate their own ideas.

5. Begin brainstorming. This step continues for a specified time period or until all ideas are exhausted.

6. Write all responses on a flip chart, blackboard, overhead projector, or other format that allows all participants to see them.

Topic: Family Member/Significant Other Perceptions of Visiting Policy in Critical Care Unit

How did you become familiar with the current visiting policy?

Have you been able to visit your family member (patient):

As often as you need?

For as long as you need?

What do you think would be the ideal visiting policy to meet the needs of you and your family member (patient)?

Do you have enough privacy during your visit?

Have you been able to get enough information about your family member (patient):

During your visit?

At times when you are not visiting?

Do you have any other comments or concerns about the critical care visiting policy?

Fig. 3-5 Example of an interview guide.

7. Allow time for discussion or clarification of ideas after the brainstorming is completed.
8. Streamline the list: you may wish to establish a plan for follow-up or action.

Nominal Group Process (or Technique)

Nominal group process, or nominal group technique, is an activity used to identify ideas and select options within a group that is quiet, reticent, or less "free flowing." Some groups may be less able to brainstorm or interrelate. These include new groups whose members are unfamiliar with each other, groups whose members do not yet trust each other, or groups that have been unable to gain consensus on an issue.

Nominal group process begins with each group member successively stating an idea. Just as in brainstorming, no discussion or feedback regarding the ideas is allowed. After all ideas have been stated, the list is condensed through discussion and multivoting until one option or the desired number of options is formulated.

To use nominal group process:
1. Identify the group leader/recorder if not already established.
2. Clarify the question under discussion. Be as specific as possible.
3. Review the ground rules for nominal group process/technique for all participants:
   - Ideas will be presented without discussion or rationale.
   - All ideas are of value. None are too abstract.
   - All ideas will be recorded.
4. Provide a brief time (1 or 2 minutes) for participants to generate their own ideas.

5. Group members take turns sharing one idea at a time. Again, no discussion or comments are allowed. If a member has no idea he or she is to pass. This process continues for a specified period of time, or until all ideas are exhausted.
6. Record all responses on a flip chart, blackboard, overhead projector, or other format that allows all participants to see them.
7. Allow time for discussion or clarification of ideas.
8. Eliminate or combine any ideas based on the discussion.
9. Use a strategy such as multivoting (described in the next section) to select the best option(s).
10. Establish a plan for follow-up or action.

Multivoting

Multivoting is a selection process used by a group following brainstorming or nominal group process. It allows the group to reduce a long list of items or responses down to a reasonable number. Several rounds of voting are required. Discussion on remaining items or responses can be entertained following the elimination of less desirable options.

To use multivoting:

1. Post the list of items or responses in clear view of all group members.
2. Number each item on the list.
3. Review each item as a group, and combine overlapping items.
4. Select a method for voting: verbal, hand, or ballot.
5. Instruct the group members to vote for one-third of the total number of items on the list. Specify the number. (That is, if there are 30 items, vote for 10.)
6. Eliminate items that received fewest votes.
7. The voting can be repeated several times until the list reaches a reasonable number.
8. Entertain discussion on items, select option(s), and, if appropriate, establish an action plan.

Run (Trend) Charts

A run chart, also called a trend chart, is a basic graph that depicts data over time. It is used to get a visual picture of trends in data. The traditional patient temperature graph is actually a run chart.

To create a run chart:

1. Draw the axes. The x axis is always horizontal, and depicts the time sequence in units such as hours, days, or months. The y axis is always vertical, and depicts the variable to be measured, such as temperature, injuries, or other specific occurrences.
2. Plot data on the graph in sequential time order.
3. Connect the data points with a line.
4. Draw a line representing the mean, or average, to provide a frame of reference. (**Note:** Experts differ over what frame of reference to use. Brassard [1989] recommends using the mean. Leebov and Ersoz [1991] recommend using the median, or the midpoint, of the data. If used consistently, either will be helpful.)
5. Analyze and use the trend data routinely to plan, carry out, or follow up with actions for improvement.
6. When seven to nine consecutive data points fall on one side of the line (mean or median), the mean has shifted, likely because of a specific change. (**Note:** Minor shifts in data may not be significant, so careful analysis and thoughtful intervention are required.)

Fig. 3-6 provides examples of run charts.

Control Charts

A control chart, just like a run chart, shows trends in data over time. Furthermore, it uses statistically determined upper and lower limits to define a range of acceptability. If data stay within the range, the process is considered "in control." Any variations in the data are likely to be the result of predictable and acceptable causes such as slight person-to-person differences. These are called *common cause* variations.

Some variations are the result of unusual occurrences, and are called *special cause* variation. Examples are an unusual error, unique client variations, or flukes.

The goal of using a control chart is to get processes of care or service "in control"; in other words, to gain consistency in their operation.

To create a control chart:

1. Draw the axes. The x axis is always horizontal, and depicts the time sequence in units such as hours, days, or months. The y axis is always vertical, and depicts the variable to be measured, such as waiting time, number of patient falls, or episodes of a specific event.
2. Plot data on the graph in sequential time order.
3. Connect the data points with a line.
4. Identify and draw a horizontal line at the mean.
5. Identify the upper control limits and the lower control limits, using statistical methods. These control limits are standard deviations, based on an organization's past performance data. Upper and lower control limits can be identified through the use of commonly available computer software or can be calculated by hand. An example of this approach is shown in Fig. 3-7 (Katz and Green, 1992, p. 111).
6. Draw upper and lower control limits onto the chart. These parameters help to identify when a process is in control or out of control. (**Note:** In manufacturing industries, control charts are sometimes called "Stop and Go" charts. Various parts of the chart are shaded red, yellow, and green like a traffic light. The area surrounding the mean is

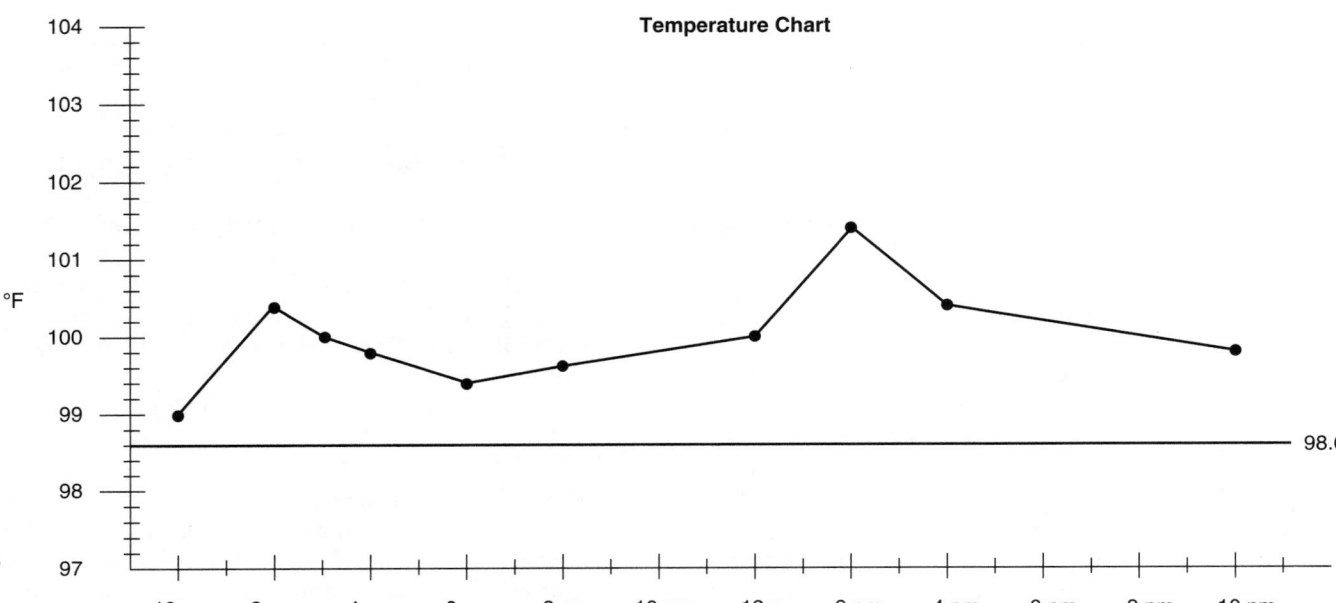

Note: In this instance, normal temperature replaces the mean.

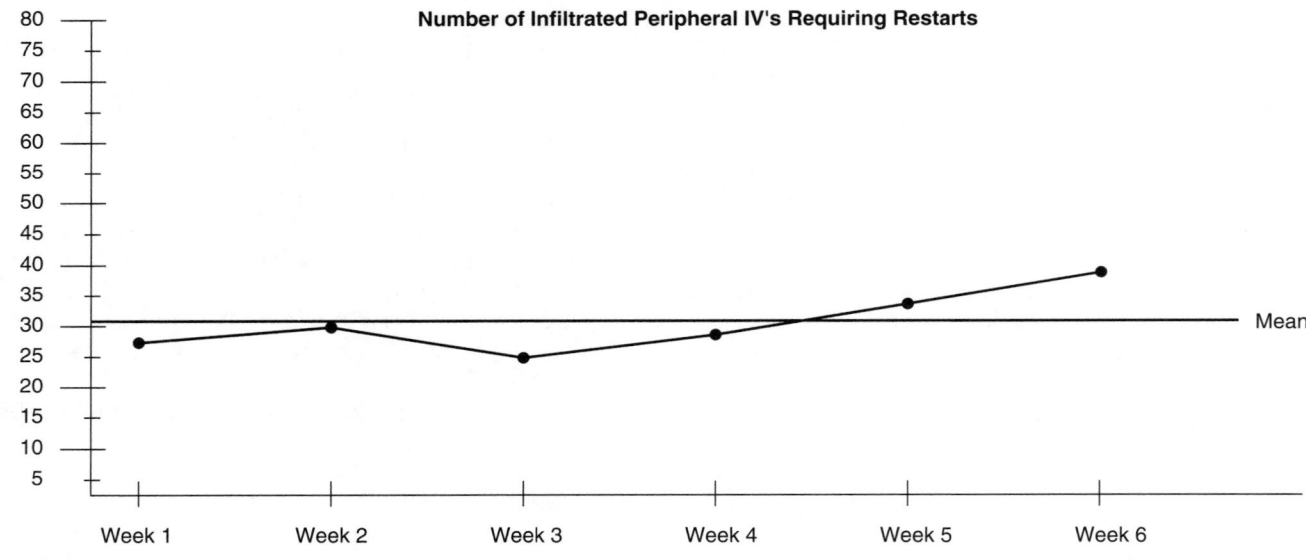

Fig. 3-6 Examples of run charts.

green, to signify that the process should keep going on this route. The control-limit area is shaded yellow, to denote a caution area, where action is required to get the process back in control. The area outside the control limits is red, to indicate that the worker should stop and make the necessary changes to gain control of the process.)

7. Analysis and actions must be carried out when data fall outside control limits. As greater consistency in the process is achieved, limits should be decreased (set closer to the mean), to further reduce process variation and streamline operations. Fig. 3-8 provides examples of control charts.

Histograms

A histogram is a visual picture, usually in the form of a bar graph, of a frequency distribution and depicts the measurement of some characteristic or variable. It is a picture of some aspect of the variation in a process (e.g., waiting time in the emergency department, number of patients with central lines on the

COL 1	COL 2	COL 3	COL 4
MONTHS	TOTAL MEDICATION ERRORS x_i	DEVIATIONS $x_i - \bar{x}$	SQUARE OF DEVIATIONS $(x_i - \bar{x})^2$
JAN	10	0	0
FEB	12	2	4
MAR	11	1	1
APR	8	−2	4
MAY	11	1	1
JUN	9	−1	1
JUL	7	−3	9
AUG	10	0	0
SEP	12	2	4
OCT	10	0	0
NOV	13	3	9
DEC	7	−3	9
TOTAL: **120**		TOTAL: **42**	

- $\bar{x} = \dfrac{\Sigma x_i}{N} = \dfrac{120}{12} = 10$

- $\sigma = \sqrt{\dfrac{\Sigma(x_i - \bar{x})^2}{N}} = \sqrt{\dfrac{42}{12}} = \sqrt{3.5} = \pm 1.9$

- Threshold parameters
   Upper limit: $\bar{x} + \sigma = 10 + 1.9 = 11.9$
   Lower limit: $\bar{x} - \sigma = 10 - 1.9 = 8.1$

(x_i = individual score; $\bar{x}$ = mean (or average) of scores; N = number of scores; σ = standard deviation)

1. Enter the number of medication errors reported each month in column 2.
2. Total the entries in column 2 to determine the annual total of the medication errors reported.
3. Divide the total calculated in step 2 by the number of months for which medication error data is available.
   Note: This quotient is $\bar{x}$, the mean, or average number of reported medication errors per month.
4. Subtract the calculated average ($\bar{x}$) from each reported number of monthly medication errors, and enter the deviations ($x_i - \bar{x}$) in column 3.
   Note: Values may be positive, negative, or zero.
5. Multiply each calculated deviation by itself, and enter the resultant products in column 4.
   Note: All values will be positive, or zero.
6. Add the products in column 4. To determine the sum of squared deviations [$\Sigma(x_i - \bar{x})^2$]
7. Divide the sum calculated in step 6 by the number of months for which medication error data is available.
8. Calculate the square root of the quotient determined in step 7.
   Note: This calculation yields σ, the standard deviation of the data entered in column 2.
9. Calculate:
   - the upper limit of the threshold parameters, $\bar{x} + \sigma$, by adding the calculated standard deviation (σ, see step 8) to the calculated average ($\bar{x}$, step 3), and
   - the lower limit of the threshold parameters, $\bar{x} - \sigma$, by subtracting the calculated standard deviation (σ, see step 8) from the calculated average ($\bar{x}$, step 3).

Fig. 3-7 Nine-step procedure for calculating a standard deviation and confidence interval. *From Katz J, E Green (1992):* Managing quality: a guide to monitoring and evaluating nursing services, *Mosby.*

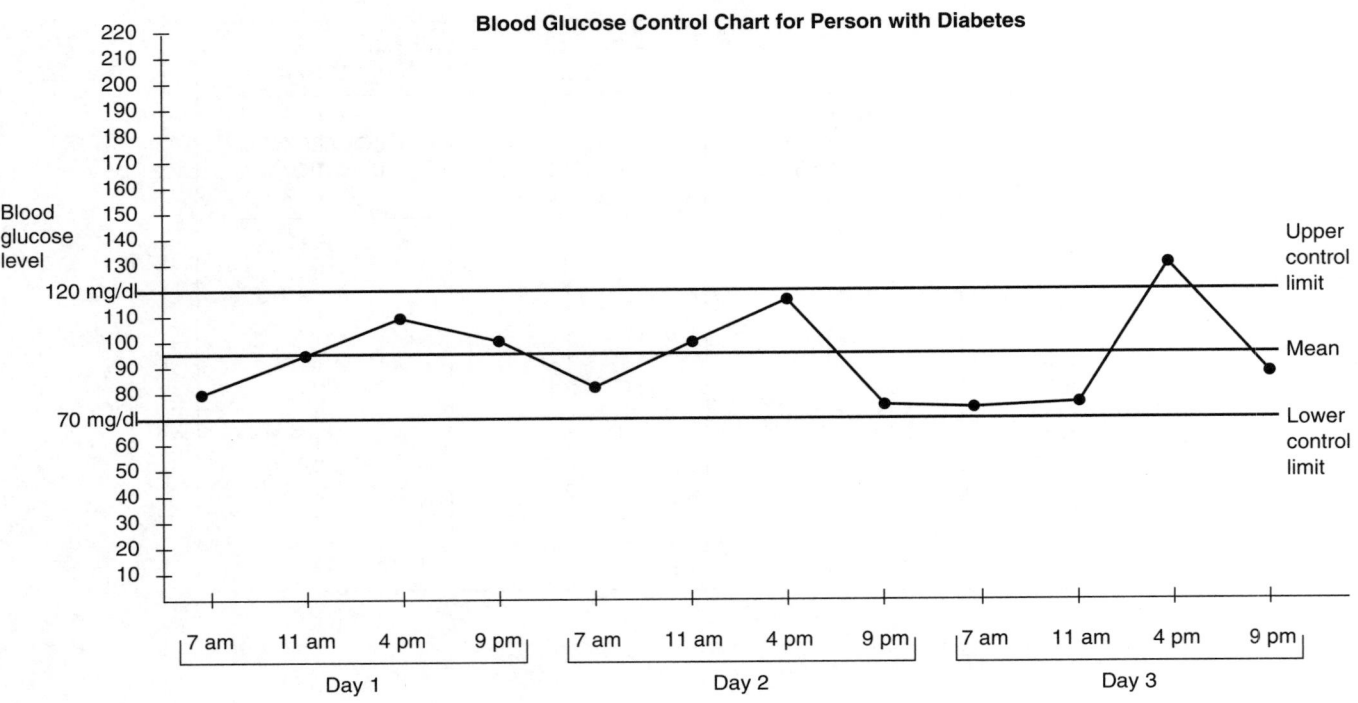

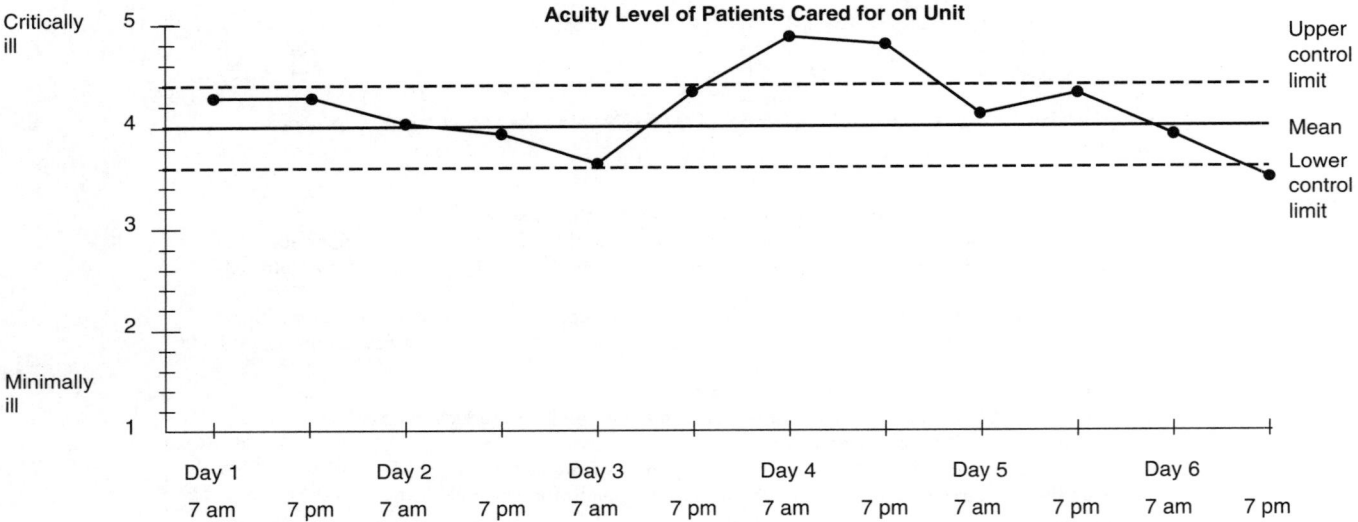

Fig. 3-8 Examples of control charts.

unit, or length of stay for a particular patient group). A histogram frequently presents data that have been organized into categories (e.g., patients waiting 10-15 minutes, more than 15-20 minutes, etc.). A graph provides more information at a glance and adds more meaningful perspective to data than does a mere list of numbers.

Histograms assume varying configurations, all ultimately useful in the task of analyzing and interpreting the data.

To create a histogram:

1. Identify the number of data points or individual observations or measurements. The histogram on the top of Fig. 3-9 reflects 216 individual data points. Organize them from the smallest to the largest.

2. Identify the range of data points by subtracting the smallest number/data point from the largest.

3. Identify the number of categories (each category will be one bar on the graph) into which you will separate the data. (Typically, 5 to 15 categories are used, with more categories used for more data

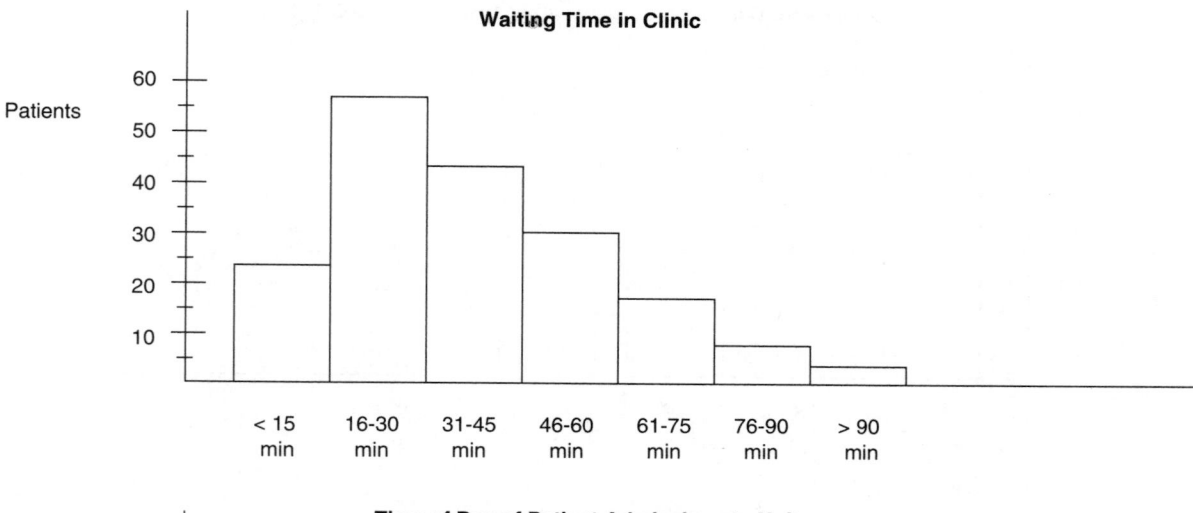

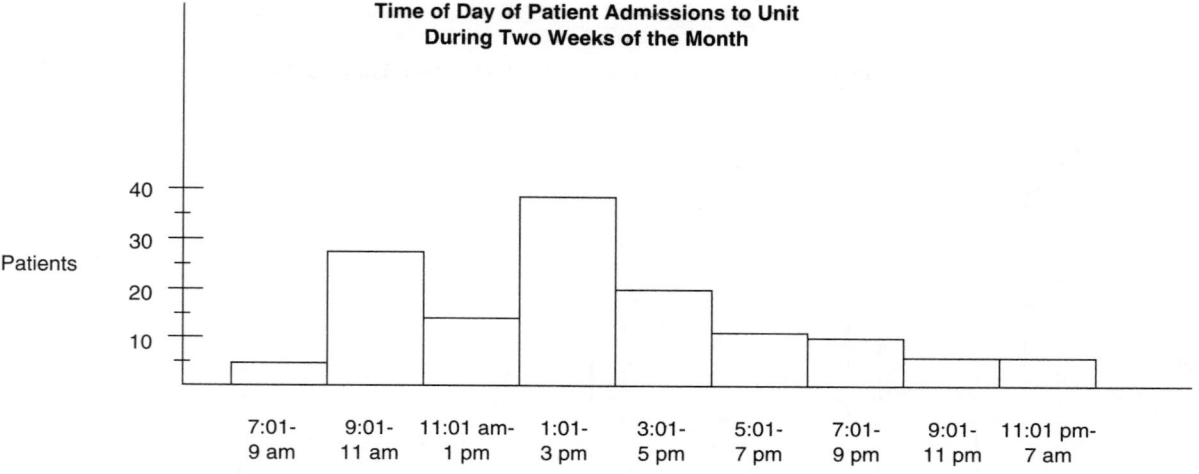

Fig. 3-9 Examples of histograms.

points.) The top histogram in Fig. 3-9 reflects seven categories of data.

4. Divide the range by the number of categories that you have decided to use. Use this result to create the category widths. The top histogram in Fig. 3-9 uses category widths of 15-minute intervals.

5. Place each data point into the appropriate category. Count the frequencies. In the top histogram in Fig. 3-9, 14 data points were identified in the < 15-minute category, 58 data points in the 16- to 30-minute category, etc.

6. Draw the axes. The x axis is horizontal, and depicts the category intervals (time periods, scores, locations, groups, etc.). Categories should not overlap. The y axis is vertical, and depicts the frequency of the variable or characteristic being measured, usually identified as numbers or percentages.

7. Plot or record data in continuous fashion, with no gaps between the columns.

8. Identify and report the mean and the range of the data.

9. Analyze these data and use them to plan strategies for process-improvement (GOAL/QPC, 1988, pp. 36-43).

Fig. 3-9 provides examples of histograms.

Pareto Chart

A Pareto chart or analysis is a tool to rank-order or prioritize problems, causes of a problem, or categories of some event or issue. It is a bar graph, ordered to reflect the highest priority on the left, with decreasing frequency (priority) thereafter. Created by Vilfredo Pareto, an Italian economist of the 19th century, it is a tool to separate "the vital few from the trivial many." Pareto charts help to prioritize efforts to identify the activities that will likely yield the greatest impact.

To create a Pareto chart:

1. Identify the categories, problems, causes, or issues to be studied, and measure the frequency of their occurrence.

2. Draw the axes. The x axis is horizontal and depicts the categories, problems or causes. The y axis is

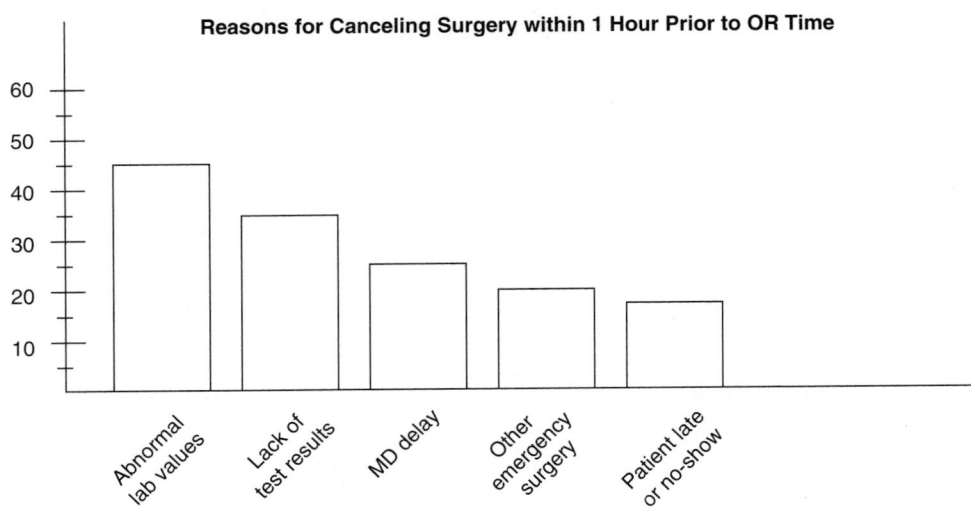

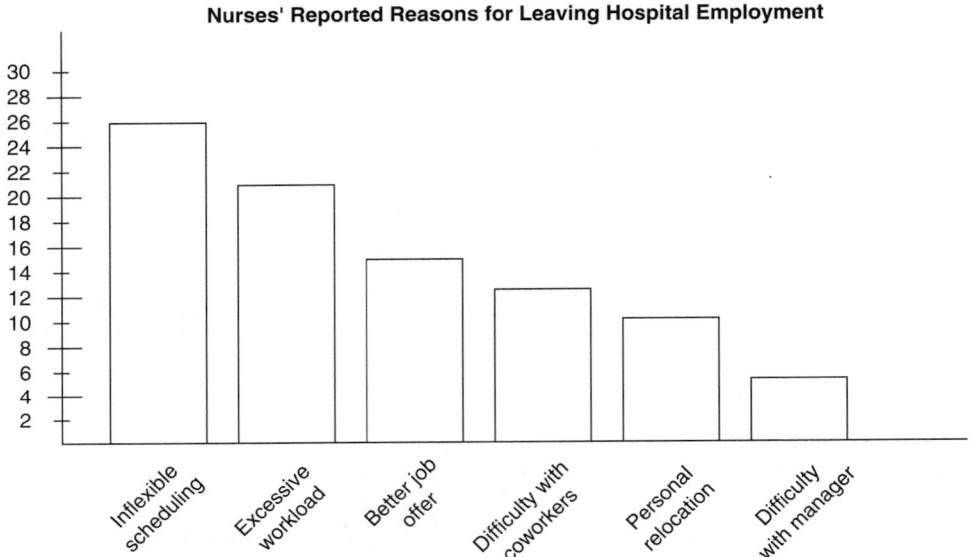

Fig. 3-10 Examples of Pareto charts.

vertical, and depicts the amount, measurement, or percentage intervals.

3. The first bar on the graph (left-hand side) is the category or cause with the highest ranking. Place other bars in descending order.

4. Keep a gap between bars on the graph, because the chart does not reflect interval data.

5. Use this chart to create a clear description of the situation, to gain consensus on the direction to pursue, and to establish an action plan for either further data collection or improvement strategies. Fig. 3-10 provides examples of Pareto charts.

Cause and Effect Diagram (Fishbone or Ishikawa Diagram)

A cause and effect diagram, also called a fishbone or Ishikawa diagram, is a tool used to identify the multiple causes of any result, outcome, or problem. It is used effectively by groups and aids in defining root causes of problems.

To create a cause and effect diagram:

1. Clearly define the end result or problem to be studied. It can be positive or negative. Write it at the end of the main arrow or spine of the fishbone (see Fig. 3-11).

2. Define the categories of possible causes to be analyzed. Write these on the bones pointing toward the spine. These categories can be generic or specially tailored to the issue and setting. For example, Brassard (1989) suggests that in a manufacturing setting, the generic categories might be manpower, machines, methods, and materials. In administration, the generic categories might be policies, procedures, people, and plant. Leebov and Ersoz (1991) suggest the generic categories of equipment, people, materials, methods, and

Possible Causes of Increased UTIs in Patients with Indwelling Urinary Catheters

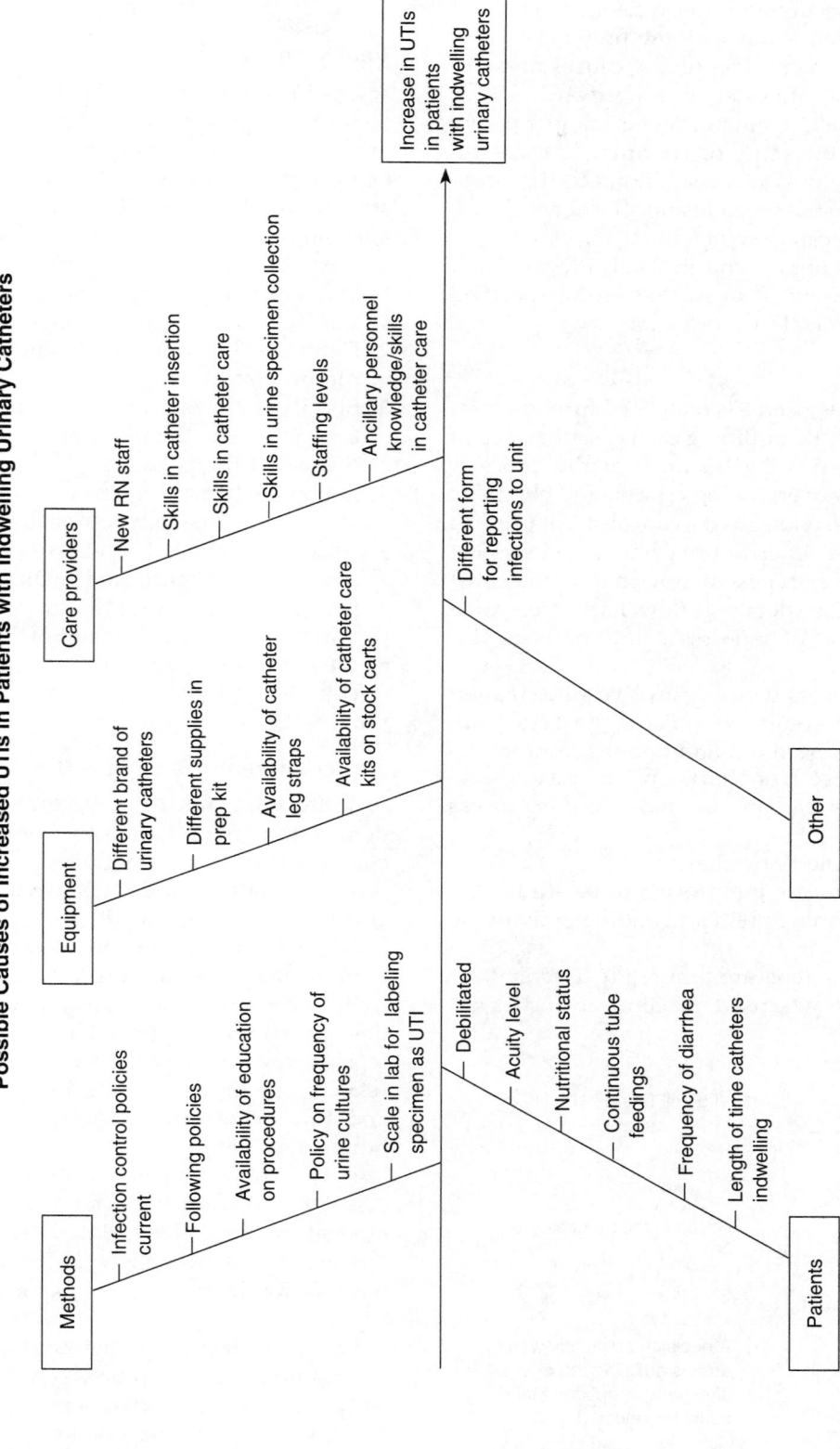

Fig. 3-11 Example of cause and effect diagram.

37

money. However defined, these categories should stimulate thinking about why the problem continues. Some recommend identifying causes first and organizing them into categories afterward.

3. For each category, brainstorm the many reasons why the problem occurs or continues. Be careful not to list symptoms of or solutions to the problem. Write the causes/reasons on short lines under the appropriate category heading.
4. This diagram is not an end in itself. Frequently it will point to the need to further study specified topic areas or to collect more data.

Detailed Flowchart

Flowcharts are tools used to create a picture of a process of care/service. By outlining each essential step in the process, it is possible to analyze the process, streamline areas of overlapping efforts, and eliminate unnecessary steps. Flowcharts can also be used to standardize a step-by-step approach to care or service.

There are several types of flowcharts, the most common being the detailed flowchart, described here. A description of top-down flowcharts is also provided.

Analyzing a process typically involves the creation of two flowcharts—one that reflects the actual approach currently carried out and one that reflects the ideal process. These two charts are contrasted, and opportunities to streamline or improve the process are identified.

To create a detailed flowchart:

1. Clarify and delineate the process to be studied.
2. Define the beginning point and ending point of the process.
3. The following symbols are commonly used in flowcharts, with arrows used to connect and direct them:

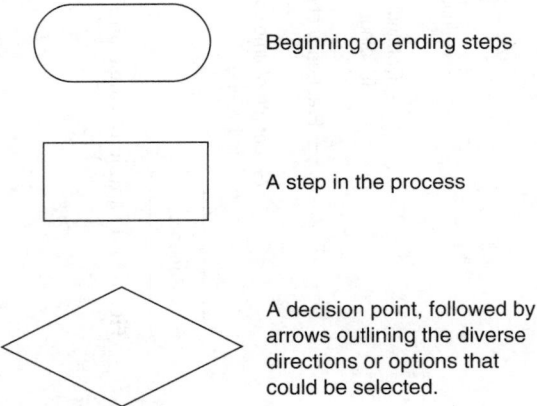

Beginning or ending steps

A step in the process

A decision point, followed by arrows outlining the diverse directions or options that could be selected.

4. Beginning at the top of a page, write the beginning step in the process. Continue down the page, highlighting each step or decision point, using the symbols. Be as detailed and accurate as possible.
5. Contrast the real and ideal processes to create plans for improvement.

Fig. 3-12 is an example of a detailed flowchart.

Top-Down Flowchart

A top-down flowchart is another tool used to create a picture of a process. In this style, the essential steps of a process form a horizontal line, with lesser steps being written underneath each major or essential step. A top-down flowchart helps differentiate major and minor steps of a process or plan, thereby highlighting where to devote greatest efforts.

To create a top-down flowchart:

1. Clarify and delineate the process to be studied.
2. Define the beginning point and the ending point of the process.
3. Specify the major, most essential steps in the process and write them in horizontal sequence across the top of the page.
4. Under each major step, detail the minor or substeps necessary to accomplish it.
5. As with a detailed flowchart, real and ideal processes can be contrasted, with the goal of streamlining and improving the process.

Or, this tool can help to plan or determine time and effort to be devoted to steps.

Fig. 3-13 provides an example of a top-down flowchart.

Scatter Diagram (Scattergram)

A scatter diagram, or scattergram, is a tool used to demonstrate the relationship between two factors or characteristics. Data are plotted on a basic graph. The resulting pattern indicates whether and how the characteristics are related.

For example, if the points run in somewhat of a line from the lower left-hand corner to the upper right-hand corner, it is considered a positive correlation. The more organized the line, the tighter the relationship. Higher "scores" of one factor are related to lower "scores" of the other factor, and improving one factor will likely improve the other.

If the points run in a line from upper left-hand corner to the lower right-hand corner, it is considered a negative correlation. Higher "scores" of one factor are usually associated with lower "scores" of the other factor. Increasing one factor will likely decrease the other.

Scattered data points without obvious pattern indicates no relationship between the two factors.

To create a scatter diagram:

1. Clearly identify the two factors to be measured— the data to be plotted.
2. Draw the axes. The x axis is horizontal and calibrates one factor or characteristic. The y axis is vertical and calibrates the other factor or characteristic. Identify intervals that will be useful for identifying patterns and trends.

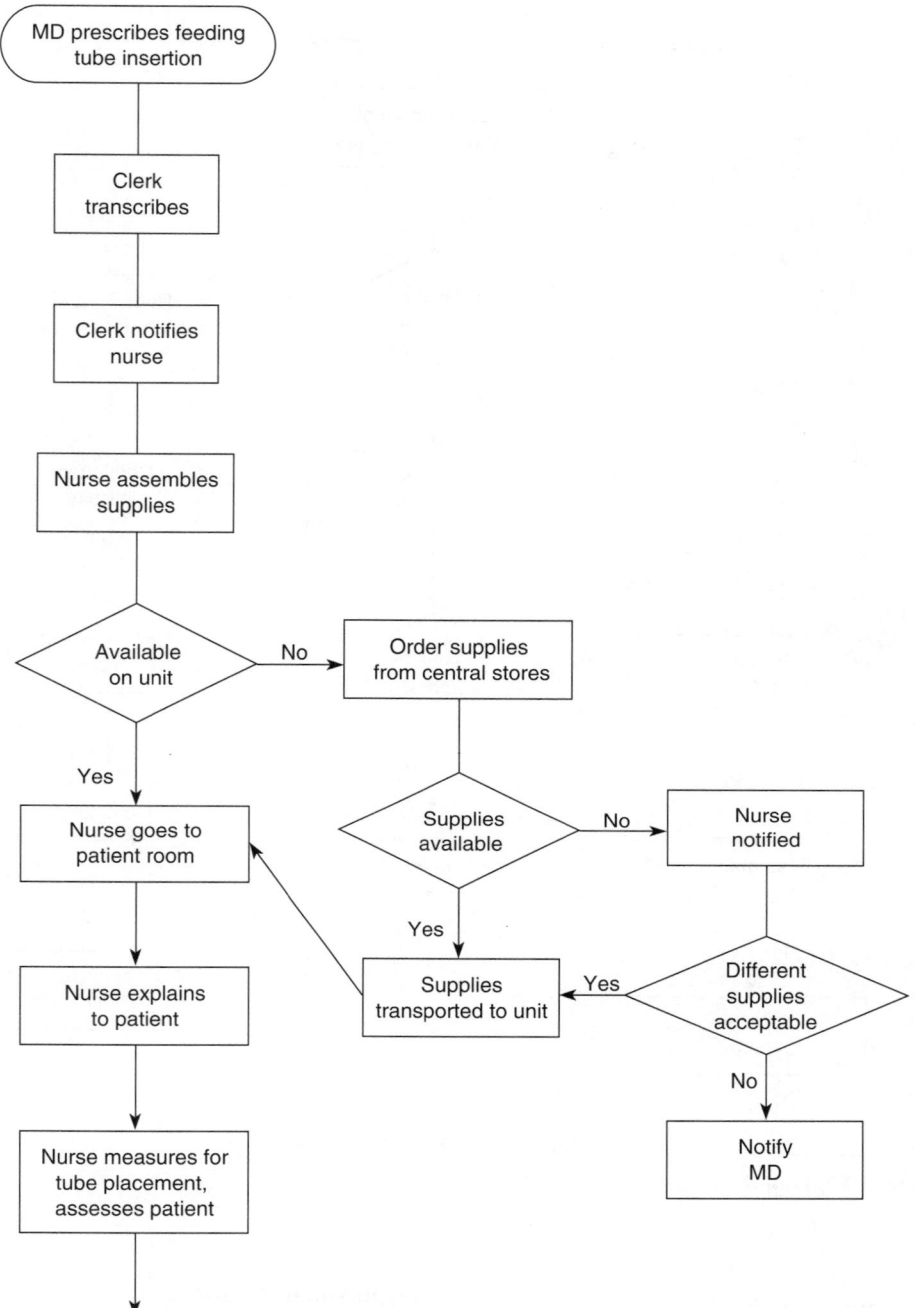

Fig. 3-12 Example of a detailed flowchart. *Continued.*

3. For each time the event occurs, plot a data point reflecting factors on both axes. Some suggest that when two data points are identical, the point should be plotted and then circled for each successive same point.
4. Analyze these data to identify patterns of relationships, and use the results in follow-up or action planning.

Fig. 3-14 provides an example of a scatter diagram.

Is/Is Not Matrix

An is/is not matrix is a tool used to identify patterns of characteristics of an event, outcome or problem.

These patterns are useful in clarifying, analyzing, and improving the problem.

To create an is/is not matrix:

1. Clarify the event, outcome, or problem statement. Keep it simple and straightforward.
2. Define the characteristics of this event. The questions who, what, where, when, and how will guide this process. Examples may include:
   - Dates of occurrence, days of week, weeks of month, months of year
   - Time of day
   - Units or departments of occurrence

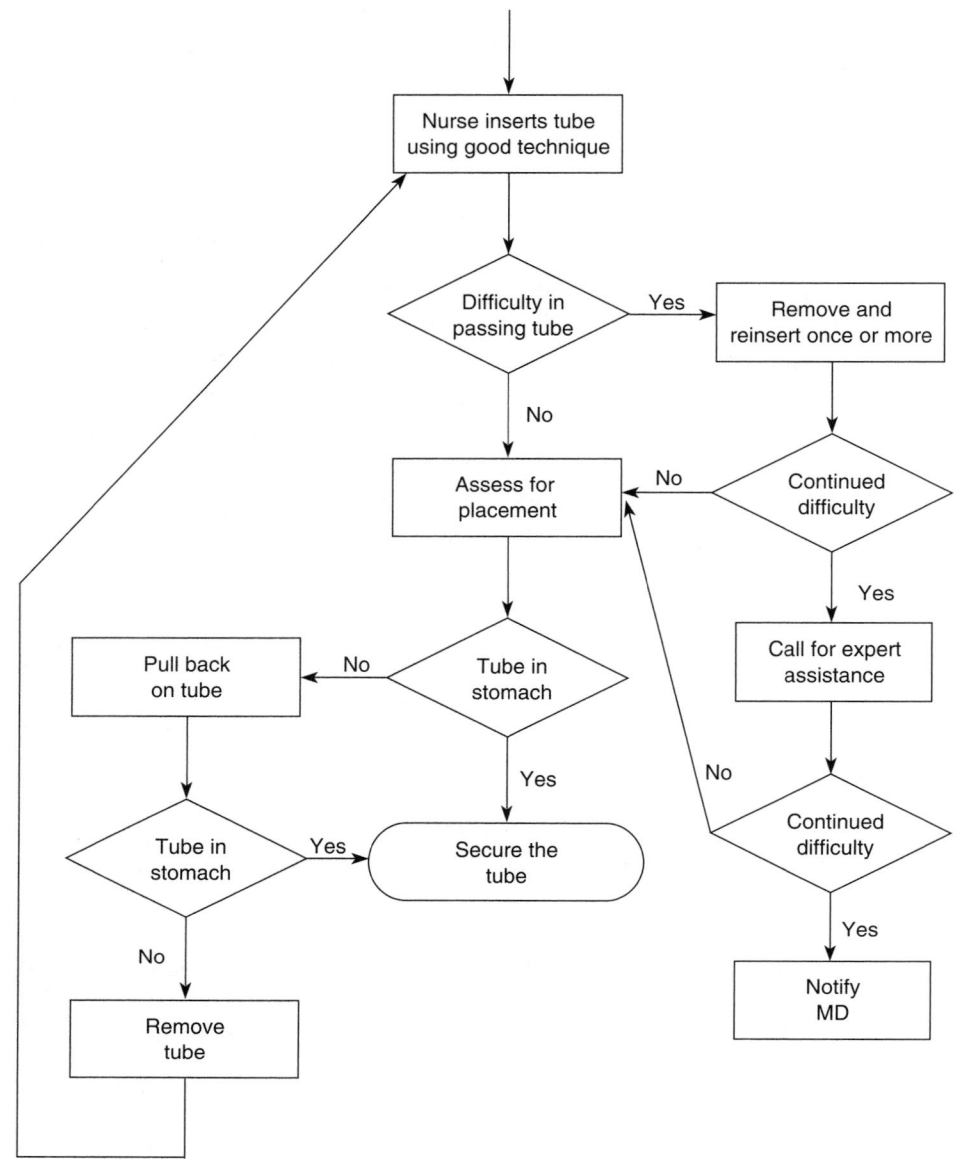

Fig. 3-12, cont'd.

- Patient/client groups involved
- Staff groups involved
- Types of practitioners involved

3. Write these characteristics in the boxes in the left-hand column of a four-column grid.
4. At the top of the second column, write "Is." At the top of the third column, write "Is Not." The final column can be labeled "Conclusions" or "Comments."
5. Fill in the boxes in the grid, noting whether each who, what, when, where, and why characteristic is or is not present, and how they differ.
6. Use this matrix to identify directions for further data collection and analysis, or to validate conclusions. Fig. 3-15 provides an example of an is/is not matrix.

Deployment Charts

A deployment chart is a matrix tool that links the steps in a process with the person responsible for it. It is useful in planning for or analyzing the flow of work.

To create a deployment chart:
1. Clarify (and set boundaries for) the process to be analyzed. It may help to establish a beginning and an ending step of the process.
2. Create a grid (see Fig. 3-16), with the left-hand column identifying the key steps in the process. Draw vertical columns to identify the individual people or groups responsible for all parts of the process.

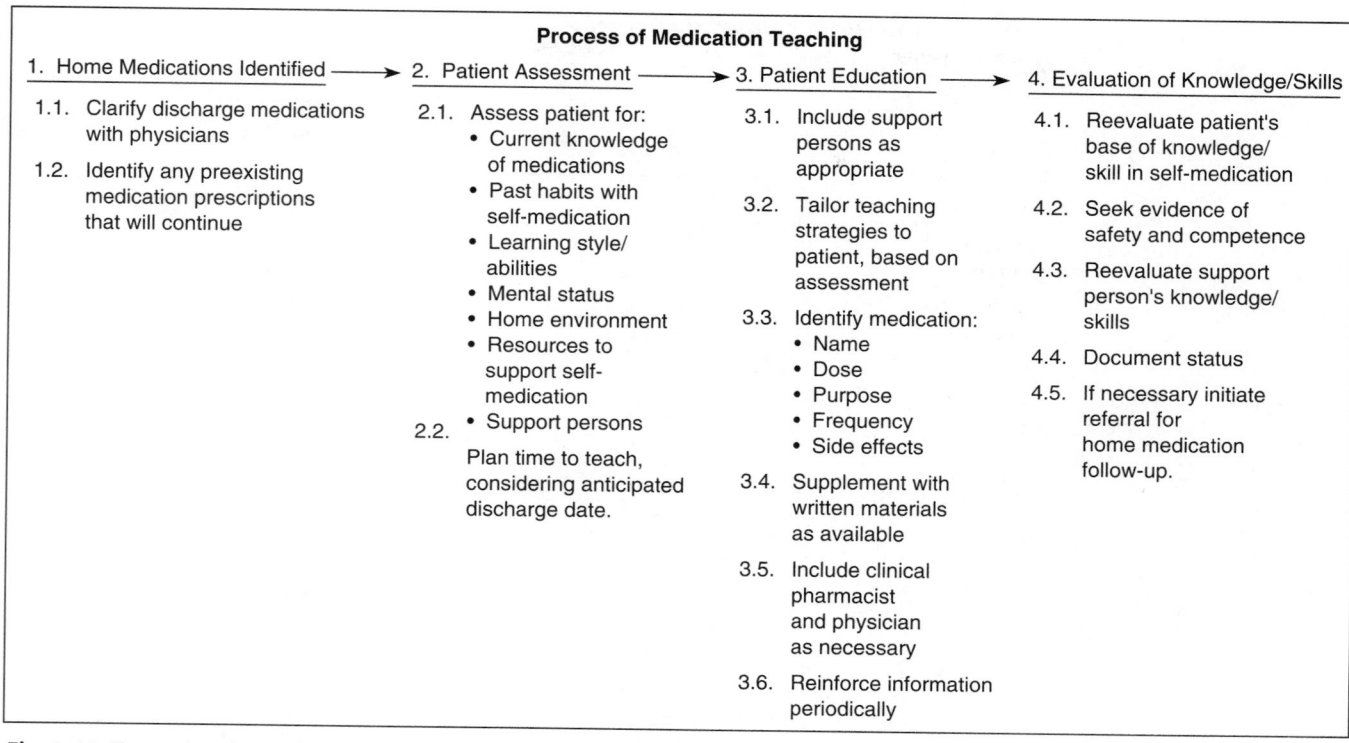

Fig. 3-13 Example of a top-down flowchart.

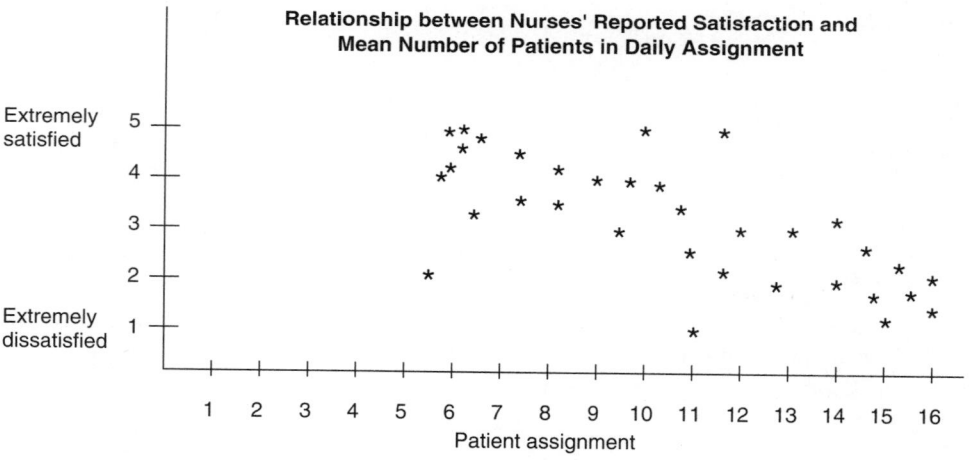

Fig. 3-14 Example of a scatter diagram.

3. Specify the people responsible for each step of the process, using the grid (matrix) boxes.
4. Some find it helpful to use a key or set of symbols to identify different types of responsibility (e.g., All are responsible for awareness, but only two must collect data, report, or carry out certain other functions).

Fig. 3-16 is an example of a deployment chart.

Force Field Analysis

A force field analysis is a strategy to analyze a situation, and/or assist with a change process. It is based on the assumption that all situations (states) are the result of restraining forces that support their being and, thus, the status quo (they restrain change). To change the situation, one must understand both what supports the current state and what are the driving forces that can help to change it. Identification of both types of forces—restraining forces and driving forces—is necessary to create planned change. To change, one needs to weaken or decrease the restraining forces and strengthen or increase the driving forces. It is insufficient to address only one or the other. This tool is more effective when used in a

Problem: Increased Postoperative Infections

	Is	Is Not	Conclusions/ Comments
What Sites of infections Types of organisms			
Who Patient groups Staff groups Types of practitioners			
Where Units/depts of occurrence			
When Dates of occurrence Days/weeks/months Time of day of surgery			

How
Characteristics of
  infection
Possible methods of
  transmission
Perioperative
  techniques involved			

Fig. 3-15 Example of an is/is not matrix.

group, and can be the focus of a brainstorming session.

To create a force field analysis:
1. Clearly define the situation or issue to be analyzed, including the current state and the desired change.
2. Create a chart with two columns: one labeled Restraining Forces, and one labeled Driving Forces.
3. Under Restraining Forces, identify the many reasons that the issue remains stable or status quo.
4. Under Driving Forces, identify the many reasons that support change.
5. Use these conditions to strategize a plan to weaken or decrease the restraining forces and strengthen or increase the driving forces.

Fig. 3-17 provides an example of a force field analysis.

Affinity Diagram

An affinity diagram is a tool used by groups to identify patterns and categories in broad or complex issues. It begins with brainstorming to identify the multiple factors related to the situation. The group then pulls into categories any factors that seem related. Categories are labeled and are then used for further analysis or action planning.

To create an affinity diagram:
1. Define the question, situation, or issue to be addressed.
2. Brainstorm the possible factors that could be related to the situation under study. Identify as many as possible.
3. Write these factors on a blackboard, flip chart, or overhead transparency. (In small groups, some

Unit Quality Assesment Functions

Steps	Amy, Chair	Michael	Liz	Tim	All Staff Members
Establish annual plan	*	*	*	*	
Define priority aspects of care/service					*
Develop indicators/data-collection tool for Aspect #1			*		
Develop indicators/data-collection tool for Aspect #2		*			
Establish data-collection time frames	*				
Collect data	*	*	*	*	
Analyze data					*

Fig. 3-16 Example of a deployment chart.

write the factors onto note cards, one factor per card. This approach helps afterward in sorting factors into categories [Brassard, 1989].)

4. Collate the factors into groups that have a common theme. After most factors have been grouped (though sometimes a few factors do not fit in the groups identified), label the categories.
5. Draw the diagram, with the question, situation, or issue at the top, and category labels flowing from it. The multiple factors can then be listed under category labels.
6. Use these perspectives for further analysis and action planning.

Fig. 3-18 provides an example of an affinity diagram.

Tree Diagram

Tree diagrams are tools used to break down a goal, problem, or idea into manageable tasks or action

NURSES' USE OF BEDSIDE COMPUTER TERMINALS

Restraining Forces	Driving Forces
Fear of computers	State-of-the-art technology
Lack of time	Rapid access to information
Lack of experience	Well-supported initiative of the organization
Few resource people for assistance	Decrease in documentation or multiple records
High patient volume and acuity	Addresses frustration/ time regarding documentation
Staffing shortages	Supports greater synthesis of data
Familiarity with chart forms	Provides cues for action and documentation
Lack of support of computers by coworkers	Supports quality assessment function

Fig. 3-17 Example of a force field analysis.

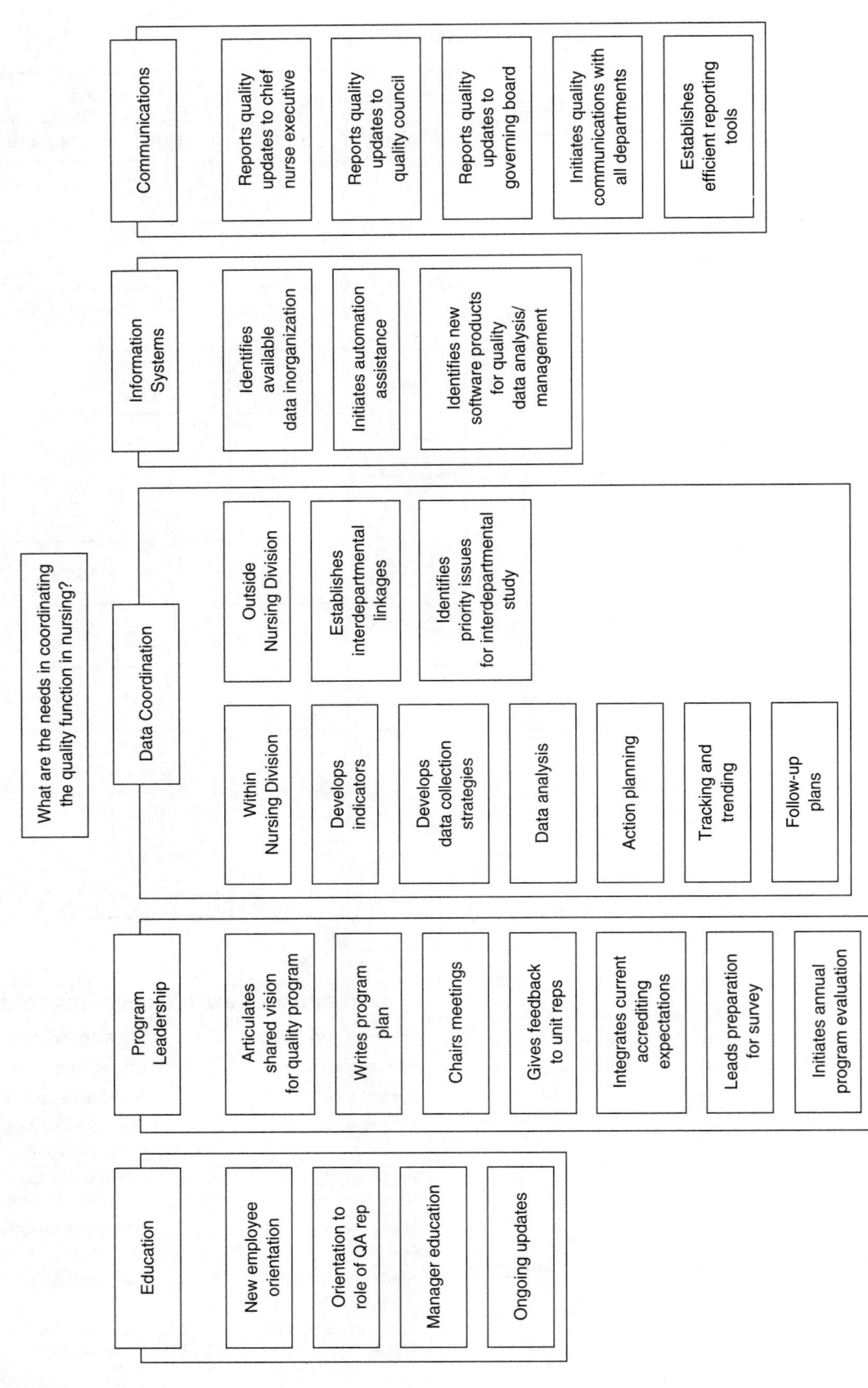

Fig. 3-18 Example of an affinity diagram.

What are the needs in coordinating the quality function in nursing?

Communications
- Reports quality updates to chief nurse executive
- Reports quality updates to quality council
- Reports quality updates to governing board
- Initiates quality communications with all departments
- Establishes efficient reporting tools

Information Systems
- Identifies available data inorganization
- Initiates automation assistance
- Identifies new software products for quality data analysis/management

Data Coordination
- Within Nursing Division
- Develops indicators
- Develops data collection strategies
- Data analysis
- Action planning
- Tracking and trending
- Follow-up plans
- Outside Nursing Division
- Establishes interdepartmental linkages
- Identifies priority issues for interdepartmental study

Program Leadership
- Articulates shared vision for quality program
- Writes program plan
- Chairs meetings
- Gives feedback to unit reps
- Integrates current accrediting expectations
- Leads preparation for survey
- Initiates annual program evaluation

Education
- New employee orientation
- Orientation to role of QA rep
- Manager education
- Ongoing updates

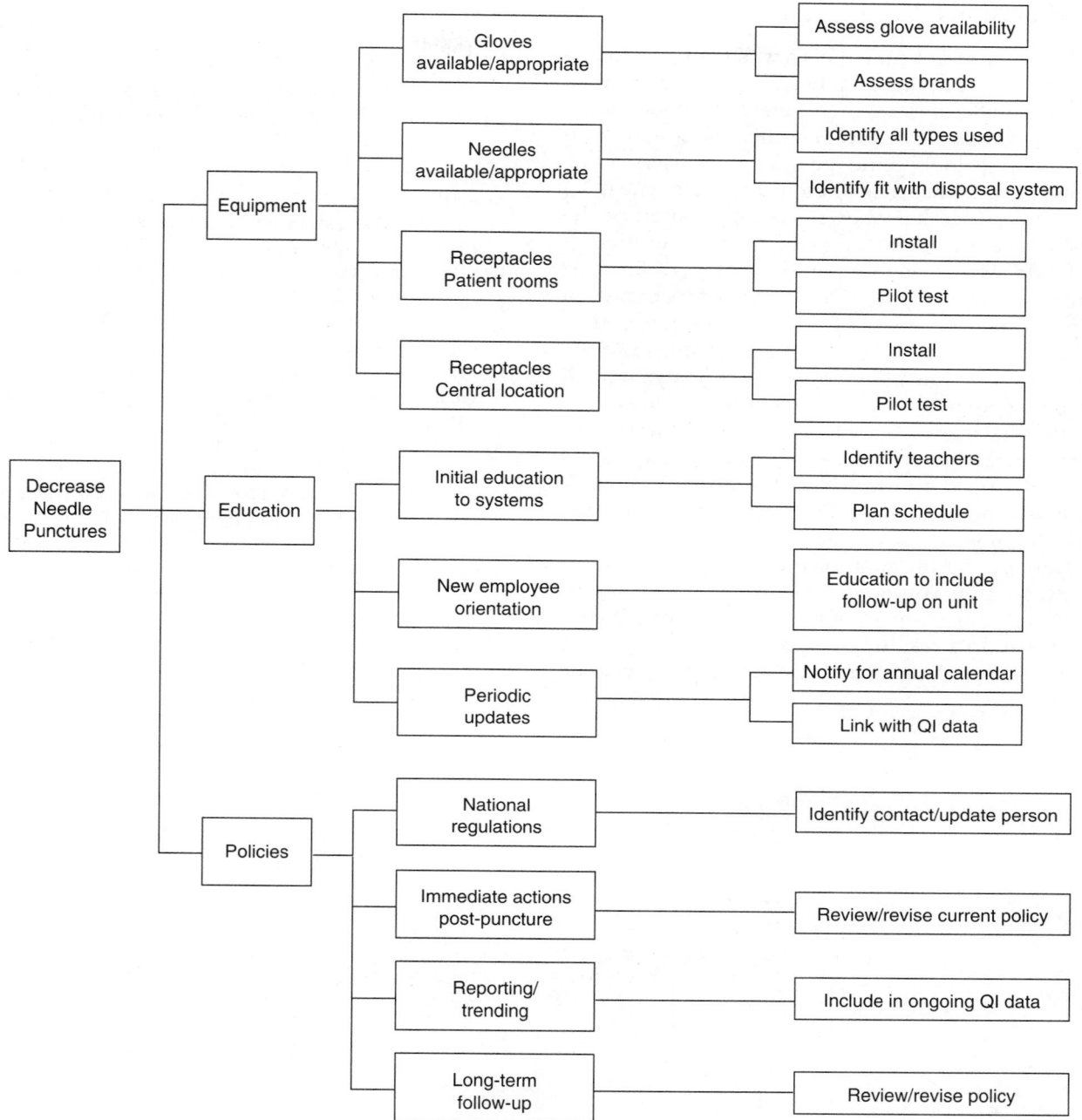

Fig. 3-19 Example of a tree diagram.

steps. They are visible models to help a group use basic logic to move from the broad situation to specific, assignable, and measurable components.

To create a tree diagram:

1. Clarify the goal, problem, or idea to be pursued. This statement is usually written on the left-hand side of a paper page, flipchart, blackboard, or overhead transparency (see Fig. 3-19).

2. Identify broad ways in which the goal, problem, or idea might be addressed. These broad strategies will flow from the focus statement.

3. For each broad strategy, identify specific tasks or action steps necessary to accomplish goals. "Branch" these action steps off to the right of the appropriate strategy statement.

4. It may be necessary to further break down the action steps until statements are in the form of manageable and assignable tasks.

5. This tool can serve as a guide for further analysis, planning and implementation of improvements.

Fig. 3-19 is an example of a tree diagram.

CONCLUSION

One's learning about the tools and techniques for assessing and improving quality and performance must not stop with a class or a reference book. Only through experience in applying them in various situations will QI tools come alive for their users. Only through experience will their true effectiveness be seen. Experience has shown that application of the tools immediately following education about them is most effective in gaining understanding. Furthermore, they are most effective when used by groups of people who are closest to the process in question.

This collection of QI tools and techniques is but a sample of the available approaches to analyzing and improving quality and performance. Other approaches have also been used successfully within organizations, and new ideas for tools/techniques are being developed and tested all the time.

Success in improving quality and performance requires the following actions:

- Careful identification of the most significant aspects of care/service
- Detailed assessment of the process of care or service and its resulting outcomes
- The collection and use of relevant and accurate data
- Aggressive analysis
- Strategic efforts to improve care/service continuously

The use of QI tools and techniques is one important and effective way to begin moving in the right direction.

REFERENCES

Berwick DM, AB Godfrey, J Roessner (1990): *Curing health care: new strategies for quality improvement*, San Francisco, Jossey-Bass Publishers.

Brassard M (1989): *The memory jogger plus+*, Methuen, Mass, GOAL/QPC.

GOAL/QPC (1988): *The memory jogger*, Methuen, Mass, GOAL/QPC.

Goldfield N, M Pine, J Pine (1991): *The health care manager's guide to continuous quality improvement*, Gaithersburg, Md, Aspen Publishers Inc.

Joint Commission on Accreditation of Healthcare Organizations (1991): *An introduction to quality improvement in health care*, Oakbrook Terrace, Ill, Joint Commission.

Katz J, E Green (1992): *Managing quality: A guide to monitoring and evaluating nursing services*, St Louis, Mosby.

Leebov W, CJ Ersoz (1991): *The health care manager's guide to continuous quality improvement*, Chicago, American Hospital Publishing Inc.

IMPROVING QUALITY AND PERFORMANCE: IMPLICATIONS FOR THE TEAM FACILITATOR/QUALITY ADVISER

Toni C. Smith

Hospitals are seeking smarter ways to do business in today's rapidly changing, competitive environment. New approaches to hospital management that emphasize *quality leadership* methods are being instituted. Quality leadership requires a shift in management style from one that focuses on limited clinical issues to one that takes on broader quality service issues of the institution. Health care organizations are now focusing on the processes used to monitor and evaluate all services provided so as to constantly improve care delivery and support systems and to meet the needs of internal and external customers. Management approach achieves improvements by using a scientific process to improve systems, basing decisions on data, and considering all customers of the hospital in planning and implementing actions. Hospitals are joining in the quality movement, and health care administrators are discovering the benefits of having people at all levels within the organization work together on project teams to improve existing operations. As health care administrators and staff recognize that inefficient production systems create the majority of quality problems, individual staff members and departments will no longer be blamed (as they often were using quality assurance approaches) for inefficiencies, negative outcomes, and variations, because these problems arise from unstable hospital processes and systems.

Strong Memorial Hospital (SMH), University of Rochester Medical Center, planned and implemented a very formal and comprehensive total quality management program (TQM) in the fall of 1991 in cooperation with the Rochester Institute of Technology Training and Professional Development Department. The hospital's TQM program is based on a written vision and philosophy statement that defines quality at the institution. This program embodies the concepts of continuous quality improvement (CQI) to assist the hospital in meeting customer requirements. The hospital has invested resources in educational/training initiatives and has established a TQM office to oversee program implementation and development.

SMH is a 750-bed acute care teaching facility in upstate New York. Hospital TQM awareness and commitment began with the training of the senior management directors of the hospital. Planning for future TQM training sessions for other hospital directors/department heads began after the hospital's management senior team members were trained. The TQM educational program was designed to provide two levels of training: basic training in TQM strategies/concepts and advanced training for selected staff in facilitator skills to guide future project teams. The role of a facilitator/quality adviser in project teams in a hospital-based total quality management program is discussed here.

DUTIES AND ROLE OF THE FACILITATOR

To help project teams function and communicate effectively, designated individuals within an institution need to receive extra training in problem solving and quality improvement strategies, project management, group-process theory/interventions, and use of statistical tools to organize data. Once trained, these individuals serve as consultants, providing technical assistance to project teams, and are known by several names, including facilitators, quality advisers, and quality specialists. For this discussion, these team consultants will be referred to as *facilitators*.

The ideal team is formed of individuals close to the process who rely on each other to work cohesively together to accomplish a specific task based on a mandate or charge. Team members need to be mutually supportive, to trust each other, and to agree to cooperate rather than compete with each other in order to get a job or project done. Facilitators help teams identify and free themselves from internal obstacles, so that the team's energy can be harmonized to focus on the pursuit of its objectives.

An individual trained as and assigned to be a facilitator must maintain a neutral position and in many ways is an outsider to a team. By maintaining a neutral position, the facilitator becomes alert for opportunities to help a team succeed in its efforts to break down barriers and improve communication among members. The facilitator assists the team to form into an effective work group by helping the team members successfully progress through the four phases of group development—orientation, interpersonal group conflict, cohesion building, and interdependence/loyalty—to emerge as a cohesive working team. A facilitator attends team meetings but is not a team member or the leader of the team. He or she may also be the facilitator for more than one team simultaneously.

The primary role of a facilitator is to help the project team members communicate within the group to avoid problems that can occur around issues of goals, roles, procedures, and interpersonal matters. Facilitators:

- Are guides but do not direct; they attend all team meetings.
- Serve as catalysts to bring about change by helping team members discover on their own new approaches and solutions to problems.
- Act as role models by demonstrating skills required to implement the problem-solving or continuous improvement processes.
- Monitor the group's application of statistical tools to be sure decisions are made on the basis of correct display and analysis of data.
- Work and meet with team leaders between meetings to plan for upcoming meetings to discuss team process issues and next steps.
- Serve as consultants to team leaders and other team members regarding TQM processes and tools.
- Provide feedback to team members on group dynamics and process issues of the team meetings that may impede or assist progress toward goal achievement. They may do so by using "group process analysis" forms that track the group's activities (e.g., monitor conversation flow/contributions of group members; evaluate structure, content and flow of team meetings, etc.).

Facilitators initially will spend the majority of their time with recently trained groups, helping them apply and practice new problem-solving skills and techniques. However, the ultimate goal of the facilitator is to guide the team in growth and development to the point where the team no longer relies on the facilitator and becomes self-supporting.

Facilitator Qualifications and Selection

At a recent seminar, Dr. Edwards W. Deming stated that individuals categorized as "best workers" have no bearing on future outcomes. He stresses that performance in a job held at present should not be the basis for prediction of performance in a new job. He says promotion or appointment of an individual to a new job or position is based on the honor system. This honor system involves the recommendation by someone who has reason to believe the person that he or she recommends will do well. This belief must come from intimate knowledge of the candidate's performance over time.

Initially, hospital administrators, directors, and department heads will recommend individuals from various departments to be trained as facilitators in addition to the TQM training that all employees will receive. Therefore, the ideal candidate to be recommended for facilitator training should be recognized as being:

- A good observer who is patient as change slowly and systematically takes place.
- Articulate and able to give constructive feedback to individuals and groups in an open and honest manner.
- Able to focus discussions for purposeful outcomes (knowing when to intercede in group discussions and when to refrain from commenting).
- Able to promote exploration, disclosure, and mutual problem solving among the diverse members of a team.
- A teacher/instructor, mentor.
- Detail and process oriented with analytical capabilities.
- Interested in learning new skills or refining existing ones.
- Willing to invest a considerable amount of time and energy into project team activities.

Facilitators should be selected from multiple clinical and support departments of the organization. Staff members who can demonstrate a working knowledge of statistical data analysis/monitoring tools should be considered. Individuals selected must receive initial training in total quality management concepts and understand how these concepts will apply to the organizational setting prior to receiving facilitator training.

Facilitator Skills

Skills needed for the facilitator role can be categorized into three observable domains of management skills as identified by Robert Katz (1974) and described by Fralic and O'Connor (1983 a,b). These three domains, technical skills, human skills, and conceptual skills, are needed by project-team facilitators. These skills will be demonstrated in varying degrees by facilitators, because of differences in team structures, goals, and objectives. Each skill domain and its definition and focus are described in Table 4-1.

TABLE 4-1 Basic Observable Team Facilitator Skills

Skill Domain	Definition	Elements
Technical	An understanding of and proficiency in a specific kind of activity involving methods, processes, procedures, and techniques (Katz, 1974)	Specialized knowledge of TQM and statistical/analytical concepts Knowledge of how to run effective/efficient meetings Facility in the use of statistical quality management tools (e.g., control charts, flow charts, Pareto charts, general statistical analysis, multi-voting, brainstorming, force field analysis) Expertise in the use of the steps in the problem-solving process or quality improvement process to address the charge of the team
Human	Individual ability to work as a facilitator of a team to build and promote flexibility and cooperation of members of the project team to unite to form an effective group. This skill is demonstrated in the way an individual perceives and recognizes the perceptions of team members (Katz, 1974)	Promotion of interactive goal-oriented communication through use and teaching of active listening skills; team coaching skills; use of a needs-based communication process Facilitating team members testing and simulating new roles and behaviors (managing emotions) during team interactions Understanding of group behavior and group dynamics to address interpersonal issues and build team commitment Ability to give feedback, to follow up, and to promote collaboration (team support of members)
Conceptual	The ability to see the entire organization as a whole by recognizing how the various functions of the organization interact and how changes in any one part affect the other parts (Katz, 1974)	Use of learning theories and stages of group/team development to promote group cohesiveness and problem solving Ability to analyze group process and apply management-theory concepts Promotion of positive interdepartmental interactions Knowledge of systems theory and concepts of profound knowledge Ability to use data management/variance analysis concepts

If individuals selected to be trained as facilitators do not possess knowledge of statistical data management strategies, these persons will need further instruction in this technical skill domain, which encompasses:

- Selecting appropriate statistical tools to prepare graphic presentations of data to show distribution of data and relationships between variables, describe data, and allow for interpretation of information correctly (data collection, description, and analysis)
- Facilitating group divergent and convergent thinking through brainstorming and consensus decision-making techniques
- Illustrating relationships between a given effect and its potential causes (e.g., with Ishikawa diagrams)

- Using control charts to monitor processes/systems over time
- Applying list-reduction strategies (e.g., weighted voting, criteria selection matrix)
- Constructing Pareto charts to differentiate the vital few causal factors from the trivial many

Facilitator Training: Content Outline

The TQM educational plan for the institution should contain a formal structure and process to train staff in TQM concepts and to train facilitators for project teams. The educational plan needs to outline short- and long-term goals of both training programs and to outline remedial, supplemental, and ongoing training activities for facilitators.

For initial training sessions it is advisable to seek outside consultation from a company or college or

---

Facilitator Training: Content Outline

Institutional Overview of Total Quality Management Concepts
Definition of TQM for institution (mission and vision)
Quality goals and objectives of the institution
Principles of quality management (processes, methods, tools, customers, variation analysis, and transformation strategies)
Training/educational plan
Communication plan (how staff will be kept informed about components of the program and program outcomes)
Employee involvement (how, who, and when)
Successful companies; benchmarking
Institutional implementation plan, timetable
Institutional quality organizational structure

Team-building Fundamentals
Purpose/function of project teams
Effective team-building strategies (goals, procedures, and responsibilities)
Interpersonal group-dynamics issues
Stages of team development
Team roles, behaviors: team leader, scribe, timekeeper, team member(s), and facilitator
How to plan, lead, and end team meetings
Theory of learning
Conflict-management strategies (diagnosing, definition, levels of conflict, stages, sources, collaboration, and resolution)

Steps/Application of the Problem-solving Process

Steps/Application of the Quality Improvement Process

Utilization and Application of Statistical Tools
(Graphs, check sheets, control charts, cause and effect diagrams, histograms, Pareto diagrams, scattergrams)

---

university experienced in training staff in health care institutions in TQM strategies. Then the institution can develop its own educational program tailored to the needs and individuals of the institution for ongoing training initiatives. The box outlines educational content for the facilitator training program.

Basic Group-management, Team-building Strategies for Facilitators

It is essential that individuals selected to serve as facilitators undergo formal training in TQM concepts prior to receiving training for the facilitator role. Persons with knowledge and skill in the use and application of statistical tools and group management techniques are desirable candidates for further training. However, programs to train facilitators need to level the content to meet the needs of people who are not experienced in the facilitator role or in the use of statistical tools. The training should provide in-depth instruction and practice in:

- Applying statistical tools of Total Quality Management
- Understanding group process and dynamics
- Understanding problem-solving and quality improvement decision-making strategies
- Promoting active listening skills
- Coaching team leaders to help plan and prepare for meetings, and coaching team members in the use of TQM tools
- Assisting the team leader in monitoring team meetings to keep the team on track and goal-oriented

Newly trained facilitators may benefit from serving as a cofacilitator with a person with facilitator experience. New facilitators need opportunities to demonstrate all the skills and techniques they learned in a controlled setting before they assume responsibility for a project team. Those with experience in the application of TQM processes and statistical tools will probably need less support and training than inexperienced facilitators. One approach to support facilitators implemented as part of the TQM program at SMH was the formation of a resource group of trained facilitators. The group's members meet regularly to support each other by engaging in mutual problem identification and problem-solving activities as they relate to the facilitator's role.

POTENTIAL PROBLEMS/PITFALLS TO THE FACILITATOR ROLE

At Strong Memorial Hospital, facilitators, as members of the Quality Resource group, meet on a regular basis to discuss issues and concerns. An interesting aspect of these meetings is the commonality of issues discussed. The issues are varied, as might be expected in a situation of many project teams addressing a variety of clinical and systems issues.

Facilitators may experience problems during initial training sessions and while working as a facilitator after initial training is completed. Specifically, the following areas may become problems or pitfalls that can hinder TQM teams. These issues need to be identified and addressed early in the implementation phase after the training process by the team's facilitator or by the department charged with implementing the TQM training program:

- Facilitators who lack experience as a team member on a trained TQM team, before assuming facilitator role
- Team members and facilitators who lack experience in the use of meeting-evaluation forms and statistical tools
- Unclear team mandate or charge from top management, or the inability of a team to identify a problem that can be solved within the specified time period

- Lack of physician and/or other staff involvement in team meetings due to poor meeting attendance or interest in the process
- Difficulty in scheduling team meetings because members will not make a commitment to make meetings a priority responsibility, and view team meetings as intrusions on their real jobs
- Team meetings where members have hidden agendas or interpersonal resentments, or lack certain shared goals and purposes
- Domination of meetings by a few members or by the leader of the department
- Strong competition between team members
- Time commitment required to have ongoing productive meetings
- Disagreement among team members over team procedures to complete tasks and make decisions
- Team feeling a lack of empowerment or direction from management which may be symptomatic of inexperienced teams or of an organization in the process of changing its culture
- Difficulty in consensus building because of diversity among members
- Confusion about the goal or purpose of the team
- One member making decisions for the entire team (this is usually found in teams in the early stages of development)
- Untrained members in the organization who lack information regarding the TQM process and feel resentment and fear due to lack of information
- Lack of interest and trust in the TQM process by team members and other hospital employees

STRATEGIES FOR SUCCESS: HELPFUL HINTS

In order for facilitators to guide and advise project teams successfully, the hospital must not only invest in initial training but provide follow-up and ongoing training to facilitators to keep them current in TQM concepts. An organizational approach and philosophy that address quality initiatives for the organization need to be created and defined. It is from this philosophical statement that TQM activities must flow. The top management group of the institution should delineate up front how and who will train staff in TQM concepts based on an established organizational vision and philosophy.

The following measures, covering a variety of areas, will help ensure the success of TQM in a health care institution:

- Institute training/educational programs in a planned manner and in manageable numbers. Avoid having too many project teams in process at the same time (seek outside support and consultation to assist in designing educational programs).
- Bring in outside experts to provide new information and review previously learned concepts to keep facilitators up-to-date in their knowledge. Continuously review established training processes to help the organization identify opportunities for improvement and barriers that may prohibit success.
- Establish a support group for facilitators to allow for networking and mutual problem solving regarding role issues.
- As part of the TQM and facilitator training process, delineate which data management tools will be taught and used initially to avoid overwhelming facilitators and team members with too much information (ideally, facilitators should demonstrate a working knowledge of data management tools before they qualify to be trained as facilitators).
- Provide a direct link for each team to the institution's management structure to review, approve, or design specific mandates for team activity.
- Establish team makeup needs based on identified mandate or charge to the team.
- Design planned communication initiatives to keep staff abreast of TQM plans and processes hospital wide.
- Follow TQM processes as taught; it is the facilitator's role to ensure that group process is used to make decisions.
- Whenever possible, avoid having untrained members on teams or having too many physicians on the same team (untrained members often impede the flow of the group and may require too much attention from the group; physician schedules may restrict their ability to meet regularly with the entire team).
- Provide group-process monitoring and analysis forms for facilitators to use to monitor group interactions and dynamics among members (train facilitators in the use of forms to evaluate group meetings, team member participation, reactions to group discussion, etc.).
- Before training of team members and facilitators, establish a process to monitor and implement the TQM program institutionwide.

CONCLUSION

To plan and implement a comprehensive quality management program requires a long-term commitment by a hospital's administration. There are no short cuts. Hospitals must pay close attention to training programs for facilitators; poorly planned programs can yield early but temporary successes because no provisions are made for continual reinforcement and support (Dixon and Swiler, 1990).

The success of project teams in an institution is critical to the success of the institution's overall quality management program and to the subsequent interest of the rest of the hospital staff in the TQM process. Facilitators in TQM programs need continuous training to help project teams in different stages of development address a variety of problems. There needs to be planned communication provided to all employees about the hospital's TQM program and the progress of established teams. Hospital staff members not involved in initial training will be curious about what is going on and will want to know when, or how they will be involved or trained. A total quality management environment requires individuals to possess a variety of specialized skills, and the guidance from individuals trained as facilitators can help team members use team-meeting strategies to improve communication as problems are identified and solved in a systematic manner.

REFERENCES

Dixon G, J Swiler (1983): *Total quality handbook: the executive guide to the new American way of doing business*, Minneapolis: Lakewood Publications.

Fralic MF, A O'Connor (1983a): A management progression system for nurse administrators, part 1, *The Journal of Nursing Administration*, 13(4):9-13.

Fralic MF, A O'Connor (1983b): A management progression system for nurse administrators, part 2, *The Journal of Nursing Administration* 13(5):32-38.

Katz RL (1974): Skills of an effective administrator, *Harvard Business Review*, 52:90-102.

CHAPTER FIVE

IMPROVING QUALITY AND PERFORMANCE: IMPLICATIONS FOR MANAGERS

Cathleen Krueger Wilson

QUALITY IMPROVEMENT AS A NEW MANAGEMENT MODEL

The move to quality improvement represents a total paradigm shift for health care managers. The implementation of quality improvement in health care organizations creates several areas of conflict for the manager. The conceptual basis of quality improvement simply runs contrary to the way in which most health care organizations are managed (McLaughlin and Kalzuny, 1990). Therefore, the way managers work now and the way they will be expected to work in a quality improvement organization are radically different. The quality improvement environment calls for changes that include a switch from individual responsibility to group or collective accountability; a shift from administrative authority for problem solving to participative problem solving; replacement of expected procedure with flexibility and spontaneity; and a problem focus yielding to emphasis on continuous improvement and entrepreneurial thinking (Gitlow and Gitlow, 1987).

New Organizational Politics

In order to replace the traditional mindsets of managers with an entrepreneurial spirit and to empower them to make the transition to quality improvement, organizational politics must be carefully scrutinized and addressed. Unfortunately, the hard reality of power and politics is sometimes overlooked, unrecognized, or deliberately avoided during the implementation of QI. The resultant conflict that arises in workplaces where politics is not addressed will be seen in manager behaviors. These behaviors are commonly mislabeled as resistance to change.

For example, in a political climate there may be managers who fail to truly empower their staff. Some managers may be obsessed with fear of losing their jobs, instead of identifying opportunities for improvement. Other managers may find it ludicrous to think of their staff as customers. These behaviors may indeed be symptomatic of resistance to change. The more likely explanation, however, is that the organizational politics have not shifted to cultivate and sustain the new brand of power relationships that is needed in a quality improvement environment. In other words, the organization does not "walk what it talks." Managers are commonly caught right in the middle of this conflict.

Organizational politics can be defined as an exchange of power and as the methods used to gain resources. A unique quality of these dynamics is that they are easy to see in others but very difficult to see in the self. Commonly practiced organizational politics fall into two types: positive and negative. Negative politics are made up of actions that serve to meet the self-interests of a manager or of the department managed. Managers who employ positive politics, on the other hand, conduct a continual self-examination of motives in order to minimize self-interest and methods that do not include coercion or manipulation (Block, 1990). Positive political skills are essential for managers who wish to succeed in quality improvement organizations.

OBSTACLES TO THE MANAGEMENT OF QUALITY IMPROVEMENT

Power and Relationships

The conflict between the old ways of doing and the new management model demanded by quality improvement is seen most dramatically when one examines the use of power in work relationships. Power in traditional organizations is a feature of manager-subordinate relationships. People behave in certain ways, not because they want to but because they have to. This *power-over* is exactly the opposite of the *em*powering relationships demanded in the quality improvement organization. It is replaced by the *power to*, which describes empowerment. Individuals choose their actions carefully, with a clear purpose in mind. There is little time spent wondering why so much energy is being expended on projects with unclear outcomes.

The empowerment of everyone to participate in a continuous search for improvement requires new power relationships at *all* levels in the organization. In traditional organizations, power comes from goal achievement, as evidenced by the popularity of management-by-objectives. In the new organization, power comes from the management of the process used to achieve the goals, as well as the outcome. Whereas individual position and status are valued in the traditional organization, power in the quality improvement organization is viewed as what Wheeler and Chinn (1991) describe as a balance between individual and group interests and expertise.

The Consequences of Hierarchy. Centralized control is a feature of traditional management structures (Mintzberg, 1979). Information is carefully guarded and deliberately communicated along the chain of command. The quality improvement organization requires that managers encourage the flow of information to all corners. There is little information that is privileged. The chain of command, with narrow subdivisions, is replaced with an accountability for the whole. Shared decision making and a network of organizational involvement in the achievement of quality are important features (Mclaughlin and Kalzuny, 1990).

Another consequence of traditionally layered organizations is the feature of polarization. Natural barriers arise as the result of the segmentation of work. Departments compete for scarce resources, and there develops a strong emphasis upon winning and losing (Bennis, 1989). This game mentality is extremely obstructive in a quality improvement organization, which will value consensus, negotiation, and integration.

The Mystification of Work. Sometimes, managers in traditional organizations think that they have to keep their work a secret, in order to gain influence (Wheeler and Chinn, 1991). They mystify the rest of the organization about what is going on "down in the basement" or behind the "closed doors." Health care organizations are particularly susceptible to mystification, because of the predominance of specialized knowledge.

Quality improvement, on the other hand, requires that the manager be open and share information readily. Dissent and criticism, sharing of information, and the active development of subordinates lead to the precise identification of quality improvement opportunities. Systems and processes are no longer hidden and can be scrutinized with intensity.

Bureaucratic Mindsets. A common experience of managers in a traditional organization is the feeling of being caught in the middle. They may believe strongly that a new direction is necessary, but they feel surrounded by people with more power, who are married to caution, control, and safety. These mind-

---

What Managers Learn in Traditional Organizations
Manipulation of events, persons or situations
Bottom-line fixations
Managing information to one's own advantage
Expedient or knee-jerk decisions
Win/lose mentality
Greed
Name-dropping
Calculation in relationships
Focus on "higher-ups" instead of the product
Success from cautious communication
Adapted from Bennis (1989) and Block (1990).

---

sets prevent an individual manager from taking responsibility for a problem and then fighting for the solution. Problem solving is left to the "higher-ups" (Block, 1990). Yet, true quality improvement demands that all parties say what they see, and then act together to resolve problems that defeat quality.

Because most managers have developed their careers in traditional bureaucratic organizations, they have developed certain beliefs about how to be successful. These bureaucratic mindsets, described by Bennis (1989) and Block (1990), are summarized in the box above.

Boss as Hero. Another trapping of traditional organizations is the notion of the boss as hero. This is a significant hazard, particularly as nursing leaders have gained national prominence. People form cults around these hero bosses, instead of entering into collective empowerment. Power and influence, then, will come from association with the hero. Information is shaded, so as to avoid directly confronting the hero's beliefs (Bennis, 1989). This dynamic subverts any attempts to tell what one knows is true—action that is required in a true quality improvement organization.

The Bottom Line Fixation. Bottom line fixations are typical in traditional organizations, where the business of health care supersedes the delivery of care. In this scenario, innovations are not encouraged unless they save money. There is little recognition of the fact that new programs always cost money to start up in the first year. There is no investment in people, or their skill development, because it costs too much (Bennis, 1989).

An overemphasis on the bottom line reflects a short-term or an immediate-gain viewpoint, which is usually most evident when monthly financial statements are reported to the management team. This orientation interferes with the long-term philosophy that befits the continuous process of quality improvement.

Managerial Uncertainty. In heavily layered organizations, such as large systems with corporate functions, the manager can easily experience a sense of helplessness and dependency on those at the top, because of the reliance on rules and the negative use of power (DelBueno and Freund, 1986). Consequently, the manager becomes obsessed with the attitudes and behaviors of executives (who can make or break a career). Searching for opportunities to improve quality will occur only if the manager perceives that the problem is a priority and the solution is favored by top management. Subordinates quickly get the message, in subtle ways, that nothing is ventured without asking approval. Change rarely occurs when managers worry about approval.

Challenges and Choices Demanded by Quality Improvement

If bureaucratic mindsets exist within the management group or the organizational culture during the implementation of quality improvement, then managers will be confronted with three sets of anxiety-producing choices (Block, 1990). First, will managers choose to hold on to what they have created, in order to be promoted? Or will they choose to design something better, something that fosters the achievement of greater quality? Second, will managers abide by the triad of safety, caution, and control rather than following an unpopular path in the pursuit of quality? Third, if in spite of confrontation, everyone ignores the real issue, will the manager be willing to put his or her job on the line (Bennis, 1989)?

It takes courage and integrity to choose innovation over the status quo, risk-taking over security, and confrontation over silence. This form of organizational bravery is particularly difficult when a problem is vaguely defined or has been ignored for a long time. Bennis (1989) refers to resignation as not only a form of organizational confrontation but an ethical imperative for leaders.

If health care organizations do not seek ways to flatten their structure, manager dependency and reliance on the chain of command will predominate the culture (Block, 1990). People will simply wait for orders, instead of acting upon opportunities to improve quality.

In order to manage quality improvement effectively, manager-leaders must choose autonomy over helplessness, courage over caution, and improvement over maintenance. These are high-risk behaviors in any work setting. For the shift to be made, organizations must be scrutinized to determine the degree to which they are infected with negative politics.

The Politics of Traditional Organizations

Manager-Subordinate Contracts. In traditional organizations, relationships between managers and those they supervise are typically based on a top-down, highly controlled, centralized transaction (Mintzberg, 1979). In the delivery of health care, managers may have many unexpressed doubts: Is that new policy really necessary? Should we continue using this equipment or should we update our practices? Why doesn't anyone notice that there are not enough resources to implement this program? However, because of an unspoken contract, decisions are not questioned. Managers submit to the authority of the supervisor, in this case (Block, 1990). For example, action teams in quality improvement organizations may unconsciously avoid tackling certain issues because of this unspoken contract.

Definitions of Success. In traditional organizations, success is defined as moving up the ladder rather than as contributing to quality. The location of one's office and parking space, the number supervised, and the level of responsibility in the organization are traditional measures of success. New people are quickly socialized into doing what it takes to succeed rather than doing what it takes to improve quality. The adage that the higher you go, the less performance matters, rings true (DelBueno and Freund, 1986).

Block (1990) argues that this definition of success creates managers who are compromised and are dependent on organizational norms rather than on their own expertise and insight. This dependency creates a tendency to control things tightly, to seek permission, to tiptoe around change, and to forbid surprises. Quality improvement suffers because it becomes a cynical joke, shared when managers gossip in private.

This definition of success focuses on the greedy accumulation of things. With this focus, it is very difficult to engage in the sharing and the equal respect demanded in a true quality improvement organization.

Manipulative Communication. Manipulation is a cluster of behaviors that serve the self-interests of some managers in traditional organizations. The ways in which managers manipulate people and situations can include saying things that they do not mean. Instead of frank appraisal, negative feedback or honesty about the merits of something, manipulative managers code their communication so as to avoid alienating anyone with power (Block, 1990). These behaviors can also occur as the result of some kinds of female socialization (Schaef, 1985).

In a manipulative culture, people use a distinct and coded message for saying no (delBueno and Freund, 1986). "No" might be communicated by sending a suggestion to an ineffective task force. It might also be communicated with a smile and the comment "Thank you for your insight on this matter." The person offering the suggestion will never hear about it again!

If communication is used to manipulate rather than to understand and respond, coded conversation is the norm. The words "I'm only telling you this because I care about you" may be coded permission to devalue a person's belief (James, 1983). Also, the phrase "I have to tell you that negative comments about you are in the organization" may really mean that the manager is not happy with the subordinate's performance. In traditional organizations, where people are focused on pleasing top management, this manipulative communication is quite effective. Subordinates will most likely change their opinions to those of their manager. Unfortunately, this change may not be in the best interest of high-quality care.

The need to appear in agreement, so that success is not jeopardized, is usually accompanied by overt or covert sanctions. Individuals who speak up may not be invited to key meetings in the future. Performance evaluations may note problems with effective communication or with tact and diplomacy. In other words, the messenger is shot (Block, 1990).

In traditional organizations, managers have had to develop a wide variety of manipulative communications, in order to garner support for projects. Mentioning top management casually in conversations has enormous influence when everyone is focused on the behaviors of those at the top. When name-dropping is combined with understating risks, influence is more easily obtained (Block, 1990).

Organizational norms that require managers to use coded and careful communications are challenged during the implementation of quality improvement. The central theme of open communication in order to improve quality will generate significant manager anxiety. People will spend energy worrying about what is "safe" to say rather than what is needed to be said in order to improve quality.

QUALITY IMPROVEMENT MINDSETS

Visible Values

Managers of quality improvement must hold certain key values and make them observable. Values and behaviors must occur together and be congruous. Moral and intellectual honesty, dedication, generosity, and forgiveness form the foundation from which all action arises (Bennis, 1989).

Evolution

Continuous improvement requires a healthy respect for the cyclical nature of things. Quality is seen as both a process and a product. Managers who hold evolution as a value see change as continuous. There are no end points, only the next phase. There are not

medication errors but opportunities for a modification of medication delivery or a chance to improve a practitioner's skills. There are not problems with the documentation system but an opportunity to bring the system up to the next level of excellence. The only constant seen is the cycle of change itself (Wheeler and Chinn, 1991).

Empowerment

A cardinal value for the quality improvement manager is empowerment. The word has been overused and misunderstood by many. The real value of empowerment is only realized when managers are aware and active in their own growth and in the development of others. Education departments are not downsized by empowering managers. Learning opportunities abound in an organization. There is a strong, easily identified belief that all human beings fulfill their potential with the right learning opportunities.

Unfortunately, empowerment has sometimes been enacted with self-indulgence and in service of the self-interests of others. Instead, empowering managers continuously seek to understand their own motivations and behaviors. They engage in careful and thoughtful listening to their inner world and that of others (Wheeler and Chinn, 1991). Criticisms, suggestions, bewilderment, fear and compliments are accepted thoughtfully and analyzed in depth by individuals and groups, *only* if they are offered with the same degree of thoughtfulness. In this way, the path to quality is not littered with quick fixes and knee jerk decisions.

The true empowerment of self and others to improve quality is the result of a manager's choice to respond to self and others, while deliberately designing structures and processes that support the delivery of quality care.

Managers who empower their staff are themselves empowered. They believe that they, not top management, are responsible for their own success. Empowered managers can describe a real purpose to their work and display a strong commitment to it (Block, 1991). In the quality improvement organization, the manager will not experience the helplessness and the vulnerability of the bureaucrat if all relationships embody the value of empowerment.

How does one recognize a manager whose value of empowerment is matched with action? Ask, does the manager consider his or her role to be a systems consultant to the staff? Are subordinates encouraged to express themselves thoughtfully, without negative sanctions? What percentage of each staff meeting is devoted to attitudes, morale, motivation, and development? Bennis (1989) recommends that at least 25 percent of every staff meeting be spent on motivation and development.

Commitment Instead of Sacrifice

A myth in traditional organizations is that part of a manager's role is to support decisions that he or she may not agree with. This expectation results in managers sacrificing what they believe or know to be true in the interests of preserving organizational harmony. For example, managers might be expected to implement programs without adequate budgets. They may be forced to implement personnel policies that demotivate staff. If, for example, a particular physician is a high admitter, the manager may have to support costly, labor-intensive practice patterns.

Managerial sacrifice on the altar of harmony must be eliminated in the quality improvement organization. Instead of this mindset of sacrifice, the manager displays constancy and choice. Poor practices are consistantly challenged. Personal and professional choice is emphasized in performance reviews and in decision making. Passivity is not accepted; indeed, it is actively confronted (Bennis, 1989). The manager consistently acts in ways that not only expect accountability but insists upon a focus on quality improvement.

Openness

Senge (1990) has aptly defined openness as comprising two parts: participative and reflective openness. One cannot exist without the other. In fact, Senge (1990) goes on to say that participation can become a kind of organizational game, without the openness of reflection. Unfortunately, the plethora of health care literature calling for participative structures and a "cult of excellence" has resulted in underdeveloped or insufficient openness. It is commonly found under the guise of participative management styles.

The quality improvement paradigm embodies much of the value system of participative structures, including beliefs about people, their work and beliefs about leadership (Wilson, 1992). Underdeveloped openness is evident when the following steps are followed in making a decision:

1. A participative group feels free to express individual ideas and . . .
2. Arrives at a greatly watered-down decision that maintains harmony and makes everybody feel good about their participation, while in the meantime . . .
3. The right decision may have been abandoned for the one that is the most conflict-free.

In this case, decision making is compromised because there has not been time spent in evaluating *why* people feel and think as they do and if the logic is sound. "Group think" is not confronted. The actual merits of thoughts and beliefs are never challenged, by self or others, whereas they would be in a climate of *reflective openness* (Senge, 1990).

Reflective openness adds the analytic review necessary for full and effective participation. This dimension of openness demands what Moss Kanter calls the presentation of "half-formed ideas." Certitude is replaced with the suspension of conviction (Senge, 1990). Cherished ideas, long-held professional mindsets, and pet peeves are put on the table and allowed to be influenced by others. Some beliefs may be inappropriate for the issue being discussed or may be based on faulty logic.

Most managers do not possess the skills needed to facilitate both participative and reflective openness. Senge (1990) recommends that the management team be involved in long-term team building, so as to develop such skills. Individuals trained in group dynamics are able to help groups process their decision making. This analysis includes differentiating between rhetoric and reality, observing for incomplete or coded communication, pointing out faulty logic, and identifying unhealthy group norms. Team-building sessions by experts will facilitate complete openness and ease some of the pressures of participative partnerships in the early stages of change to a quality improvement environment (Wilson, 1992).

Consider the following example:

A participative planning group was evaluating the design of a nursing case manager role. The group was made up of head nurses, human resource experts, staff nurses, and a clinical director. The head nurses just recently had been moved into exempt positions, a change that they were not very comfortable with. When the status of the case manager role, as an exempt position, came up for discussion, several head nurses expressed concern. They stated that the organization was not ready for this leap. Others argued that no staff nurse would apply for such a position, because of the loss of overtime. A few lone voices expressed a belief that the exemption of the case manager role identified it as a clinical leadership role in the organization. One person observed that a hospital she had visited was changing its exempt case manager role back to a nonexempt one.

After much discussion, the group came to consensus that the role should remain nonexempt. The group leader applauded everyone for their openness and honesty. However, if the group members had thoughtfully challenged their assumptions, they may have observed that the head nurses were unhappy about their loss of overtime and were transferring that unhappiness to the staff nurses. Second, they might have recommended an alternative; for example, the case manager could work extra hours at a different rate of pay. Third, they might have reexamined the grading of the position in relationship to the overall goal of nursing case management.

The combination of participative and reflective openness is a strong antidote to the faulty logic and the self-interests that plague traditional organiza-

---

Sources of Knowledge in Quality Improvement Organizations

Knowledge of self and others
Recognition of a person's "ways of knowing"
Knowledge of true intent
Knowledge of the here and now
Knowledge of systems
Experience and wisdom
Expertise

---

tions. The manager who takes the time and makes the commitment to implement a prevailing openness will lead the organization to decisions that flow from knowledge, vision, values, and commitment.

New Power Relationships

Participative Partnerships. The effective managers of quality improvement will form partnerships with others in order to remedy systems problems or to stimulate innovation. A partnership implies equality in a relationship, where individuals have the same authority for decision making. This is in contrast to the manager-subordinate relationship, where one person has power over the other. Partnerships reflect the authority to act equally in the pursuit of quality. Participative partnerships can be extended into four areas of an organization: peer relationships, manager-subordinate relationships, departmental operation decisions, and multidisciplinary decision making. The implementation of these participative partnerships can be phased in, one group at a time, until the whole organization functions in partnerships (Wilson, 1992).

It is very important to take the time to determine both the location and the degree of participation expected at each step in the implementation of quality improvement. Failure to provide this definition can result in power conflicts, role confusion, and poor decisions.

Knowledge and Power. The quality improvement manager recognizes the central role of knowledge in the development and maintenance of quality health care delivery systems. Several kinds of knowledge are valued and therefore are actively solicited before a decision is made. These are summarized in the box above.

True quality improvement organizations demand that systems and the people functioning in them are given continuous opportunities to improve. Outmoded systems are replaced by new ones, and the actual problem is identified and matched with the best solution. Such optimum outcomes can only be achieved when power relationships shift from the power of position to the power of knowledge. It is not who you are but what you know that results in in-

fluence. Leadership will shift from person to person, depending on knowledge, expertise, skill, or the nature of the problem. Power, in this context, is *not* used for self-promotion but to take responsibiltity for action. In turn, action involves managers choosing to really know themselves and others, to comprehend the reality of the moment, and to understand both intent and motive (Wheeler and Chinn, 1991). The manager who views knowledge as power does not operate under the bureaucratic mindset of hoarding that knowledge. Instead, in combination with the value of empowerment, knowledge is diffused across the organization. Sharing is encouraged, as something healthy and desirable. Information flows are lateral and extensive. Therefore as many people as necessary have the knowledge (and power) to act on quality issues (Gitlow and Gitlow, 1987).

The Power of Design. If the power of position is diminished in the quality improvement organization, it must be replaced with something else if it is to be given up willingly. The search for continuous improvement requires that the power of position be replaced with the power of design. Managers who operate from the power of design study the system, its internal and external influences, and the culture of work and its respective socialization processes. They then design new systems, which improve the quality of thinking, thoughtful reflection, participation, and team learning (Bennis, 1989; Senge, 1990).

When managers are encouraged to develop their skills in systems design, they are able to let go of a feeling of giving away their power to other groups. Instead, they perceive that they have chosen to give power to an entity that they have created themselves. This shift in perception makes the development of action teams much easier (Orsburn, Moran, Musslewhite and Munger, 1990).

Finally, the manager-architect develops a mastery in the design and testing of mental models (Senge, 1990). "What if" is the calling card of this activity. Proposals are designed and recommendations trialed on a regular basis. There is no such thing as a bad idea. Mistakes are seen as learning opportunities. The entrepreneurial spirit flourishes!

New Definitions of Control. Clearly, the quality improvement organization requires that managers replace systems that control people with systems that bring people together in action. What happens to control? Managers are used to being the ones responsible for outcomes and will worry about how to control for good outcomes (Senge 1990). In the quality improvement environment, control is achieved when managers make sure that every decision is analyzed from a systems and a long-term view. What core resources of the organization might be quickly depleted if we aggressively pursue this direction? Are any aspects of patient care compromised in the future? What could be built into the design in order to negate this influence? How will other departments be influenced by the change? For example, an expansion of health care services into rural areas may look financially lucrative in the short term. However, the costs of maintaining such services over time may drain the organization of needed dollars to replace capital equipment.

A key role of the manager in quality improvement is to evaluate each decision in relationship to its effect upon the viability of the system as a whole. In addition, this systems thinking must be taught to the participative groups, with the manager's help. In this way, poor decisions arising from inexperience or faulty logic are avoided (Senge, 1990).

QUALITY IMPROVEMENT AND POSITIVE POLITICS

The predominance of positive politics will stimulate a pioneering spirit in an organization. All participants feel in charge of their own destiny and a part of creating something which they own (Block, 1990). Quality improvement demands new manager-subordinate relationships, a different definition of success, and positive forms of communication.

New Manager-Subordinate Contracts

Under quality improvement, managers and their subordinates enter into partnerships for quality. It is an entrepreneurial agreement, which views the most reliable source of information as that coming from the expertise of the person. Thinking and ideas are valued and expected. Action occurs without "touching bases" or "sending up trial balloons" (Block, 1990). While mistakes are not punished, there are sanctions for failure to carefully think about an idea, challenge it, and then examine it in relationship to the system.

New Definitions of Success.
In traditional organizations, success is seen as a collection of outcomes. In the quest for continuous improvement, the *process* of goal achievement is equally valued. Managers who achieve outcomes while developing others will be successful. Compensation programs will value knowledge at all levels, so that individuals can choose to grow and develop in clinical positions and reap rewards. This will eliminate the "brain drain" occurring when people forsake clinical work in favor of the greater rewards associated with management roles. Success will be defined as the quality of the journey to outcomes (James, 1983).

Positive Communication Modes.
Much has already been said here about the communication modes that must be in place in order to support quality improvement. What is central to all the discussion is that communication must be authentic and be grounded in a recognition of the value of another. This means that it is OK not to know the answer, to wait and think before giving an opinion, and to communicate intuition or instinct. There are no secrets, only incomplete information or information which is not in a condition to be shared. Name-dropping, "lip service," and approval-seeking communication modes are confronted as inauthentic and self-serving. The process of communicating is as valuable as its content.

CHARACTERISTICS OF QUALITY IMPROVEMENT MANAGERS

How do you differentiate between lip service and a true commitment to quality improvement? Effective manager behaviors, as described by various authors, are summarized in the box on page 60.

Avoiding Suicide

Many of the attitudes and behaviors described as desirable for the quality improvement manager require organizational courage and significant risk taking. When should the manager slow down or abstain from making these shifts, so as to avert political suicide and loss of any influence upon quality care? Block (1990) recommends that managers avoid risk-taking when they are new to the job or the organization, when the organization is on the brink of financial disaster, following periods of risk and growth, and when the politics are so negative that trust has been eroded.

The manager can also avoid catastrophe during the transformation to a quality improvement organization by building in certain precautions. These include recruiting new workers with honesty. Tell them both the flaws and the strengths of the organization, the difficulties they will face and the state of the change. Make sure that their *mindsets* and their skills match the quality improvement philosophy. Know your territory and avoid underestimating the influence of organizational culture. Identify the old guard and give its members the time to digest your ideas. This will decrease the likelihood of frightening them and stimulating caution and control. Plan from a conceptual base, not a rhetorical one, and make sure that the planning is not dominated by agitators rather than change agents (Bennis, 1989).

CONCLUSION

In summary, the new paradigm for management in quality improvement organizations can be conceptualized in an acronym. Each letter of the word *quality* represents the mindsets and intents from which

---

Characteristics of the Quality Improvement Manager

Bennis (1989)
Holds each person accountable for his or her work
Encourages subordinates to call and chair meetings
Devotes 25 percent of each staff meeting to morale
Makes commitments instead of sacrifices
Acts as a consultant to staff
Introduces choice

Orsburn et al (1990)
Does not value one role over another
Hands authority to others with comfort
Does not undercut persons in new roles
Gives concrete suggestions to stimulate thinking

Senge (1990)
Acts as a guide and nurturer of ideas
Displays a commitment to truth and inquiry
Practices openness
Invests in self and others
Tests mental models

Wheeler and Chinn (1991)
Knows who his or her group is
Pursues realistic purposes
Understands the relationship between professional
  values, beliefs, and quality of work
Recognizes the wide range of personal needs that
  influence process
Clearly communicates expectations
Protects the integrity of the group

Block (1990)
Employs positive politics in the pursuit of quality
Chooses improvement, courage, and autonomy
Confronts manipulative communication
Engages subordinates in entrepreneurial contracts
Empowers self and others

---

manager actions arise in the quality improvement organization. "Q" represents the questioning mind-set needed to understand the relationship between systems and quality. The letter "U" symbolizes the understanding of self and of others, which is critical to telling what is known when seeking quality improvement. "A" stands for the accountability for reflective and participative openness. "L" represents what Senge (1990) refers to as the concept of localness, or extending authority for decisions to where the work is performed. "I" symbolizes the integration that occurs when people are encouraged to act. It also characterizes the systems designed by the manager architect. "T" represents the thoughtfulness brought to bear on all decisions and the different forms of knowledge applied in thinking. And "Y" symbolizes the yielding that occurs in quality improvement organizations. The yielding to the influence of a partner and the yield in terms of outcomes are represented in the letter "Y".

REFERENCES

Bennis W (1989): *Why leaders can't lead*, San Francisco, Jossey-Bass, Inc., 69-136.

Block P (1990): *The empowered manager*, San Francisco, Jossey-Bass, Inc.

delBueno D, CM Freund (1986): *Power and politics in nursing: A case book*, Owings Mills, Md, Rynd Communications, 10-12.

Gitlow HS, SJ Gitlow (1987): *The Deming guide to quality and competitive position*, Englewood Cliffs, NJ, Prentice-Hall Publishing, 111-129.

James J (1983): *Success is the quality of your journey*, New York, New Market Press, 68.

McLaughlin P, AD Kalzuny (1990): Total quality management in health: Making it work. *Health Care Management Review* 15(3): 7-14.

Mintzberg H (1979): *The structuring of organizations*, Englewood Cliffs, NJ, Prentice-Hall Publishing, 330-333.

Moss Kanter R (1989): *When giants learn to dance*, New York, Simon and Schuster, 154.

Orsburn JD, L Moran, E Musselwhite, JH Zenger (1990): *Self-directed work teams*, Homewood, Ill, Business One Irwin, 95-98.

Schaef AW (1985): *Women's reality*, San Francisco, Harper & Row, 40-42.

Senge PM (1990): *The fifth discipline*. New York, Doubleday/Currency, 274-363.

Wheeler CE, PL Chinn (1991): *Peace and power. A handbook of feminist process*, New York, The National League for Nursing.

Wilson CK (1992): *Building new nursing organizations*, Gaithersburg, Md, Aspen Publications Inc., 50-141.

IMPROVING QUALITY AND PERFORMANCE: IMPLICATIONS FOR STAFF EDUCATION AND DEVELOPMENT

Rita S. Fogel
Elaine L. Smith

The paradigm shift from quality assurance (QA) to quality improvement (QI) has tremendous implications for the health care industry in general and nursing staff development (SD) departments in particular. Quality improvement as compared with QA is a much more comprehensive process and as such holds much promise for improving health care quality. As facilitator of learning for new employees, incumbent staff, and in many cases the community, the SD educator has a great deal of influence on the practice of nursing and quality health care. The involvement of SD departments in the QI process is an issue that must be examined. This chapter will explore different levels of involvement and describe the experience of an SD department that also has responsibility for QI in the nursing department.

Organizing and educating for QI and the role of SD departments will most likely be different in every institution. Regardless of the institution or chosen methodology there will be an impact on SD. What that impact is depends on management's expectations of SD involvement, the size of the organization, the size of the SD department, the history of involvement with the quality process and the attitudes of the SD educator.

Relationships between QI and SD Roles and Responsibilities

When QI is introduced into an organization, ongoing education of all employees is essential. The SD department may not be involved at all in this new initiative; it may be overlooked; it may be involved in both the educational aspect of implementation and QI in the SD department; or it may be responsible for directing QI in the nursing department.

Nonparticipating Departments. The idea of becoming involved with QI on any level may sometimes be perceived as overwhelming. Members of the SD depart- ment may avoid any involvement with the process. The decision not to participate on any level should be examined very carefully. Hiding in the shadows has many ramifications for SD and the nursing depart- ment.

The Forgotten Department. Staff development depart- ments may be overlooked entirely when QI is intro- duced in an organization. Many agencies hire exter- nal consulting groups that supply "trainers"; or the agency creates a rollout plan that requires top man- agers to train the next level down and the next level to train the middle level in a cascade effect until every level in the organization is educated, with little or no role for staff development initially. At some point in time, the trainers will leave and managers may dele- gate the responsibility of education. As staff educa- tors know only too well, many times the department will be called upon to take over the educational as- pect.

Staff Development and QI

Staff development departments may be involved with the QI process in several ways. The department may be considered a key player in the implementa- tion of the QI plan and be very involved in educating the staff about the QI process. In addition, staff de- velopment departments may also be affected just the same as every other department and begin to pursue quality with others in new ways.

Staff development educators have a much more comprehensive role beyond educating for QI. There are two dimensions that are to be considered: quality in the institution, especially in the nursing depart- ment, and quality in the staff development depart- ment (Katz, 1992).

In addition to the education program in QI con- cepts, quality must be inherent in every aspect of staff development activities and offerings, including orientation, ongoing staff development, in-servicing of new products, and continuing education.

Staff development departments should be involved with their own quality assessment processes. It is important to evaluate and improve services provided to customers, the nursing staff, and other departments. Documenting the impact of staff contributions to quality, cost issues, and high-quality outcomes validates the important role the SD department plays in the quality improvement process (Katz, 1992).

There are several resources available to help staff development educators organize and implement a program of continuous quality improvement in their department.

Almost required reading is the chapter "Managing the Dual Dimensions of Quality" by Katz (1992). Katz provides a comprehensive theoretical and practical discussion of the role and responsibilities of the staff development educators in the quality process.

In 1990, the American Nurses Association (ANA) published *Standards for Nursing Staff Development*. The standards provide an organizing format for staff development departments. *Quality Indicators for Nursing Staff Development* (Jeska, Fischer, and McClellan, 1992) is a manual that uses the ANA standards as a basis for quality indicators and is helpful in integrating QI improvement principles into SD practice.

Integrating QI into Traditional Staff Development Roles

When an SD department embraces QI, it affects every area of the department's responsibilities. Typically included under the SD umbrella are orientation, staff development, continuing education, and in many instances involvement with schools of nursing using the hospital for clinical practicums.

Orientation. The orientation period is a critical time for the new employee and the organization. It is the time to introduce the concepts of QI in addition to policies, procedures and necessary skills. It is an opportunity for orientees to familiarize themselves with the mission and culture of the organization and their role, responsibilities and accountability for the quality of patient care. Staff development educators can assist new employees in this endeavor. Simple things such as discussing the organization's mission statement, philosophy of nursing service, and job descriptions enable orientees to get a "feel" for their new organization.

In many facilities, senior-level nursing administrators meet each group of new employees and share their plans and visions for the department. This communicates a sense of commitment and often inspires orientees to become part of the team. Perhaps one of the most convincing and effective ways of learning

the culture is to work with a preceptor or mentor. This experienced practitioner can share invaluable tips and insights with newcomers to help them become familiar with a unit's culture and values.

Orientation is foremost a period of assessment. What knowledge and skills are needed to fulfill job responsibilities? Is the orientee competent to fulfill these responsibilities? Staff development educators are in a pivotal position to assess and document the competence of new employees. Patient outcomes are improved when a competent staff member delivers care according to established standards of care and practice and to policy and procedure, in a manner pleasing to the patient. It is important to note that competence assessment is not a one-shot procedure. It is an ongoing process that begins before hiring and continues throughout the duration of employment.

The principles of QI can affect the way staff development departments plan and implement their orientation programs. Crucial to the success of any program is leadership commitment. For existing orientation programs this may mean ensuring that managers are knowledgeable about the programs' scheduling, content, and evaluation results. In the planning of a new system of orientation, it would be imperative to include managers in the identification of critical competencies needed by practitioners in their areas of responsibility. Managerial input can be solicited via focus groups, targeted questionnaires, or personal discussions and dialogue. Inviting and involving nurse managers to participate in planning helps to solidify commitment when implementation time rolls around.

Customer satisfaction with orientation can be addressed from two perspectives: the satisfaction of the orientee with the quality of the program and the satisfaction of the managers with the end product—a competent staff member. Evaluation tools can provide useful data on the employee's perception of modules, audio-visuals, lectures, and demonstration. Some staff development departments choose to conduct retrospective evaluations; this provides employees with the opportunity to evaluate how beneficial the orientation program was to the establishment of their practice. From an administrative perspective, orientation programs need to be evaluated for cost effectiveness and efficiency. Are results being achieved with the most efficient use of time, people, and money? Which teaching strategies provide the best outcomes? By establishing clear standards, performing accurate employee assessments, providing targeted educational strategies, and concisely documenting initial competence, staff development departments can provide high-quality orientation programs.

Staff Development and Continuing Education. Learning does not end with the completion of the orientation program. It is naive to assume that once QI is introduced in orientation, educational responsibilities are fulfilled. To sustain the momentum, educational offerings must be ongoing. When programs or classes concentrate on clinical issues, "quality elements" and the effects on patient outcomes should be included. Classes for managers and staff should also focus on what QI is and how to put its tenets into action. Knowing about the process, knowing how to look at methods, and having systems for improvement are important in motivating personnel to become involved in improving care, process, and systems. People need the tools and information on how to use them.

The QI process provides an automatic assessment for identifying educational needs. The monitoring process can target areas for improvement. The astute staff development educator will be able to diagnose which areas require educational remediation and which do not. Recognizing the difference is indeed a challenge. Educators can lend their assessment and problem-solving skills to unit managers as members of the quality team. In most cases improving quality requires more than a Band-Aid inservice. A combination of managerial and educational strategies and, in some cases, system changes will be required.

In QI cultures the role of nurse educators goes beyond simply "inservicing." Educators can assist managers and staff in improving their skills with the process of communicating QI program results. From offering tips on public speaking to teaching about audiovisual technology, staff development departments are rich resources for more effective presentations. Clear, concise, visual data displays can have a powerful impact. Often, SD departments provide programs on the use and applications of computer software packages for quality data management and display.

Continuous improvement should become the watchword of the education department's program of staff development and continuing education. Rich data on customer satisfaction can be retrieved by use of well-designed evaluation tools. Feedback on the quality of the presentations, audiovisual media, and handouts and an environment conducive to learning are critical for future programming efforts. Beyond measuring customer satisfaction, staff development educators must evaluate the clinical outcomes of the programs provided. That is, as a result of educational experiences, has the clinical performance of the staff improved? It is imperative to link staff development programming with the quality improvement initiatives of the organization, department, and unit. This keeps the department in touch with some of the priority issues affecting nursing practice. Educators can increase their perceived and actual value to the organization by directing their time and energies toward improving outcomes with high volume, high risk, problem prone and high cost indicators.

Student Affiliations. New graduates are not always familiar with the concepts of QA/QI. A survey of selected schools of nursing indicated that these were not included in the curriculum. This finding has been corroborated by Crosby, Finnick, and Ventura (1991), who reported "that preparatory education was rarely a source of QA information." Working together, education and service can provide this information to undergraduate as well as graduate students. Staff development educators can share current organizational quality trends with affiliating faculty and students. Information can be shared in a variety of formats. Participating in curriculum advisory committees enables SD educators and faculty to conduct dialogue about practice patterns and future directions. Through these meetings the emergence of the quality culture within hospitals can be explored and implications for curriculum content addressed. Another strategy for staff development to consider is serving as adjunct faculty at affiliating colleges and universities. Guest lecturing on quality issues can be an exciting opportunity for educators and promotes interest and awareness among students. In return, faculty may be able to share their research knowledge and expertise. This bartering of resources can promote collegial relationships, maximize quality initiatives, and ultimately improve patient care.

Within their own department, staff development educators can evaluate and improve the quality of the affiliation process. Issues such as contracts, faculty orientation, student orientation, preceptor assignment, and problem resolution should be looked at periodically.

Within the traditional roles of staff development departments there is room for quality improvement. Through the services it provides, a staff development department can promote an organization QI program and at the same time improve its own performance.

Nontraditional Roles for Staff Development in QI

While some nursing departments separate SD and QI, others have or are in the process of combining these functions into one area. Assuming the responsibility for QI is indeed a challenge. Yet it is a logical acquisition. It places the department in a pivotal position within a health care organization and gives the department the opportunity to be involved with organizationwide quality improvement activities.

The assumption of the responsibilities of QI may require some restructuring and shifting of responsibilities. Quality assurance programs certainly are not a new concept or activity in health care settings. Positions and committees do not have to be dismantled when reporting mechanisms change. What does have to change is the mindset of the personnel, the committee members, and the members of the nursing department. For so long we have looked to identify problems, collect data, and recommend corrective action plans to remedy deficiencies that in many cases we lost sight of why we were doing "quality assurance." Changing the name from quality assurance to total quality management or to quality improvement starts the momentum, but there is much more to do than changing words. Making quality improvement work in a health care setting takes the efforts of many people who truly value customer service and the concept of continually improving process and outcome. Most important is support from top-level management.

When an SD department takes on the responsibility of QI, consideration must be given to the impact on personnel, finances, space, and time. Taking the time to address these areas and planning for the changes helps to make a smoother, more effective transition. Some questions to examine are:

- Is the change viewed as an opportunity to the SD department leader and educator?
- Is there ongoing support from the leadership?
- Is there financial support or do priorities have to shift in order to make the accommodation?
- Will any existing personnel be reassigned to the SD department?
- Is there enough space in the department to physically accommodate the personnel and the many records?
- Is there enough secretarial help to support the increased volume of work?
- Is there a computer available for data storage and retrieval, for analyzing and publishing reports?

Quality improvement efforts require a positive collaborative manner among departments. Existing committee structures may provide the vehicle for multidisciplinary interactions and improvements. These include committees within the nursing department specifically involved with QI as well as nurse practice and policy and procedure committees. Most important, nursing must be represented on organizationwide quality improvement teams/committees. These committees represent part of the communication network that is essential.

ONE INSTITUTION'S EXPERIENCE

Long Island Jewish Medical Center (LIJMC), 15 miles east of New York City, is a voluntary, nonprofit, tertiary care teaching hospital with 825 beds. It employs approximately 1500 registered nurses and 320 ancillary nursing personnel. More than 600 students a year from 12 schools of nursing come to LIJMC for undergraduate and graduate experiences.

The Medical Center has three hospitals on one campus:

- Long Island Jewish Hospital (425 beds), an internationally known tertiary care hospital for adults
- Schneider Children's Hospital (150 beds), the New York area's only hospital built just for children
- Hillside Hospital (223 beds), a renowned psychiatric hospital with inpatient and outpatient programs

Since 1990, coordination of nursing quality assurance/quality improvement activities has been the responsibility of the Department of Nursing Education, QI and Research. The heart of the program consists of unit-based committees coordinated by unit-based QA reps and an assistant director of nursing for QA. The associate administrator for education, QI and research assumed the chair of the Corporate Nursing QA Committee and became a member of the Hospital Wide QA Committee (physicians) and Patient Care Services Committee (all other hospital departments).

The Corporate Nursing Quality Management Committee was originally formed for the purpose of directing the overall systems and structure for nursing QA activities throughout all divisions of the medical center. Membership includes nursing representation from all clinical divisions, nursing education, the Nursing Procedure Committee, and the Nurse Practice Committee. All decisions are reviewed with the vice president for nursing and the associate administrators of nursing for all divisions. The organizational framework is shown in Fig. 6-1.

The meeting of the committee generally consists of progress reports on various projects, the impact of findings from surveys, and recommendations for change that would impact policy, procedure, nurse practice, or nursing education. Because of the diverse membership, communication to other committees and groups is achieved.

The professional development of the nursing staff at LIJMC is supported by the Department of Nursing Education, QI and Research. The members of this department provide educational resources for orientation, staff development, continuing education, and student affiliations. Linking QA and education has proven to be an opportunity for staff development. First, educators are targeting issues for programming. Second, the education department has the talent, skills, and resources to "spread the word" and communicate the mission of quality improvement activities. To reap the benefits of the quality improvement movement, all participants require educational preparation. The nursing education department has a responsibility to its internal customers from the vice president for nursing to the nursing assistant to facilitate learning on quality improvement concepts, techniques, and outcomes. Quality is the key to organizational survival. Nursing education departments must impart the message at every level of programming.

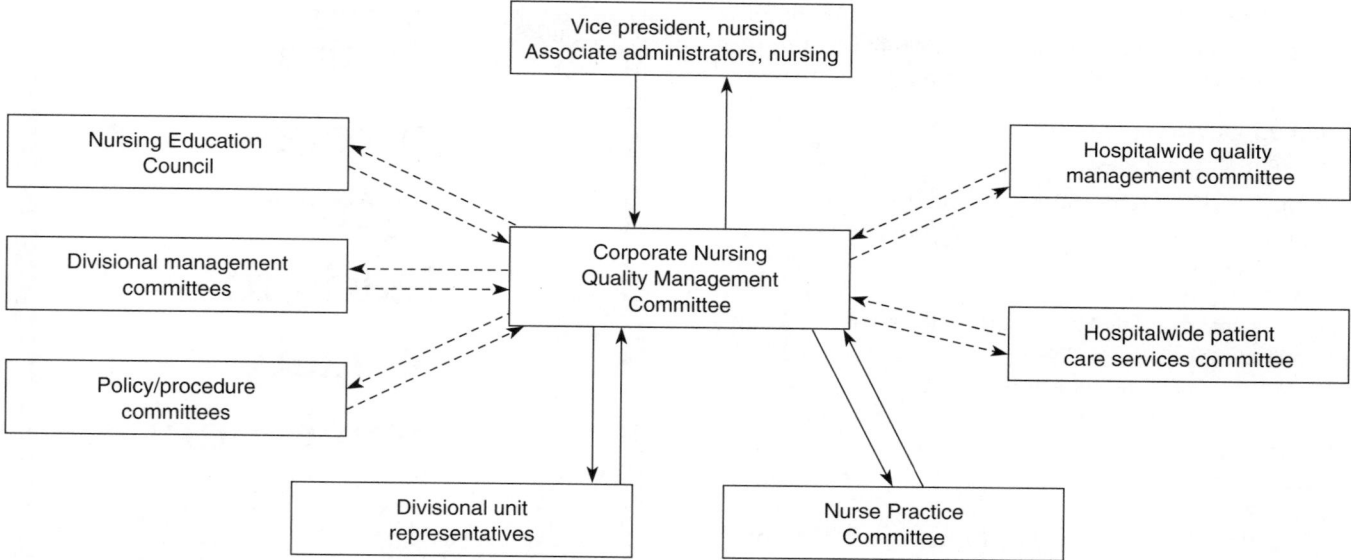

Fig. 6-1 Organizational chart for nursing quality improvement.

A Program for Orientation and Staff Development

Impetus for Starting the Program. Educational activities on quality assessment and improvement were undertaken for three reasons. First, there was a renewed commitment to and interest in quality. Second, there was a clear need to better prepare managers and staff to participate in quality activities. Third, education for quality flowed with the changes in the Quality standard of the JCAHO. The Department of Nursing Education at LIJMC embarked on a dual approach to quality education:

1. Reaching the grassroots through orientation and staff development programs
2. Enhancing the performance of unit-based quality improvement representatives

Reaching the Grassroots: Orientation Strategies. A system of competency-based orientation has been in place at LIJMC since January 1989. A competency-based orientation "is a method that focuses on the end results of orientation," write Abbruzzese and Quinn-O'Neal (1992, p. 257). Orientees must master generic as well as unit-specific competencies. Competency statements and critical behaviors are formatted into an orientation contract. The contract also contains a listing of learning resources such as policies, standards of care and practice, audiovisual aids, and self-study modules. A space is provided on the contract for a validation signature and the date the critical behavior was achieved. In an attempt to promote participation in quality activities, it was included as a generic competency required of all registered nurses.

Learners attend a brief lecture by the orientation coordinator. The presentation comprises:

- Overview of the QI plan at LIJMC
- Responsibilities of the registered nurse related to QI activities
- Completing a chart documentation survey

A self-study module is another resource available to the new employee. Modules are effective and efficient mechanisms for facilitating learning. Nurses can review the information at their own pace, spending as much time as needed to learn the material. The development of the module will be discussed later in this chapter.

After participating in the lecture and in a review of the module, nurses are asked to put the information into action. Once on their unit of employment, nurses participate in the QI survey process. Experience has shown that it is more practical to involve orientees with generic, corporatewide indicators such as documentation rather than try to survey a unit-based indicator. This method allows for greater flexibility by not locking into each unit's particular data-collection and analysis cycle. The added benefit of using documentation indicators is that nurses also familiarize themselves with the documentation policies, forms, and layout of the medical record.

The building of quality into the orientation program sensitizes new employees to the significance of this process to their professional practice and the organization.

Staff Development Strategies

Although the Nursing Education Department had incorporated quality specific content into general orientation, it had not been aggressive in educating the incumbent staff. A major staff education program on quality was initiated in January 1991, aimed at reaching 1100 nurses at all three divisions. Information presented on quality would be at a basic level to provide a foundation for future programming.

Program Development

An ad hoc committee was developed to direct the creation and implementation of the quality education program. The working committee consisted of the assistant directors of nursing education, assistant director of nursing quality improvement, and nurse educators from the OR, neonatal ICU, CCU, ED, and pediatrics. At initial meetings, target dates for implementation and determined educational strategies were established. The committee allotted three months for preparation time. Meetings were held for approximately one hour every two to three weeks to achieve the goals.

Selecting the educational format required much thought and discussion. What would be the most effective and efficient way to do this? Which methods would reach the largest number of people? How could constancy and consistency of information be ensured when multiple instructors with varying degrees of expertise in quality improvement would be involved? The outcome of discussions resulted in the decision to create a self-study module for every RN in the facility and to offer a one-hour class as a review of the material. To give the efforts a high profile and identity, the title "Quality Assurance Reflects Caring" was selected. Its logo was a single long-stem rose. To keep the momentum alive after the program, the committee felt a theme button that could be worn by participants would help. A tasteful button that reflected the rose logo was designed. A novelty-supply company manufactured 1,500 buttons at a modest charge.

Course/module content reflected two principles: "keep it simple" and "make it real to the practicing nurse." The JCAHO Ten Step Plan was selected as the framework to build upon. The intent was to focus on the potentials and positive outcomes of QI. A glossary of quality terminology was developed to guide the education process. This was a critical step. In general, nurses were not familiar with many of the terms used. A foundation for future learning efforts was dependent on understanding the language.

Committee members were given individual assignments to complete to speed content development. Information was gleaned from literature, the existing quality plan, and JCAHO Standards. All work was coordinated by the assistant director of nursing education.

The next step was to determine the module design. Each page of the packet presented a minimal amount of information and used large type for easy, quick reading. The committee was fortunate to have an artist as part of the team. The artist illustrated each

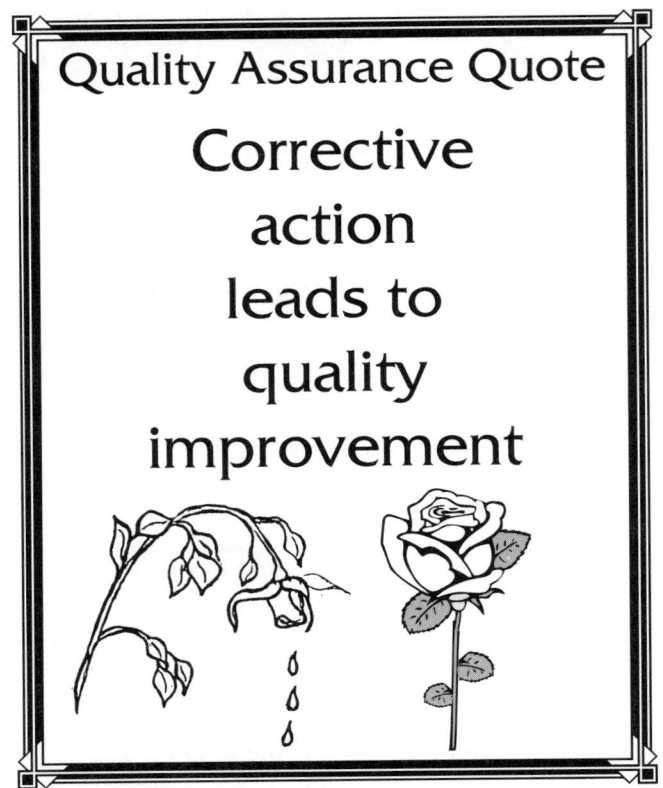

Quality Assurance Quote

Corrective action leads to quality improvement

step of the Ten Step Plan to add richness and diversity to the work. It was important to design an attractive product that would hold the audience's attention. Interspersed throughout the module were "QA Quotes"—major points that required emphasis or clarification (see the box above). The completed package is 50 single-sided pages including pretest and posttest questions. The print shop at LIJMC replicated and bound 1,200 copies for distribution. Normally the staff development department reuses modules. It was decided that in this case each nurse should be able to have her or his own copy for reference.

The development of the accompanying course outline flowed smoothly once the module was completed. The committee wanted to use this one-hour time frame to review both cognitive quality information and to address nurses' attitudes toward quality activities. The goal was to make the course as interactive and positive as possible. Experience indicated that most nurses dread QA programs; they often found them dull and boring.

To encourage thinking and discussion the class opened with a Mind Map exercise. "QA" was placed on the frontal lobe of a diagram of the brain, and participants were asked to free-associate, jotting down their first thoughts. The notations were shared, and the instructor used them to initiate discussions on attitudes and beliefs held by nurses about quality. Most reported QA as an important professional re-

```
                Long Island Jewish Medical Center
              Department of Nursing: Nursing Education
                  Quality Assurance Reflects Caring
                         Attitudinal Survey

Directions:  Please circle the number which best corresponds to your opinion.
        5   strongly agree
        4   agree
        3   neither agree or disagree
        2   disagree
        1   strongly disagree


  1. Quality assurance is an important              5   4   3   2   1
     professional responsibility.

  2. Quality assurance is an effective and          5   4   3   2   1
     efficient method of problem solving.

  3. Quality assurance activities are               5   4   3   2   1
     punitive in nature.

  4. Quality assurance activities take away         5   4   3   2   1
     from my ability to provide patient care.

  5. Quality assurance is a high priority.          5   4   3   2   1

  6. Nurses should be more involved with            5   4   3   2   1
     quality assurance.

  7. The class and module helped me to              5   4   3   2   1
     understand the QA process.

  8. I will participate in QA activities            5   4   3   2   1
     on my unit.

  9. Patient care will improve as a result of       5   4   3   2   1
     the QA process.

 10. QA gives me control over my practice.          5   4   3   2   1
```

Fig. 6-2 Post-program survey.

sponsibility that is an effective and efficient method of problem solving. Nurses shared their observations of the quality process on their respective units and were able to describe the positive impacts on patient care. Overall, the feeling about quality assurance among the staff was a positive one. It became the challenge of the Nursing Education department to keep the momentum going. The ad hoc committee determined that careful evaluation of the program was needed. It was decided to use both a generic program evaluation tool and to design a post program attitudinal survey as shown in Fig. 6-2.

Program Implementation

A matrix model was used to coordinate program implementation. It was designed to include every unit of the medical center. Units were grouped together to form four cohorts. Each cohort was allotted a two-

week time frame within which to schedule attendance at the program. The self-learning modules were delivered to the units two weeks before their scheduled start-up time. This enabled the nurses to review the content and complete the pre- and posttest questions.

A series of classes was established for each of the four cohort groups. The objective was to provide sufficient opportunities for attendance on work time. It was clear from the outset of program planning that overtime costs could not be accrued. To achieve both objectives, classes were scheduled around the clock and on weekends. The typical matrix offered classes at the following time frames:

3 AM-4 AM
4 AM-5 AM
11 AM-12 N
3 PM-4 PM
4 PM-5 PM

These times were most convenient for scheduling staff members who predominantly work 12-hour shifts. A total of 111 classes would be needed. Obviously such a rigorous schedule would require a cadre of instructors. All the resources of the Nursing Education department—about 20 instructors—needed to be tapped. Before they could educate others, they needed to educate themselves. At LIJMC, the nurse educators meet together on a twice-monthly basis. These meetings were used as "train the trainer" sessions for the Quality Assurance Reflects Caring program. Every educator received a module and class outline. The quality class was presented to the educators in the same format they would be using with the staff. This process allowed for a dry run of the content outline and enabled the educators to ask any questions they had about the material. It was at this meeting that the established class schedule was circulated. Each educator was asked to sign up to instruct at least five classes. Once this step was completed the master matrix of classes, indicating date, time, location, and instructor, was distributed to all nursing managers and educators.

Program Evaluation

Because much time and energy and many resources were devoted to the development and implementation of the Quality Assurance Reflects Caring program, evaluation of the classes was a priority. Overall analysis revealed the following:

Total number of classes offered: 111

Total number of classes not completed due to no show: 5

Total number of RNs completing class: 986 (88.2%)

Total number of program evaluations received: 978

Total number of attitudinal surveys received: 880

The analysis of generic evaluation forms revealed that most participants believed that the course and presenters were well prepared and met their needs. The topic was a realistic one and was presented at an appropriate level. Eighty-seven percent of the nurses rated the program good to excellent.

Table 6-1 illustrates data from the attitudinal survey. These responses were used for future program planning and refinement. The SD department was pleased to see the overall positive beliefs and attitudes about quality reported by staff. Continued effort would be needed to shift the perception of quality assurance away from the punitive and toward the positive.

A Program for Unit-Based Quality Improvement Representatives

Encouraged by the success of the grass-roots program, administrators planned the next phase of quality education. For a number of years, LIJMC had espoused a unit-based approach to QI. Staff nurses and unit managers served as unit-based QI representatives. These individuals formed the backbone of the nursing QI program. The responsibilities of this position included participation in indicator selection, survey-tool development, data collection and analysis, and feedback to the unit. It became evident that this pivotal cadre of people needed additional education to fulfill their role expectations. As the hospital organization has become more and more decentralized, the QI representative position has expanded. The rate of turnover among unit representatives has increased. Nurses would be involved with quality activities for a few months, then ask for reassignment. Many representatives considered their assignment to be a thankless job, adding to their workload without sufficient impact or reward. To address these concerns, the Nursing Education department's objectives were:

1. To develop an efficient, effective mechanism of QI representative education
2. To send a message of recognition and appreciation to the incumbents
3. To assist QI representatives in becoming more effective in improving care and service

Program Development

As with all major programs, a subcommittee of educators was formed to develop this educational program. Again, representatives came from the three hospital divisions. In retrospect, membership on the committee should have included key unit representatives, nursing managers, and a representative from the Quality Department outside of Nursing. Many of the original members of the Quality Assurance Reflects Caring team were asked to lend their skills to this new project. The committee allotted itself two months to develop and implement the Quality Improvement Representative Program.

Selecting the educational format was the first objective. A decision was reached to offer an interactive one-day workshop, providing time for review of key content points and for small group work. To simplify scheduling issues, the committee designed the offering to be provided in one full day. This structure worked best in the institution; however, the course could also be designed as two half-day classes or a series of one-hour programs over time.

With the format established, course content and method of instruction needed to be set.

The finished product consisted of the following:

• The Year in Review: successes of our QI program
• QA/QI terminology
• The LIJMC Quality Improvement Plan
• QI Representative Role Definition
• Indicator selection
• Developing Monitoring Tools

TABLE 6-1 Review of 800 Attitudinal Surveys

	Number	Percent
1. *Quality assurance is an important professional responsibility.*		
Total number of *strongly agreed* [5]	673	76
Total number of *agreed* [4]	201	23
Total number of neither *agreed* nor *disagreed* [3]	4	
Total number of *disagreed* [2]	1	1
Total number of *strongly disagreed* [1]	1	
2. *Quality assurance is an effective and efficient method of problem solving.*		
Total number of *strongly agreed* [5]	468	53
Total number of *agreed* [4]	377	43
Total number of neither *agreed* nor *disagreed* [3]	31	
Total number of *disagreed* [2]	1	4
Total number of *strongly disagreed* [1]	3	
3. *Quality assurance activities are punitive in nature.*		
Total number of *strongly agreed* [5]	45	5.1
Total number of *agreed* [4]	122	13.9
Total number of neither *agreed* nor *disagreed* [3]	182	20.7
Total number of *disagreed* [2]	326	37.0
Total number of *strongly disagreed* [1]	205	23.3
4. *Quality assurance activities take away from my ability to provide patient care.*		
Total number of *strongly agreed* [5]	48	48
Total number of *agreed* [4]	93	10.6
Total number of neither *agreed* nor *disagreed* [3]	134	15.2
Total number of *disagreed* [2]	359	40.7
Total number of *strongly disagreed* [1]	246	28
5. *Quality assurance is a high priority.*		
Total number of *strongly agreed* [5]	355	40.3
Total number of *agreed* [4]	418	47.5
Total number of neither *agreed* nor *disagreed* [3]	90	10.2
Total number of *disagreed* [2]	12	1.4
Total number of *strongly disagreed* [1]	5	0.6
6. *Nurses should be more involved with quality assurance.*		
Total number of *strongly agreed* [5]	377	42.8
Total number of *agreed* [4]	429	48.8
Total number of neither *agreed* nor *disagreed* [3]	63	7.2
Total number of *disagreed* [2]	7	0.8
Total number of *strongly disagreed* [1]	1	0.4
7. *The class and module helped me to understand the quality assurance process.*		
Total number of *strongly agreed* [5]	331	37.6
Total number of *agreed* [4]	469	53.3
Total number of neither *agreed* nor *disagreed* [3]	63	7.2
Total number of *disagreed* [2]	14	1.6
Total number of *strongly disagreed* [1]	3	0.3
8. *I will participate in quality assurance activities on my unit.*		
Total number of *strongly agreed* [5]	313	35.6
Total number of *agreed* [4]	476	54.1
Total number of neither *agreed* nor *disagreed* [3]	85	9.6
Total number of *disagreed* [2]	4	0.5
Total number of *strongly disagreed* [1]	2	0.2
9. *Patient care will improve as a result of the quality assurance process.*		
Total number of *strongly agreed* [5]	406	46.1
Total number of *agreed* [4]	411	46.7
Total number of neither *agreed* nor *disagreed* [3]	51	5.8
Total number of *disagreed* [2]	9	1.1
Total number of *strongly disagreed* [1]	3	0.3
10. *Quality assurance gives me control over my practice.*		
Total number of *strongly agreed* [5]	250	28.4
Total number of *agreed* [4]	418	47.5
Total number of neither *agreed* nor *disagreed* [3]	180	20.5
Total number of *disagreed* [2]	25	2.8
Total number of *strongly disagreed* [1]	7	0.8

- Basic Statistical Analysis
- Taking a Look at Systems
- Presenting Results

Teaching methods used included lecture, discussion, overhead transparencies, handouts, role playing, and group exercises and presentations.

The program was developed for an audience that would be drawn from the three hospital divisions. The curriculum needed to be applicable to everyone but not so generic as to be meaningless. Endeavors were made to include a variety of examples from each setting. The QA/QI systems at each hospital have much in common; however, some points of departure exist. In the end, the differences did cause some confusion among the participants. The seven faculty persons, as members of the Program Planning Committee function, were able to resolve any questions or confusion that arose during the day. The conference room was set up with tables seating five to six people to encourage and support interaction. Participants had the opportunity to select an indicator, develop a survey tool, and perform a basic statistical analysis. Each group selected a reporter, who presented the outcomes to the class at large. Comments, critiques, and questions were fielded by both the reporter and course faculty. Each group was rewarded with a warm round of applause for its accomplishments.

Program Results

A total of 50 QI representatives attended the inaugural program. The majority found the class beneficial to their role. It was particularly surprising to learn that most of the representatives found the review of terminology very helpful. Participants gave the committee feedback on content that needed more or less emphasis. In general, attendees were looking for practical tips and "how to's." The small group exercises were very successful. Many respondees requested further programming efforts along these lines.

Program evaluations also reflected that most participants would have preferred to be in classes specifically designed for their division. It was also noted by consensus that fewer faculty would have been better. Participants found the differing perspectives and examples more confusing than helpful.

Course faculty met about one week after the program to review the evaluations and refine the content and timeframes.

CONCLUSION AND RECOMMENDATIONS FOR THE FUTURE

Now that LIJMC has completed the technical aspects of quality education, it is planning to move on to the all encompassing concepts of QI. This does not necessarily mean reinventing the wheel or discarding current QA programs. It does mean developing and

implementing programs that educate the staff about the basic principles and applications of QI. Other related topics that are planned include customer/guest relations, team building, communication skills, time management, and delegation. One of the programs, customer/guest relations, is being planned in collaboration with the Nursing Department, Social Services, the Training Department, Security, and Housekeeping. The multidisciplinary team will present the program to all departments of the Medical Center.

Staff development educators must take a positive position within their organization. If you are not already involved with the quality improvement initiatives, become involved. Read the literature about quality improvement. Attend programs and seminars so that you are an educated consumer. Look at your own department first: do you have a philosophy and standards for education? Move out of your department and become involved with a QI team. Educators should be in on the planning process of new programs. They should not be called upon only to educate. Network with SD and QI departments in other organizations. Most colleagues are quite willing to share, and you can learn from the exchange of ideas.

Staff development educators are creative and motivated individuals who have much to offer the QI process. In addition to being educational resources, they are a support system for the nursing staff. Participation in continuous quality improvement endeavors will help the educator now and in the future.

Shifting the paradigm from QA to QI will require different operational and educational strategies for SD departments. Continuous quality improvement is more than a process, it is a change in the value and beliefs of all participants. There is no end point, only ongoing assessment and improvement. It will take time, effort, and perseverance and flexible, committed, knowledgeable educators working as part of the larger team to bring this undertaking to fruition.

REFERENCES

Abruzzese R, B Quinn-O'Neal (1992): Orientation for general and specialty areas. In R Abruzzese, editor, *Nursing staff development: strategies for success*, St Louis, Mosby, 244-270.

American Nurses Association (1990): *Standards for nursing staff development*, Kansas City, Mo, American Nurses Association.

Crosby F, M Ventura (1991): Needs of nurse educators and clinical nurses regarding quality assurance education, *Journal of the New York State Nurses Association* 22(1): 4-7.

Jeska S, K Fischer, M McClellan (1992): *Quality indicators for nursing staff development*, Pensacola, National Nursing Staff Development Organization.

Katz J (1992): Managing the dual dimensions of quality. In R Abruzzese, editor, *Nursing staff development—strategies for success*, St Louis, Mosby, 293-316.

SECTION II

IMPROVING QUALITY AND PERFORMANCE

Applications and Examples

The heart of improving quality and performance lies not so much within theory as it does within the strategic efforts of people, working together to make things better. Section II tells those stories. Chapters provide a spectrum of examples of early QI efforts and the work of specific project teams. Topics on which the teams focus are likewise diverse, addressing such issues as wheelchair access in the hospital lobby, skin care management, and prompt delivery of patient medications.

The hospitals featured in this section have varying levels of experience. Some have just started their QI initiative, while others have several years' experience, providing a scope that runs from the simple to the sophisticated.

Chapters in this section have been organized to begin with hospitals in early stages of QI efforts: nurses carrying out projects with the involvement of one or two other departments. As chapters progress, examples reflect more organization-wide involvement.

Chapter 7 begins the progression with a description of the early transitions to QI at Lakeland Regional Medical Center in Lake-land, Florida. The nursing quality program initiated the shift at Lakeland by folding QI concepts and early projects into the preexisting QA structures. These projects included scheduling for rehabilitative therapy, increasing education and communication regarding quality, enhancing patient education, improving nutrition, and addressing patient satisfaction.

The QI efforts at Bon Secours Hospital in Grosse Pointe, Michigan, are described in Chapter 8. This chapter describes the hospitalwide program structure and reports in depth on the hospital's effort to improve skin care management.

At St. Vincent Medical Center in Toledo, Ohio, the QI effort focused on patient identification. Admission of patients through multiple hospital admission routes has created the need to improve methods for patient identification, to assure the provision of safe and appropriate treatment. St. Vincent's experience in this area is reviewed in Chapter 9.

Chapter 10 focuses on the challenging issue of patient satisfaction. The Cleveland Clinic Foundation supported multiple, unit-specific efforts to improve patient satisfaction. This discussion provides perspectives on empowering staff members to tailor efforts to their unique people, resources, and situations.

In Green Bay, Wisconsin, Bellin Hospital used a QI initiative to address interunit transfer of patients. As is described in Chapter 11, the "transfer tug-of-war" battle was won by both patients and staff members through collaborative and strategic QI efforts.

The universal hospital issue of incident reporting is discussed in Chapter 12. Staff members of The New York Hospital worked to create a tool that would meet data-collection needs of the organization without prompting finger pointing (assignment of blame) as the action for resolution.

Chapter 13, reporting on the QI initiative at Boston's Beth Israel Hospital, describes a project that addressed missing and unavailable intravenous medications. Work of the task force assembled for this problem is covered in depth, from assessment through analysis and on to process improvement.

The organization-wide transitions implemented at the Medical University of South Carolina Medical Center in Charleston are described in Chapter 14. The center's Quality Redesign Task Force serves as an example of creating change to improve quality. Also described is a project focusing on laboratory studies as ordered in the ambulatory areas.

The unique model for QI implemented at Froedert Memorial Lutheran Hospital in Milwaukee is the subject of Chapter 15. This model for 100 percent employee involvement is examined through the description of several projects, including improving wheelchair availability in the lobby.

Chapter 16 looks at early experiences in the total quality management process at the Johns Hopkins Hospital in Baltimore. The overall transformation process is described, and the project team that worked on the transportation process for inpatient care and radiology is discussed in detail.

The implementation of the TQM process at the University of Iowa Hospitals and Clinics in Iowa City is covered in Chapter 17. The work of several project teams is also briefly identified.

Finally, Chapter 18 summarizes the lessons learned from collective perspectives on these experiences.

The authors of these chapters and their respective clinical agencies are to be congratulated and recognized as trailblazers who are striving toward excellence in new ways and sharing the early lessons with the profession. Readers are encouraged to scrutinize and learn from both the outcomes and the impact of their efforts, as well as the process and experiences of living through these transitions.

CHAPTER SEVEN
FROM QA TO QI
People, Materials, and Methods Bridge the Transition

Mimi Jenko
Mary E. Geary

In Fort Myers, Florida, one can tour the Thomas Edison Winter Home. The laboratory there and the neighboring museum are filled with a vast collection of inventions, from the electric light bulb to the phonograph. Many lives were enhanced as a result of Edison's achievements, and his efforts are a testimony to humanity's quest for improvement.

The nursing profession has similarly made meaningful and lasting contributions, both in clinical practice and in academic spheres. Florence Nightingale was made an honorary member of the American Statistical Society for her work in developing statistical graphical techniques to analyze and improve health care quality (Binns and Early, 1989). Additionally, many care providers were not encouraged to take an active role in collecting and analyzing data. Many were never given opportunities to collaborate with peers regarding corrective actions necessary for improvement. Today's quality revolution, however, is providing unique opportunities for the direct care provider, and the role of the staff nurse and the front-line care provider has changed significantly and forever.

Despite potential long-term benefits, change of any sort is often viewed suspiciously. Events may become institutional stressors because they require considerable restructuring of goals, behaviors, and expectations. Yet, as Beck, Rawlins, and Williams (1984, p. 365) write, "change is less disruptive when it occurs at a reasonable rate and does not drastically alter strongly held beliefs, values, or patterns of behavior." Based on that premise, one institution chose to make a gradual change by building on an existing program's assets and strengths. This chapter describes one institution's early injection of quality improvement (QI) principles into a traditional quality assurance (QA) program.

HISTORY OF THE LAKELAND REGIONAL MEDICAL CENTER (LRMC) NURSING QUALITY PROGRAM

Before 1988, quality efforts at Lakeland Regional Medical Center (LRMC) in Lakeland, Florida, con-

sisted of isolated audits, which were performed by persons outside the unit or department. Staff nurses had little, if any, understanding of the purpose of these efforts. The chart audits typically reviewed documentation issues and were viewed by the staff as a useless and sometimes punitive activity. Under these conditions, quality activities would never become any part of daily nursing practice at the staff nurse level.

In 1987, LRMC hired a new chief nurse executive (CNE), who brought with her a strategic vision for nursing. Naisbitt (1982, p. 98) defined a strategic vision as a "clear image of what you want to achieve, which then organizes and instructs every step toward that goal." The CNE's vision of nursing staff involvement in and ownership of clinical practice guided the restructuring of all nursing quality activities. Consistent with total quality management (TQM) literature, this vision is described as "workforce empowerment" (Williams and Howe, 1991, pp. 14-15), which includes the ingredients of "natural participation . . . top to bottom involvement within the organization from the start," and "influence without authority," which allows workers to make meaningful contributions to business decisions.

The restructuring of all nursing quality activities occurred in three essential areas previously described in the literature: *people* (staff able to educate about QI principles), *materials* (educational materials, books, and copies of reports), and *methods* (such as data measurement) (Caplan, 1970).

Restructuring of People

In the spring of 1988, several part-time clinical nurse specialists were hired and reported directly to the chief nurse executive. The clinical nurse specialists (CNS) functioned in a consultant/educator role to staff nurses and managers regarding quality issues. Based on extensive literature reviews, the CNS's made recommendations of ways to implement unit-based quality assurance at LRMC. Using the expertise of the clinical nurse specialist as consultant/educator, each unit chose aspects of care that were important in their area of practice and of interest to the staff. This

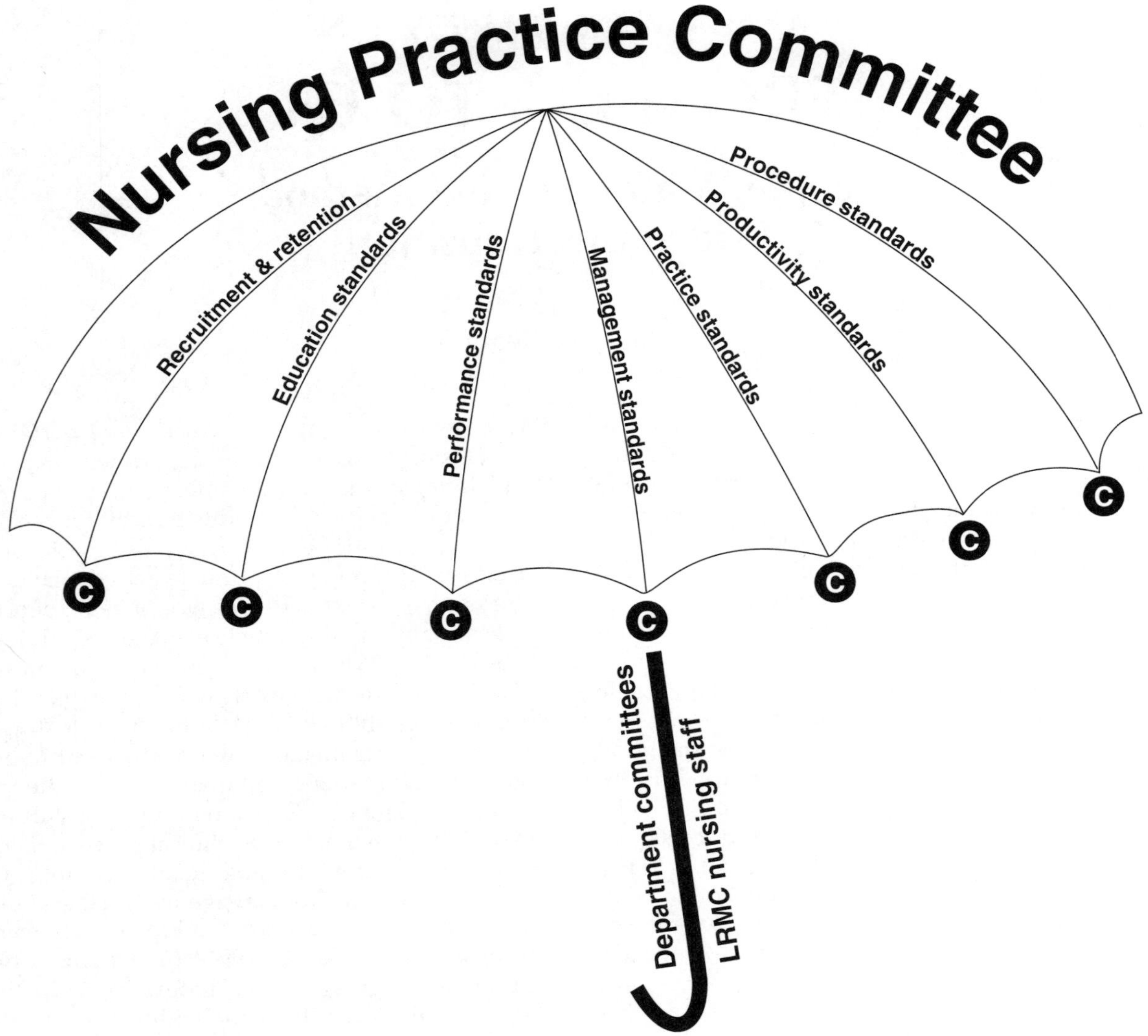

Fig. 7-1 The NPC is the umbrella committee for LRMC's participative governance structure for nursing practice.

represented the beginning of nurses' ownership in quality assurance activities. Throughout the first year, one-to-one consultation was provided at the staff nurse level. By using Caplan's definition of *consultation* as a "process of interaction between two professional persons . . . where the consultant exercises no administrative or coercive authority over the consultee," (Johns Hopkins, 1991, pp. 19-20) the role of the CNS was positively received and well utilized.

By October 1988, each of the 21 nursing units/departments formed a QA committee and elected a chairperson, who serves as the unit's liaison to the newly created Nursing Practice Committee (NPC). The NPC is the umbrella committee for Lakeland Regional's participative governance structure for nursing practice (see Fig. 7-1). By annually reviewing standards of practice and care, departmental plans for improving quality, and quarterly reports of all quality activities, the Nursing Practice Committee es-

tablishes a planned, systematic, and ongoing process to assess and improve quality. Minutes from the NPC are reported directly to the hospital QI/RM Committee, which ultimately reports to the board of directors. The Nursing Practice Committee is chaired by a staff nurse and is composed both of staff nurses, senior-level management, and ad hoc clinical nurse specialists.

Monthly meetings of all quality committee chairpersons were initiated after the first year's unit-based QA activities were appraised. The appraisals overwhelmingly noted that the chairpersons want both support and exchange of information from their peers. Held in an informal morning coffee format, the meeting was both an enjoyable activity and an effective method of gradually teaching QI principles. Facilitated by the clinical specialists, the group often applied quality tools and QI theory to a common theme. This active learning process coupled with practical problem solving is congruent with adult learning theory (Redman, pp. 95-97) and is illustrated in the following example.

Improving a Faulty Process

The Rehabilitation Services department at LRMC was receiving numerous late-arriving patients from various nursing units. When a patient was late for an in-house physical therapy appointment, it was important for several reasons. First, the patient would not receive the benefit of a full and complete treatment time. Additionally, the physical therapists were idle while waiting for the arrival, creating chronic waste of professional time. Traditional communication methods between physical therapists and individual nursing units had not been effective in improving the late-arrival problem because the entire process was faulty.

Poor planning has been described as the root of many quality problems. When goods and services fail to meet customer expectations, they fail. Problems are created for internal customers; they include lengthy delays and redoing prior work (Binns and Early, p. 14). In order to plan a more efficient process, the director of the rehabilitation services department was invited to a nursing chairperson's meeting. The group discussed the issue and first created a cause and effect, or "fishbone," diagram, listing all the possible reasons for late patient arrivals. Since there were no wrong or right ideas, this approach proved to be a nonthreatening way to discuss the problem. No one department or discipline was blamed for the late-arriving patients. Fig. 7-2 illustrates the cause and effect diagram that was constructed by the group.

The next task was to analyze all the steps of the process, beginning with scheduling a patient for therapy to the patient's arrival in Rehabilitation Services. Two units were chosen; the processes are illustrated in a flowchart diagram (Figs. 7-3 and 7-4). It became apparent to the group that unit A and unit B had different steps in the process, as well as different outcomes. Unit A received the Rehabilitation Services schedule on the prior afternoon; this allowed the nursing staff time to plan the patient's following day. In contrast, unit B received the schedule via a telephone call that morning, leaving the nursing staff less time to organize the patient's day. Transportation of patients was also handled differently on the two units. Unit A, which had a high volume of patients receiving rehabilitation, had one person responsible for transportation. This transport person was a key communicator between the nursing unit and Rehabilitation Services, often preventing miscommunication and patient delays. On unit B a low volume of patients was transported by various personnel from Central Transportation Services (CTS) and a consistent communication link did not exist. While unit A was not having difficulty getting patients to rehabilitation on time, unit B was having difficulty.

Analysis of these data, including the QI tools and techniques used, revealed that unit B's process was faulty. A task force/quality team of all involved departments and disciplines was created; it included nursing, transport services, unit coordinators, Hospital Information Services (HIS), and rehabilitation services. Forming such a group had a distinct advantage: all departments that affected the process were represented. A single-discipline task force/quality team would not have had all the information necessary to make a feasible corrective action. For example, the Central Transport representative explained why it was cost-effective for unit A, and not unit B, to have an assigned transport person.

Representatives on the task force/quality team based their evaluations on the previously designed flowcharts and fishbone diagram, and they made a formal recommendation for improvement. Within a week, every nursing unit in the organization began receiving the next day's Rehabilitation Services schedule on the prior afternoon. The corrective action has been implemented for six weeks at the time of publication, and data on patient arrival times are being gathered. Collaboration between departments, part of the QI philosophy, was possible because the involved departments focused on the complex steps involved in the process instead of who had the blame. Arrival times at Rehabilitation Services will be continuously monitored in order to improve service to the patient.

Restructuring of Materials

One of the keys to a successful QI program is an "open, educational philosophy about QI" (Bush, 1991, pp. 175-176) where the practices and underlying theories are presented in a straightforward manner and made easily accessible to all members of the institution. At LRMC, the clinical nurse specialists promoted educational opportunities in three specific modes:

- A monthly mailing of pertinent articles
- An in-house bimonthly newsletter, called *Quality Concerns*
- An annual educational conference, open to all LRMC employees

The clinical nurse specialists recognized that few unit-based QI chairpersons have the time to scour the literature. Yet they wanted to be kept informed. Each month, the CNS's would send two or three short articles, along with a cover memo announcing future events, to each unit-based QI chairperson. The cover memo was always signed "from M and M" (the initials of the CNS's) and the mailing sometimes included a bag of M & M's candies. Seemingly corny, this small gift helped the QI chairperson feel appreciated and special. Additionally, the cover memo was always sent to the unit manager, so communication was consistent at all levels of the organization.

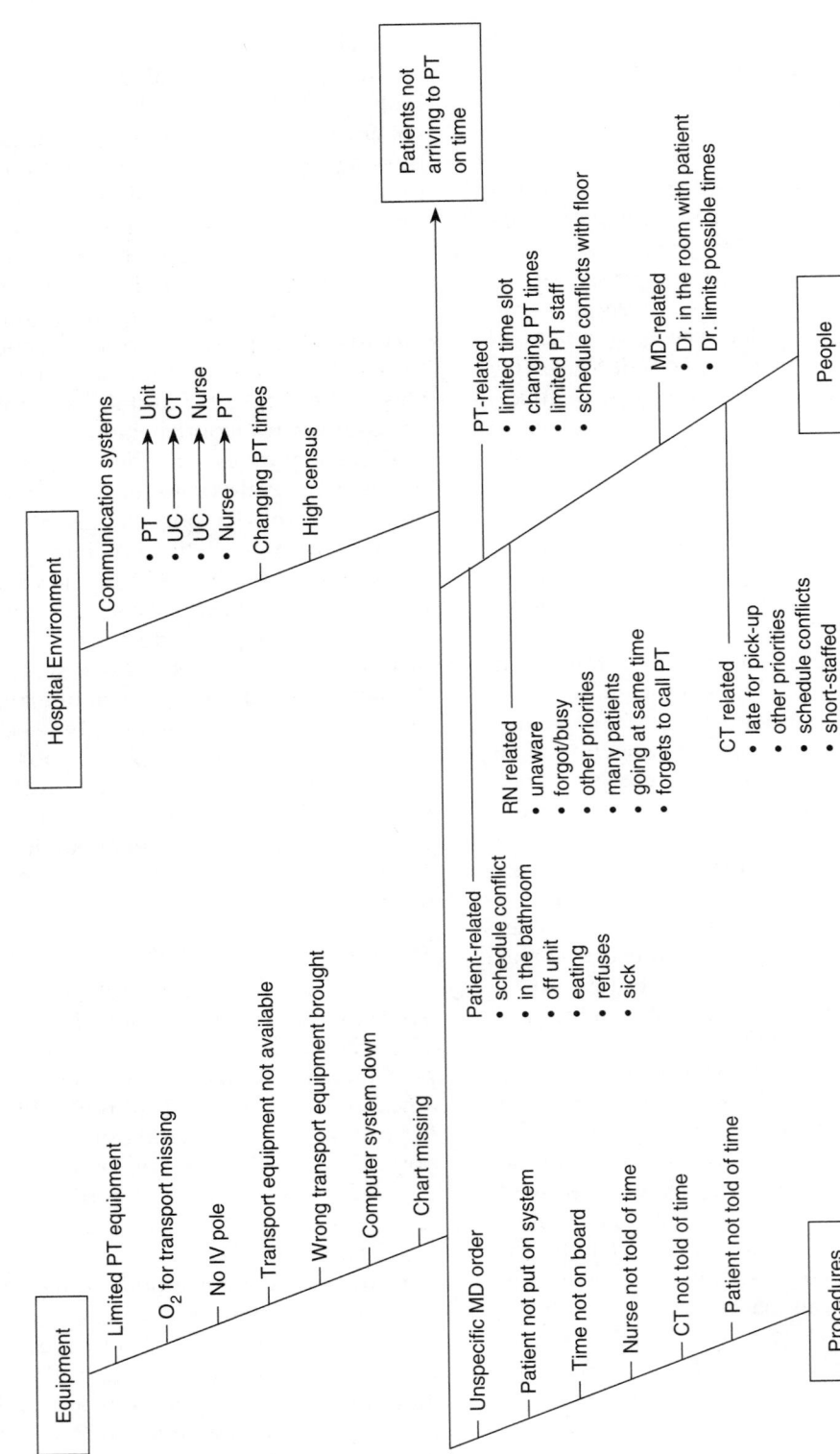

Fig. 7-2 Fishbone diagram: late-arriving patients.

76

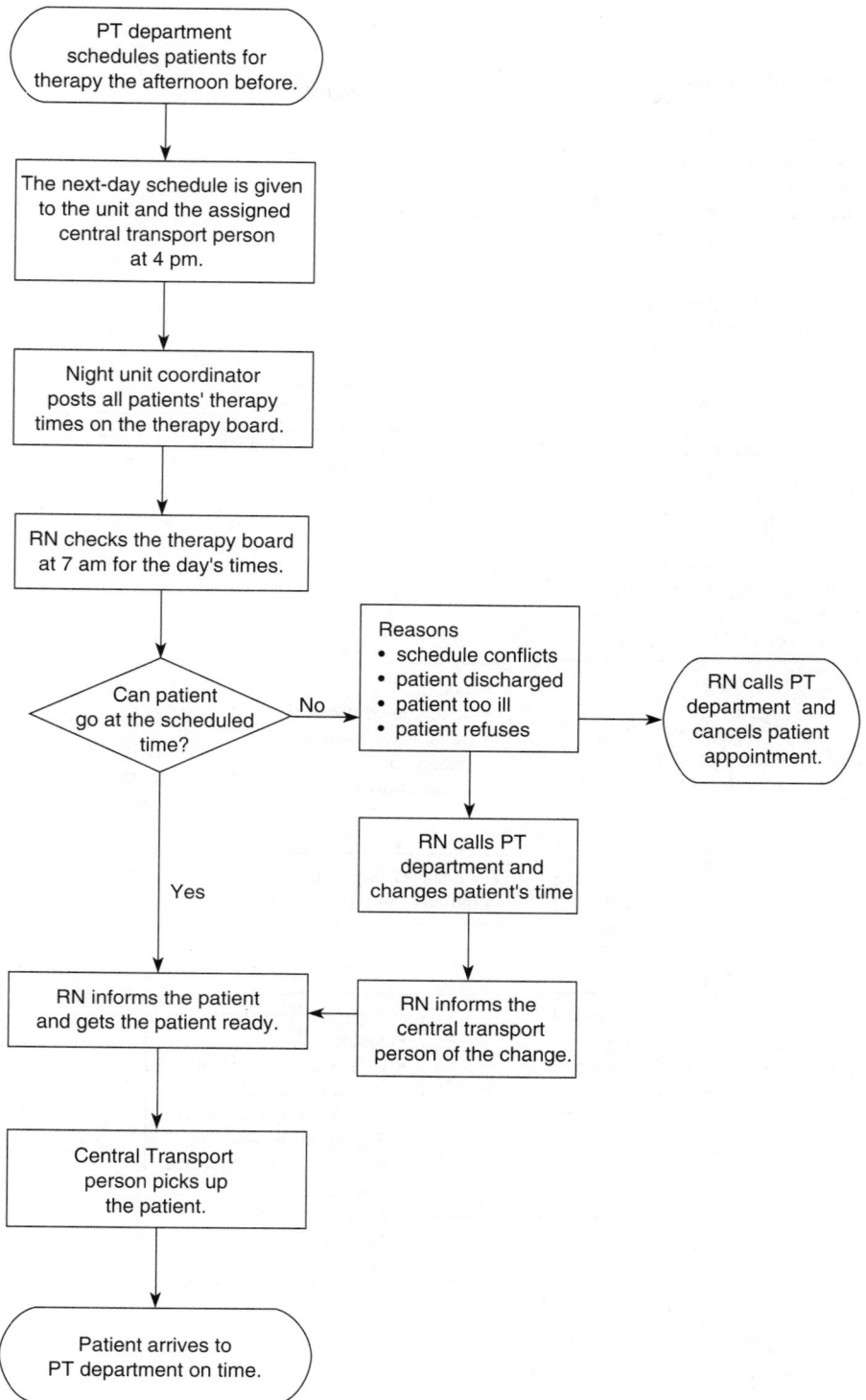

Fig. 7-3 Flowchart of process on Unit A.

At times, a particular topic required the synthesis of many articles, as well as concrete examples to enhance the explanation. In that case, a summary article would be written and published in the bimonthly newsletter. Such articles featured research findings in quality improvement, the changing requirements of various regulatory agencies, the major clinical func-

tions for nursing, and concepts of customer-supplier relationships. The newsletter also included several units' QI activities: their identified areas needing improvement, their unique ideas for corrective action, documented improvements in care, and the names and professional titles of all the quality committee members and chairperson. In addition to providing

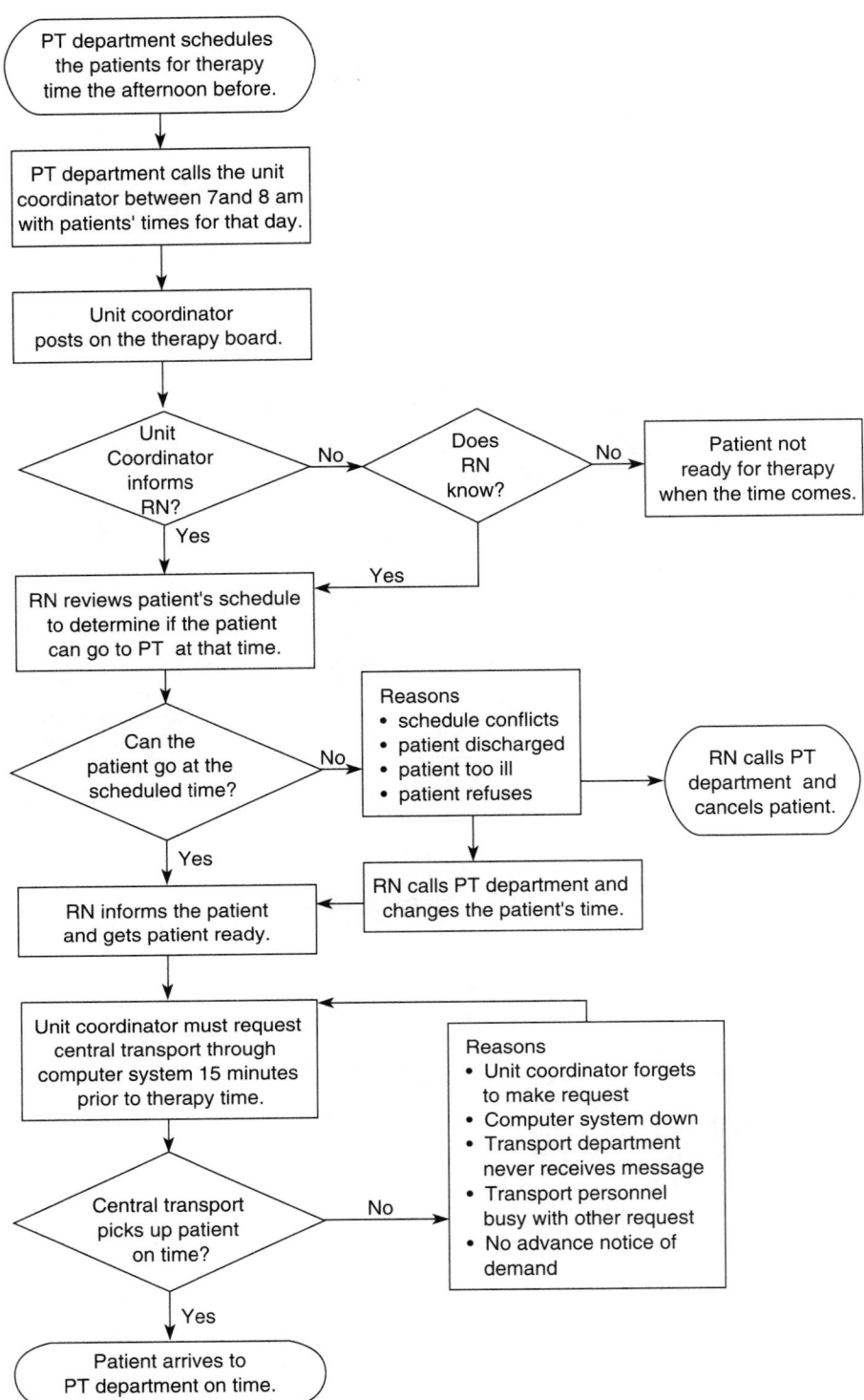

Fig. 7-4 Flowchart of process on Unit B.

recognition of unit-based efforts, the ideas served another vital service. In a large institution, there are many practitioners who never interact with each other in the course of a normal working day. Ideas from a featured unit often "pollinated" other areas within the institution, thus enhancing interdepartmental communication and collaboration. The LRMC

newsletter began in 1988 and has been well received by the staff.

When a particular topic became of great and sustained interest, the topic was presented in an annual conference format. Open to all members of the institution, topics at the day long event are tied into quality improvement efforts. The first annual conference was held in 1989 and has gradually captured the interest of other clinical disciplines involved in quality improvement efforts. Topics for keynote addresses have ranged from changes in the JCAHO standards and the concepts of discharge planning to the theory and principles of research utilization in clinical practice. The conference also included a notebook of speakers' handouts and small breakout sessions. For newer chairpersons, a favorite breakout session was the one presented by three experienced unit-based QI chairpersons, who shared their successes. They each discussed for 20 minutes how interest in QI was generated on their unit and how other practitioners, such as dietitians and physicians, were involved. The information-sharing session gave the newer chairpersons ideas for the future and fostered an esprit de corps among all chairpersons.

Restructuring of Methods

It became evident, after the first year's unit-based quality assurance activities were appraised, that a method was needed to define and organize divisionwide nursing functions. When feedback from the unit's self-appraisals was compiled, several themes were noted:

- Most of the activities were based on medical diagnoses and on process indicators.
- Staff nurses related frustration integrating daily clinical practice with QA activities.
- There was a lack of divisionwide consistency in quality activities, resulting in duplication of efforts in drafting measurable indicators and thresholds that reflected a single standard of care (Gillette and Jenko, 1991, pp. 20-24).

In the book *Quality Is Free,* Phillip Crosby (1979) addresses the cost of quality as the expense of doing things wrong. Throughout the institution, hours of valuable nursing time were spent redrafting pertinent aspects of care, corresponding indicators, and recollecting data. The lack of a simple, yet efficient, method was casting a negative shadow on the unit-based program.

Clinical nurse specialists coordinated these bits of feedback and began a literature search. This search yielded a single reference pertinent to nursing, in which a major clinical function was defined as:

An end product (or service) that a department is responsible for delivering. . . . Without a list of principal functions you cannot decide whether a particular function is significant enough to require formal quality assessment, nor know how adequate is the scope of your quality assurance program (Wilson, 1987, p. 53).

A nursing task force, composed of six staff nurses and one CNS, was formed. The task force based its work on Wilson's definition, as well as previously published definitions of outcome, process and struc-

ture (Marek, 1989, Lower and Burton, 1989). Members of the task force agreed that a major clinical function should:

- Express the diversity of clinical services provided at a comprehensive acute care facility
- Account for 10 to 20 percent of a nurse's time
- Provide a framework for monitoring the outcomes of nursing care, yet include process and structure indicators when they demonstrate an impact on outcome (Larson and Oram, 1989)
- Reflect the institution's nursing standards of practice and standards of care

LRMC's five Major Clinical Functions, approved and adopted in May 1990, are Patient/Family Education, Facilitation of Self-Care, Symptom Distress Management, Provision for Patient Safety, and Enhancement of Patient Satisfaction. To highlight the framework's usability in various clinical settings, Table 7-1 provides a concise overview and integrates the concept of major clinical functions with patient outcomes (Gillette and Jenko, 1991).

The original purpose of defining these functions was twofold: "to maximize the staff nurse's time spent in QA activities, thus reducing the cost of quality, and to provide a unifying framework around which any clinical area's monitoring and evaluation activities could revolve" (Gillette and Jenko, 1991, p. 24). Yet over time, these functions enabled nursing staff members to visualize their patient care activities in a broader scope. For instance, patient/family education is not unique to a single unit or department. Additionally, several units may be providing patient safety for the same population, such as elderly women admitted either to a medical or a psychiatric unit.

Furthermore, LRMC's Major Clinical Functions provided a familiar vehicle to educate staff about the key functions, defined as "cross-departmental processes" (ANA, 1973). Major clinical functions forced the staff nurse to look beyond strictly unit-based, compartmentalized activities, thus recognizing similarities in practice across the division of nursing. For example, nurses manage pain regardless of the pain source (e.g., labor pains vs. pain from cancer). Efforts to improve pain management may lead a staff nurse to collaborate with an internal resource, such as the pharmacy, or an external resource, such as a hospice program. Such features are hallmarks of quality improvement.

Each Major Clinical Function provides the opportunity for the development of both outcome and process indicators. The following actual examples demonstrate the ways by which LRMC staff nurses broadened traditional quality assurance activities, using Major Clinical Functions as the bridge.

Patient/Family Education

Education of patients and their families has been a long-standing interest of the nursing profession, as

TABLE 7-1 LRMC's Five Major Clinical Functions, with Examples

	OB/GYN	Medical/ Surgical	Pediatric	Psychiatric	Critical Care
Clinical Function					
Patient/Family Education	Patient is able to demonstrate care of the infant's umbilical cord	Patient is able to demonstrate proper insulin administration	Patient/family are able to identify signs and symptoms of sickle cell crisis and when to seek medical attention	Family members are able to identify alcohol codependency behaviors	Patient/family comprehend and cooperate with post-PCTA orders of strict bed rest for 18 hours
Facilitation of Self-care	Post-op GYN patients are able to ambulate the length of the hall with assistance by the 2nd post-op day	Hypertensive patient monitors and maintains blood pressure within normal limits	Juvenile-onset diabetic monitors blood sugar and administers own insulin	Anorexic able to gain weight and/or maintain weight within normal limits	While confined to strict bedrest, patient begins to work on ROM exercises with nursing and physical therapy
Symptom Distress Management	Labor pains are effectively relieved	Postoperative pain is relieved through use of pharmacologic agents and comfort measures	Patient's nonverbal cues of pain (facial expression, crying, body position) are assessed and relieved	Patient is able to partially relieve anxiety through use of relaxation therapy	Patient's difficulty in breathing is assessed and relieved
Provision for Patient Safety	Laboring patients are properly placed and maintained in stirrups without injury	Absence of hospital acquired decubiti	Absence of patient falls from cribs	Absence of suicide attempts	Absence of infection from central line
Enhancement of Patient Satisfaction	Post-op GYN patients feel that they were offered adequate comfort measures	Families of terminally ill patients feel that they were treated with dignity and respect	Parents perceive that they are included in the patient's plan of care	Patients were satisfied with the quality of the various group therapies	Family satisfied with the degree of information from the ICU staff regarding patient's condition

evidenced by the 1973 edition of the American Nurses Association Standards for Nursing Practice (ANA, 1973). Using these standards as a basis, the Same Day Care (SDC) staff focused improvement efforts on inconsistent preoperative instructions and education. Nurses felt that many patients were arriving at the unit with too little preparation. Many patients were unprepared for the experience and had never even considered such issues as parking the car or securing a ride home. Last-minute specifics regarding laboratory requests or procedure-related questions sometimes led to delayed or prolonged procedures. Traditional QA methods might focus on documentation—for example, which nurse did not document the preoperative teaching. However, the Joint Commission (1991, p. 7) advises that "care will be improved by not focusing primarily on outliers or bad apples but by looking at the complex series of activities that compose any key function in the hospital." Such advice led the committee on a different quest.

Following a QI approach, members of the Quality Improvement committee first needed data to validate their concerns. All scheduled SDC patients (169 patients) were interviewed over 2 weeks. Both outcome and process indicators, in the form of interview questions, addressed the following areas:

- Does the patient understand the reason for the admission?
- Are preoperative orders on the chart?
- Were preoperative procedures (lab, x-ray, etc.) done prior to admission?
- Were the preoperative procedure results on the chart?

Data revealed generally inadequate preparation regarding:

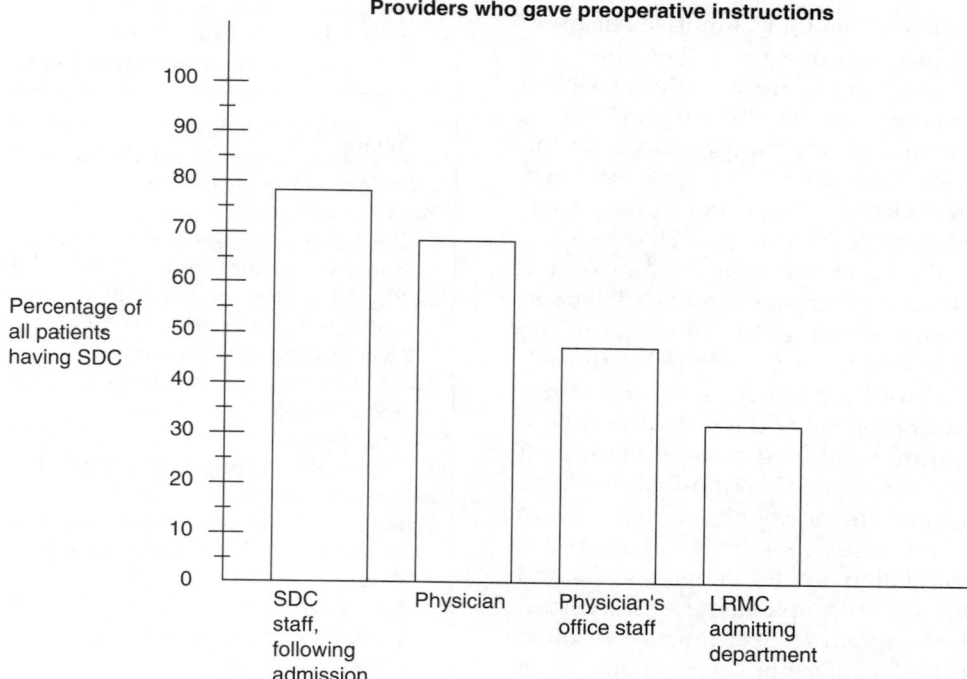

Fig. 7-5 Pareto chart showing which practitioners were providing preoperational instructions to Same Day Care (SDC) patients.

- Instructions about operation and the associated permit
- Diagnostic testing done prior to the day of the operation
- Instructions for pre- and post-operative care

These data were then organized into a Pareto chart by the QI Committee, as shown in Fig. 7-5. The nursing staff determined several causes of inconsistent patient education, despite the existence of a comprehensive "Outpatient Information" booklet published by LRMC. Because the physician/office staff was determined to be the combined major source of preoperative teaching prior to admission, corrective actions were aimed in this area.

Often, implementing a corrective action leads one out of one's specific unit, department, or even institution. Great care must be made to present a total attitude of cooperation: that is, let's work together to improve patient care. Guided by a cooperative spirit, the QI Committee made a list of all 40 admitting physicians. Individual committee members were assigned to a particular physician/office staff. With the "Outpatient Information" booklet in hand, these people paid personal calls on the physician's office, in order to identify and establish rapport with a so-called contact person. Because lengths of stays have shortened, the importance of preoperative teaching before admission was stressed in order to achieve a better patient outcome.

After the initial contact was made, periodic phone calls made to the "contact person" served both as a reminder to the office staff to use the "Outpatient Information" booklet and as a means to maintain communication channels. Remonitoring revealed a dramatic 68 percent improvement. The initial evaluation found that only 20 percent of the patients received written preoperative instructions. Even though 88 percent of the patients are currently receiving written instruction, a continuous effort to improve is in effect. Although productivity is not quantified, clearly the improved process led to a decrease in wasteful staff time. Procedures and surgeries now are no longer delayed or canceled because of patients' misunderstanding. Also, patients are no longer delayed searching for a parking space or arriving without a proper preoperative prep.

The major clinical function of patient/family education remains an aspect of care on Same Day Care. This continuous monitoring is consistent with QI philosophy, which strives to maintain improvement over time.

Provision for Patient Safety

Patient safety has been previously defined as absence of any harm that could have been prevented by reasonable means (Reames, 1988, p. 72). The Medical Intensive Care Unit (MICU) nurses recognized a patient safety issue of increased urinary tract infections (UTI) among their patient population. In a traditional QA framework, the responsible nurses might have been counseled about the risks of infections or required to attend additional in-service sessions on the prevention of UTIs. Yet, the QI Committee began by addressing the processes of care rather than the performance of individual nurses. Retrospective data, regarding many facets of the patients' conditions, were gathered and analyzed to focus on the processes of care. After data were gathered and analyzed, common characteristics were discovered. The majority of the patients with a UTI were on a ventilator and were receiving tube feedings as a nutritional supplement. Common findings included diarrhea and the cultured organism of e. coli in the patient's urine. The MICU staff, intrigued with their findings, then reviewed the literature regarding nutritional needs and problems of the COPD/ventilator patient. The literature supported giving intermittent bolus tube feedings instead of continuous feedings in order to decrease the incidence or severity of diarrhea. Based on research, the QI Committee made a recommendation to the general staff, and bolus tube feedings were implemented as a corrective action. This change in clinical practice resulted in a decrease in the incidence of diarrhea and in an absence of UTI's for a 9-month period.

An additional, yet unexpected, benefit occurred from the literature review. The nursing staff now had an increased awareness and interest in the nutritional needs of ventilator patients. The literature recommended the review of laboratory values in order to determine nutritional status. Because patients on ventilators require additional calories, they are a high-risk population for unmet nutritional needs. The MICU's Scope of Service included a high volume of ventilator-dependent patients, thus warranting "The Nutritional Management of the Critically Ill Patient" as an important aspect of care. The QI Committee began a concurrent review of all MICU patients who had been under NPO instructions for three days. Indicators were (1) Were parenteral or enteral feedings initiated? and (2) If enteral feedings were stated, was the patient tolerating the feedings without diarrhea?

After monitoring this aspect of care, the QI Committee reported its conclusions to staff members and the involved physicians. Data demonstrated that not all ventilator patients were being adequately supplemented, as measured by various laboratory values. Second, the sample of ventilator patients directly admitted from home, versus those admitted from another unit, had laboratory values that demonstrated malnutrition. In addition, data revealed that many obese patients had unmet nutritional needs, showing that patient weight was not always an adequate measure of nutritional status.

The review of these conclusions led to the involvement of other clinical disciplines and departments. The restructured QI Committee, which is multidisciplinary, continues to monitor the nutritional manage-

---

MICU Multidisciplinary Approach to Assessing and Improving Quality

Major Clinical Function: Provision for Patient Safety
Aspect of Care: Nutritional Management of the Critically Ill Adult Patient

Physician Indicators

1. Physician will assess and document patient nutritional status after third day NPO—100%
2. Physician will order lab work to assess nutritional status of patients who are NPO or on parenteral/enteral feedings per protocol—100%
3. Physician will adjust nutritional intake to correct metabolic deficiencies—100%

Nursing Indicators

1. Nurse will weigh patient daily and report variances of 5 pounds to physician—100%
2. Nurse will evaluate nutritional needs of patient and initiate nutritional consult of patient NPO longer than 3 days—100%
3. Nurse will notify physician of patient intolerance to parenteral or enteral feedings—100%

Nutritional Indicators

1. Well-nourished patients receive nutrition within 3 days of admission—100%
2. Patients who are NPO or have one or more of the "malnourished" criteria will receive automatic Nutritional Support Service (NSS) consultation to evaluate appropriate nutritional therapy—100% ("Malnourished" criteria: Inadequate oral intake at home, anticipated inadequate oral intake 5 days or more; weight loss 10% or greater; albumin less than 3.0)
3. Patient receiving enteral nutrition will be assessed by NSS within 24 hours of receiving order for optimal nutritional support appropriate for patient's clinical status—100%
4. Patients receiving enteral nutrition will be monitored by NSS every 5 days for prevention, detection, and management of complications—100%
5. Patients receiving enteral nutrition will receive appropriate energy and protein in order to attain nutritional goals—100%
6. An NSS consultation will be complete on each patient managed by the NSS team within 24-48 hours of receiving the consultation—100%

---

ment of the critically ill adult patient. In addition to nursing indicators, physicians and nutritional-support services have indicators that assess their practice and contribution to this aspect of patient care. Using the major clinical function of *Provision for Patient Safety* as a foundation, the narrow picture of a strictly nursing problem expanded to a broader approach. The box illustrates the MICU multidisciplinary plan, which continues to guide all quality improvement efforts.

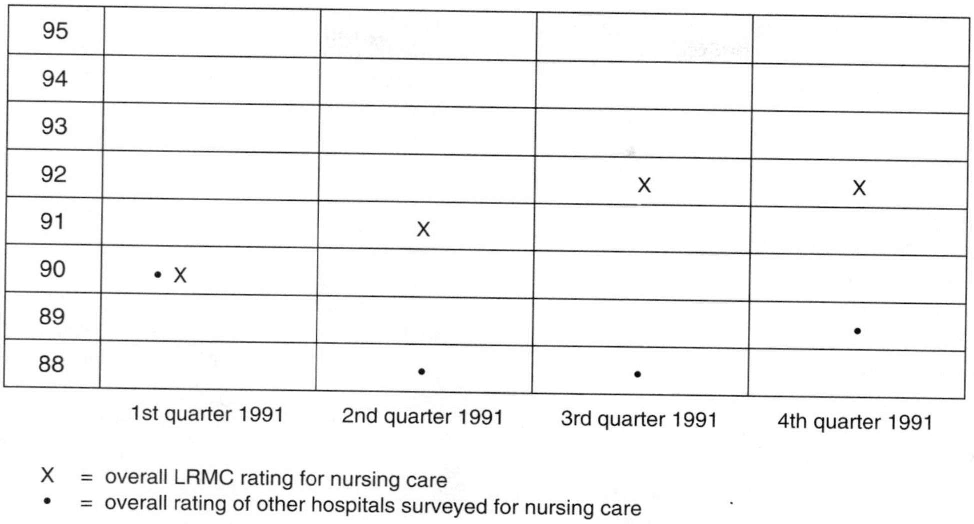

	1st quarter 1991	2nd quarter 1991	3rd quarter 1991	4th quarter 1991
95				
94				
93				
92			X	X
91		X		
90	• X			
89				•
88		•	•	

X = overall LRMC rating for nursing care
• = overall rating of other hospitals surveyed for nursing care

Fig. 7-6 Run chart demonstrating overall patient satisfaction with nursing care at LRMC, as compared with similar institutions.

ENHANCEMENT OF PATIENT SATISFACTION

Formerly, nurses have concentrated on what they thought patients should have and how patients' needs should be met. According to Bader (1988, p. 11) today's patient (i.e., *health care consumer*) wants to be involved in his or her own care, and "health care consumerism is related to perceived quality of care." Hospitals often are judged by the quality of the nursing care since nurses are highly visible and intimately involved with direct patient care.

Using Risser's framework, patient satisfaction is conceptualized as "the congruency between a patient's expectations of ideal nursing care and the patient's perception of the nursing care actually received" and is considered a legitimate measure of the quality of care. Three areas of nursing actions that constitute nursing care were identified:

1. Interpersonal relationships and the personality of the provider
2. Professional competence of the provider
3. The nurse's ability to provide information to the patient (Bader, p. 12)

At LRMC, the concept of benchmarking is used through a housewide patient satisfaction survey. Benchmarking is defined as:

the ongoing process of measuring products, services, and practices against the toughest competitors of those known as leaders in their fields. Benchmarking means a constant search for the best business practices that will ultimately lead an organization to superior performance. (Tackett, p. 14)

Administered by a national consulting firm since 1990, survey data are gathered from the entire inpa-

tient, same day care, and GI unit populations, as well as a representative sample of emergency department patients. The resulting information is compared with data from similar hospitals across the country.

In addition to general hospital data, each nursing unit/department receives specific data. An individual unit can track and trend its ratings over time, as well as its ratings compared with the divisionwide threshold for patient satisfaction and its ratings compared with those of similar institutions. In order to represent these data visually, a run chart is used to identify significant trends in data averages. The run chart (Fig. 7-6) demonstrates overall patient satisfaction with nursing care at LRMC, as compared with other, similar institutions.

Information regarding satisfaction with specific nursing behaviors, such as nurse promptness or noise levels on the nursing units, is also provided. Each QI Committee monitors trends of at least one behavior or service that had a consistently low score. By using the major clinical function of *Enhancement of Patient Satisfaction* as a foundation, corrective actions have focused primarily on systems problems. One unit that implemented a corrective action installed a new call-light system, in which beepers instead of announcements over an intercom transmit messages for nurses. This systems change resulted in a quieter unit and increased patient satisfaction over time.

On the OB unit, the QI committee members used the patient satisfaction data, gathered from July to October 1991, as a foundation for working with two specific departments within the institution. From the analysis of patient complaints about "messiness of bathroom in terms of linens and trash," Environmental Services was invited to help improve the system. By working together, two changes were implemented: trash cans were emptied more frequently by Environmental Services, and linen disposal bags were placed in the patients' bathrooms every morning by nursing personnel. These corrective actions resulted in a 5 percent ratings improvement over a 6-month period.

Additional patient complaints that were analyzed provided an opportunity to collaborate with the dietary department. The QI Committee recognized that new-mother patients were extremely hungry after delivery. For patients giving birth after the hospital kitchen was closed, the unit didn't have any food except soda pop and packaged crackers. A joint corrective action involved the dietary department providing the OB unit with a supply of frozen dinners. These dinners can be prepared in the microwave by the nurse and provided at any time to the patient. This simple corrective action contributed to a 3 percent ratings improvement over a 6-month period.

Since its inception in 1990, the Major Clinical Functions framework has given nursing units a common ground, along with a means to collaborate with other departments and disciplines.

CONCLUSION

Many institutions share the goal of a strong QI program based on multidisciplinary involvement. This goal, however, cannot be instantly attained. It requires patience and an investment of time and energy, in order to nurture the necessary professional growth. To use a garden analogy, many attentive hours must be spent in soil preparation, as well as watering and weeding, before vegetables grow and flowers sprout. The resulting bounty, far exceeding what could be purchased in a store, can be a source of pride and delight.

At Lakeland Regional Medical Center, such an investment was made. Through the commitment of people, materials, and methods, aided by strong and continued support from senior-level management, a gradual bridging of traditional quality assurance to quality improvement occurred. Because staff felt ownership in the quality program, it was eager to build on the strengths of the past, as well as to evaluate objectively all opportunities to improve. Through this approach, the future will be nonthreatening and will offer vast opportunities for continuous improvement in patient care.

REFERENCES

American Nurses Association (1973): *Standards of nursing practice*, Kansas City, Mo, ANA.

Bader MMM (1988): Nursing care behaviors that predict patient satisfaction, *Journal of Nursing Quality Assurance* (2)3: 11-17.

Beck CM, RP Rawlins, SR Williams (1984): *Mental-health-psychiatric nursing*, St Louis, Mosby.

Binns GS, JF Early (1989, Autumn): Hospital care frontiers in managing quality, in *Juran Report*, 10, Wilton, Conn, Juran Institute.

Bush DL (1991): *Quality improvement in healthcare organizations*, Blackwood, NJ, Diversified Business Associates.

Caplan G (1970): The theory and practice of mental health consultation, New York, Basic Books.

Causey WB, editor (1991, October): Surveys will change with JCAHO key function process, *Hospital Peer Review* 16(10): 141-143.

Crosby PB (1979): *Quality is free*, New York, McGraw-Hill.

Gillette B, M Jenko (1991): Major clinical functions: a unifying framework for measuring outcomes, *Journal of Nursing Care Quality* 6(1): 20-24.

Johns Hopkins University School of Hygiene and Public Health (1991, Summer): Integrating QA and QI: marriage or mayhem?, *Quality Exchange*.

Joint Commission on Accreditation of Healthcare Organizations (1991): *Using CQI approaches to monitor, evaluate, and improve quality*, Oakbrook Terrace, Ill, JCAHO.

Larson E, LF Oram (1989): From process to outcome in infection control, *Journal of Nursing Quality Assurance* 4(1): 18-26.

Lower MS, S Burton (1989): Measuring the impact of nursing interventions on patient outcomes—the challenge of the 1990s, *Journal of Nursing Quality Assurance* 4(1): 27-34.

Marek KD (1989): Outcome measurement in nursing, *Journal of Nursing Quality Assurance* 4(1): 1-9.

Naisbitt J (1982): *Megatrends*, New York, Warner Communications Company.

Reames K (1988): Ensuring patient safety, *Journal of Nursing Quality Assurance* 3(1): 72-75.

Redman B (1988): *The process of patient education*, ed. 6, St Louis, Mosby.

Tackett S (1991): Benchmark matrix and guide:part 1, *Journal of Quality Assurance* 13(5).

Williams TP, RS Howe (1991): *Applying total quality management: a nursing guide*. Chicago, Precept Press, National Association of Quality Assurance Professionals.

Wilson, CRM (1985): *Hospital wide quality assurance: models for implementation and development*, Philadelphia, W.B. Saunders.

CHAPTER EIGHT

MONITORING SKIN INTEGRITY WITHIN A QI STRUCTURE

Geri Day
Judy Malinowski
Beatrice Hessen

Bon Secours Hospital is a 311-bed community health care facility in a well-established residential area of Grosse Pointe, Michigan. It offers the community a wide range of both inpatient and outpatient services. Of the adult inpatient admissions (excluding obstetrical admissions), 52 percent are patients over the age of 65.

QUALITY ASSURANCE STRUCTURE

Bon Secours has had an active hospitalwide quality assurance department for many years. This department facilitates the data retrieval of medical staff indicators and compiles reports for the divisions within the medical staff. It is also responsible for assisting the ancillary departments in their quality assurance activities. All departments in the hospital report twice a year to the hospital quality assurance committee.

The nursing department has had an active quality assurance program since the early 1970s. In 1985, the program became decentralized, with unit-based quality assurance councils for every unit, consisting of staff nurses, with the clinical nurse manager as chairperson.

Each unit council reports on its quality assurance activities through a central nursing council, and the report is given twice a year to the hospital committee. The nursing quality assurance program at Bon Secours is coordinated by the quality, standards, and research specialist.

THE MERGING OF QA AND QI

In the late 1980s, the hospital began to explore the concept of continuous quality improvement, which was gaining much attention in health care facilities across the country. As noted previously, terms such as continuous quality improvement (CQI), total quality management (TQM), and continuous improvement process (CIP) were considered different names for the same basic concepts adapted from industrial quality control theory (Andrews, 1991). Total quality management has been defined as a management system for continuously improving performance at every level of every business function by focusing on maximization of customer satisfaction (Fifer, 1990). As in many other health care facilities, the question was raised as to how quality improvement and quality assurance were going to integrate and function simultaneously.

At Bon Secours Hospital, the newly appointed director of continuous improvement, the director of hospital quality assurance, and the nursing quality, standards, and research specialist agreed that it was important that they meet every two weeks to keep lines of communication open and to develop a model of how quality improvement and quality assurance would integrate. They agreed with Labovitz's statement (1990) that TQM and quality assurance are complementary.

Many hours of education and brainstorming went into the development of a visual model for QA/QI at Bon Secours Hospital. Continuous quality improvement is the cultural change that is taking place (see Fig. 8-1). This cultural change will affect every employee on every level and in every department. Total quality management is the management process that supports and nurtures this cultural change. TQM adopts Deming's 14 Points and emphasizes the need for top and middle management to delegate as much authority as possible to subordinates (Casalou and Walton, 1986). The system of organization in place at Bon Secours Hospital includes both traditional departments and service lines. The indicators that are in place to measure quality are derived from professional and service standards, customer satisfaction measurements, data for appropriate utilization of services, and regulatory body requirements.

The methods of pursuing improvement in these indicators include activities that focus on quality control (technical measurement and correction of deficiencies), quality assessment (indicator measurement and action based on professional evaluation of deficiencies), and quality improvement teams (focus groups chartered by the newly formed Hospital Quality Improvement Council). Much of the CQI method-

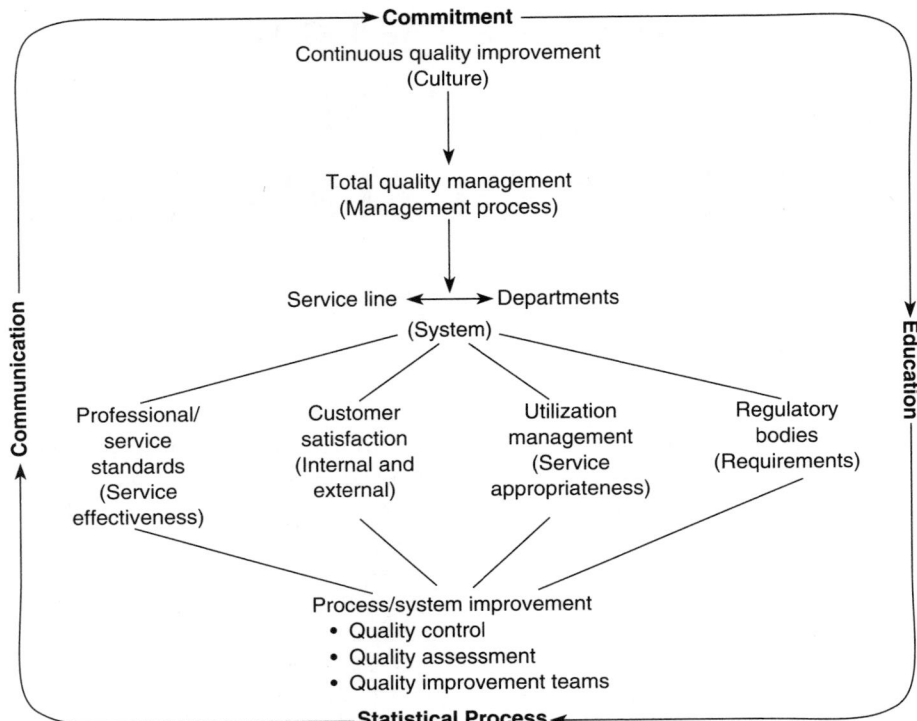

Fig. 8-1 A model for the integration of QI.

ology is being used by all groups, which wish to have a better understanding of the issue under question. This entire model is supported by commitment, education, statistical process and communication.

As part of the collaborative efforts to link quality assurance and quality improvement, it also became necessary to decide how information would flow between the Quality Council and the Hospital Quality Assessment Committee. The Quality Council decided that it was a steering committee and would not get involved in hearing reports of the quality activities. It did, however, want to be given a summary of what activities were going on for quality improvement. This summary would be provided by the Hospital Quality Assessment Committee. It was also decided at this time that the quality improvement teams that were forming throughout the hospital would report to the Hospital Quality Assessment Committee. Their reports would then be included in the regular routing of quality improvement information (Fig. 8-2).

Nursing Department Involvement

As all of these activities were going on in the hospital, the nursing department was also considering how it could begin to adopt some of the QI methodology and still adhere to the Joint Commission on Accreditation of Healthcare Organizations standards for Quality Assessment and Improvement (1992). These standards require identification and monitoring of important aspects of care. It was decided that a "team" approach would be used to identify indica-

tors and conduct professional evaluation related to the important aspects of the nursing department as a whole. In the past, the indicators had been decided upon by the central nursing quality assurance council, which consists of nursing management and education. It was also recognized that another way to make the transition from traditional quality assurance to continuous quality improvement would be in the use of tools such as flowcharts, run charts and Pareto diagrams. These tools can facilitate objectivity and help teams understand the causes of observed performance (JCAHO, 1991).

Nosocomial Decubiti as an Indicator

Since decentralization in 1985, the nursing department quality assurance program has identified a certain number of department wide important aspects of care in nursing. These aspects were always generic enough to be monitored on almost every unit and were in addition to those important aspects chosen by individual units.

Skin integrity has always been identified as a nursing department important aspect of care. There is evidence that this aspect of care is recognized nationally as one of those most important to nurses. At the annual National Quality Assurance Conference held in 1990, nurses from across the country and representing 11 specialty areas identified maintenance of skin integrity as one of the universal important aspects of care (Schroeder and Katz, 1992). Skin integrity is cited as one of the most frequently occurring outcome in-

Bon Secours Hospital
Grosse Pointe, Michigan

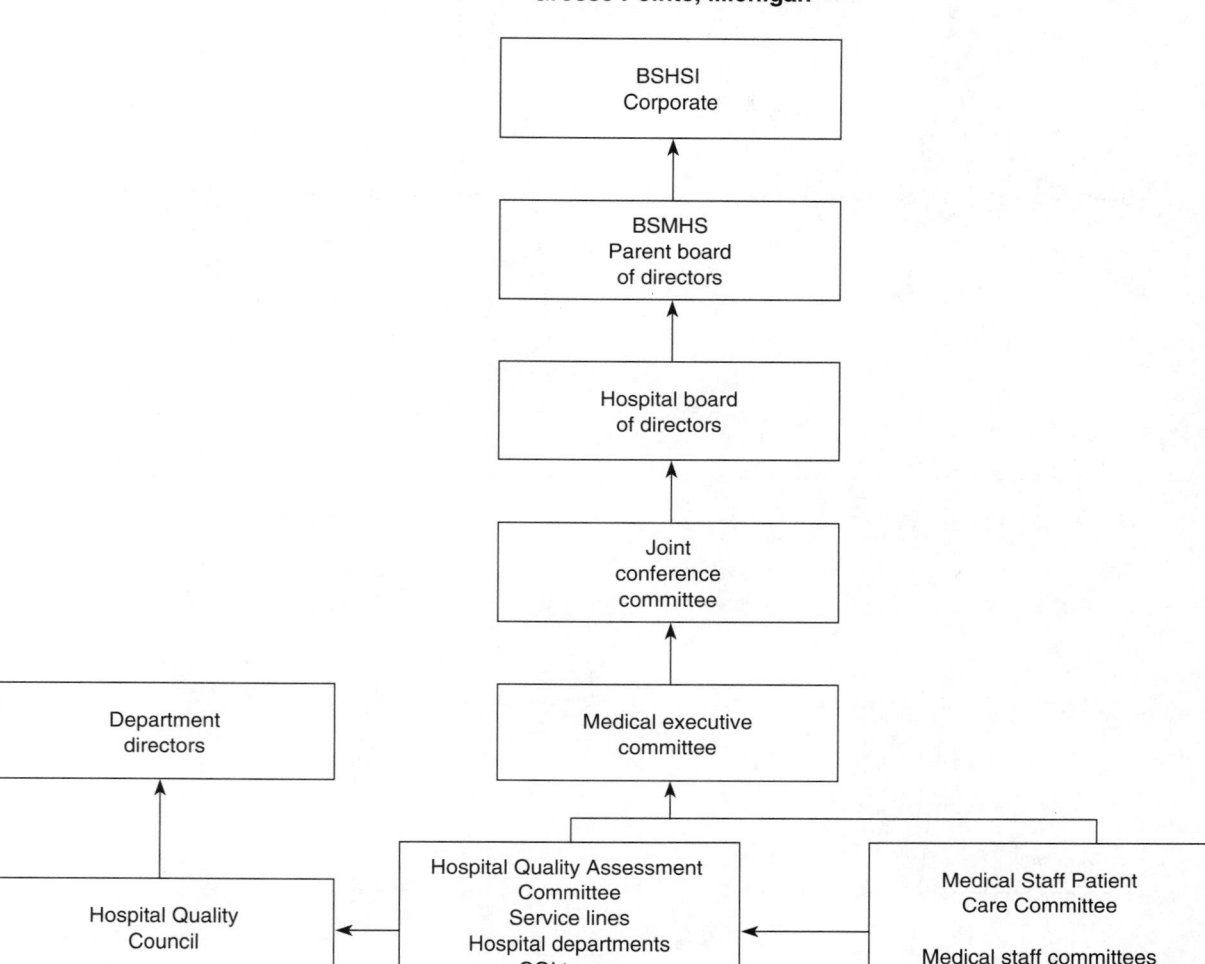

Fig. 8-2 Quality assessment information flowchart.

dicators when quality of nursing care related to physiological status is measured (Marek, 1989). The federal Agency for Health Care Policy and Research has also identified this issue as one of the three areas in which it will develop guidelines. More than three million persons in the United States, most of them elderly, suffer from decubiti (Arikan, Kingery, Beall, and Abbott, 1990). After skin integrity was identified as a departmentwide important aspect of care in nursing, nosocomial decubiti was selected by the nursing department as the indicator.

Data Collection

Data was first collected on this indicator in 1988. The data-collection method was not reliable. It was a tool filled out and sent to Nursing Quality Assurance by registered nurses when a nosocomial decubiti was discovered. It was difficult to ensure that each decubiti was reported. Nonetheless, the information that

was collected was compiled for both departmentwide and unit-specific totals. Variables that were tracked included age, immobility, incontinence, and nutrition, as well as treatment modalities. This information did give the nursing department some idea of the numbers of nosocomial decubiti that were occurring. No specific protocol for treatment of decubiti existed at that time.

In 1990, the collection of data on nosocomial decubiti became the responsibility of a staff person in the hospital Quality Assurance Department. Nosocomial decubiti information was collected during total chart review, which was done retrospectively for other medical indicators. It was felt that now the number of nosocomial decubiti identified would be reliable as every chart was reviewed for decubiti. Professional evaluation regarding the variables that were involved was left up to each unit's quality assurance councils.

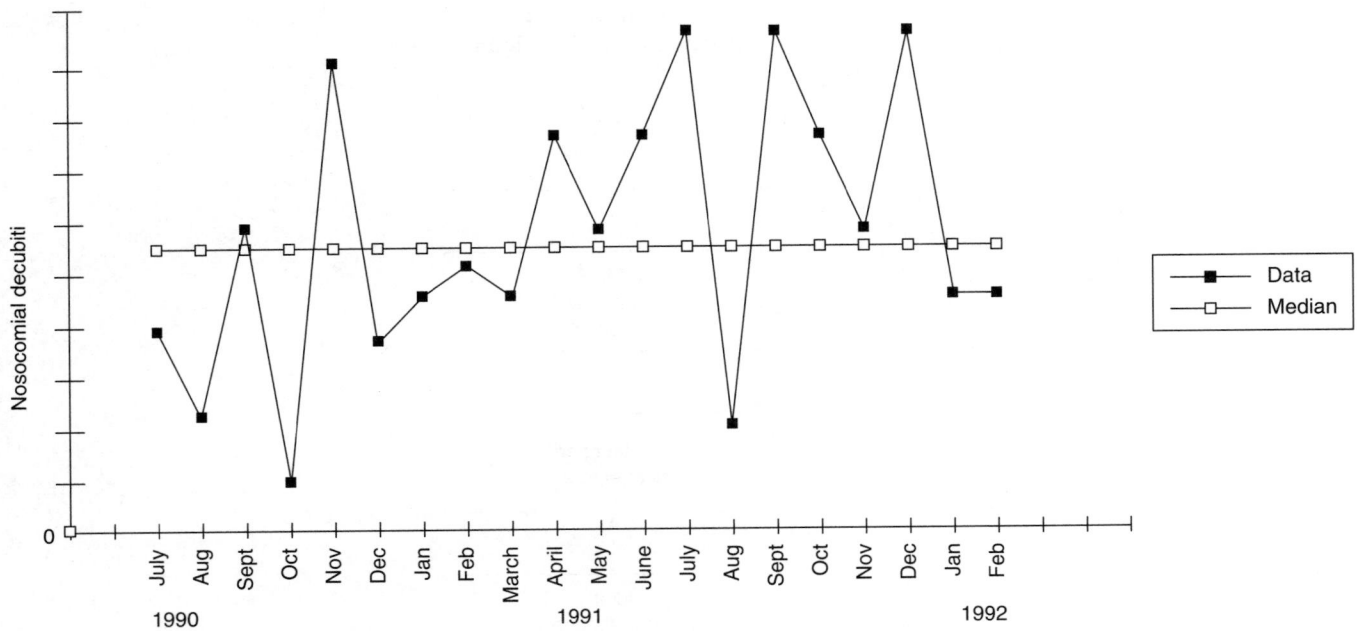

Fig. 8-3 A run chart showing the number of nosocomial decubiti per month.

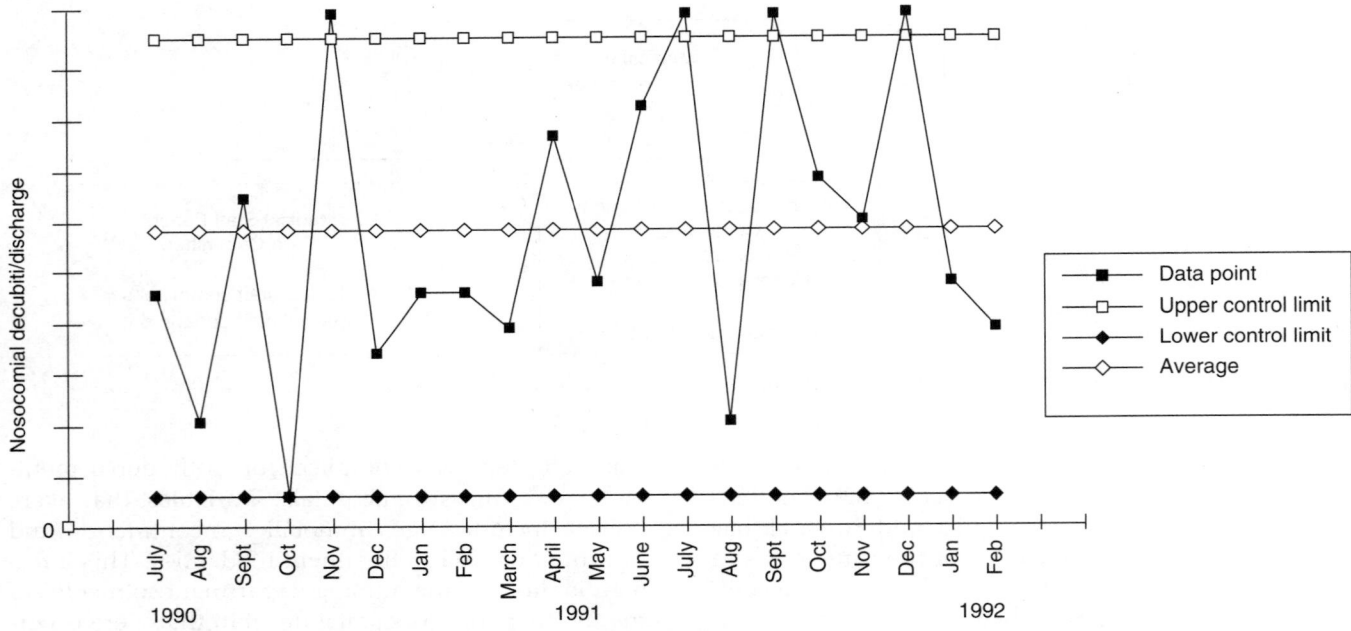

Fig. 8-4 A control chart showing the percentage of nosocomial decubiti per discharges per month.

QI Tools Used

In 1991, the nursing department decided to begin to trend the nosocomial decubiti statistics using some of the quality improvement tools. The hospital director of continuous improvement was asked for assistance in this effort. The first tool to be employed was the run chart. One of the most valuable uses of the run chart is to identify meaningful trends or shifts in the average (Brassard, 1989). The total number of nosocomial decubiti per month since July 1990 were dis-played on the run chart (Fig. 8-3). Run charts were also compiled for each individual unit's results.

The next tool used was the control chart. A control chart is simply a run chart with statistically deter-mined upper control limit and lower control limit lines drawn on either side of the process average (Brassard, 1989). This chart was also developed for the nosoco-mial decubiti (see Fig. 8-4) and was constructed so that the number of decubiti was calculated as a percentage of discharges. It was felt that this made the data more comparable from month to month.

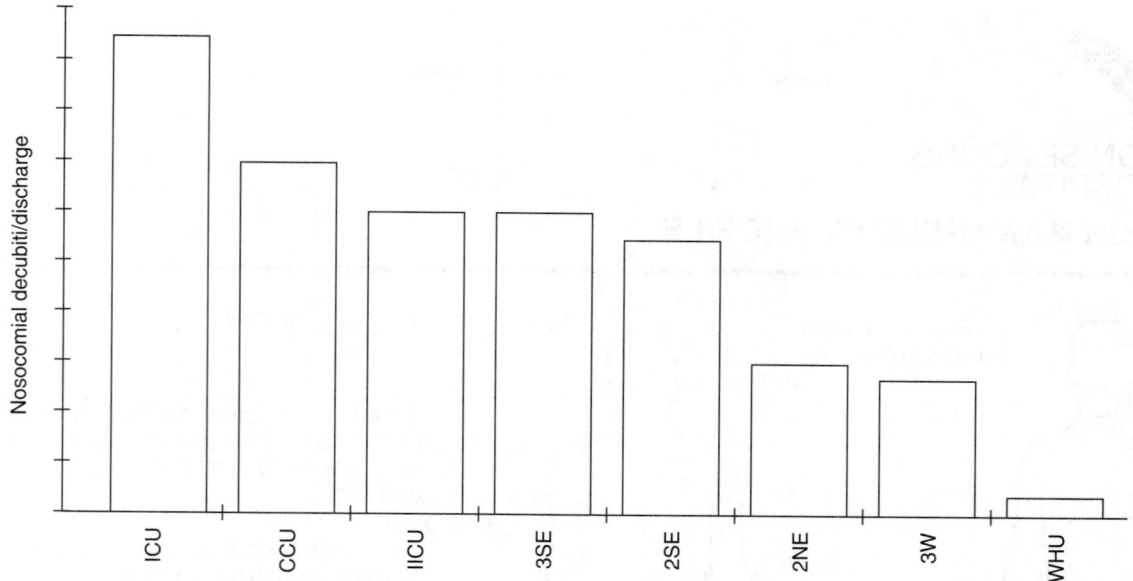

Fig. 8-5 A Pareto diagram showing those units with the greatest number of nosocomial decubiti per discharges.

Using several months' worth of data, a Pareto diagram was assembled in order to compare the number of decubiti on various units. A Pareto diagram is a special form of vertical bar graph that helps to determine which problems to solve and in which order (Brassard, 1989). In this instance, areas with very low discharge rates appear to have the greatest problems due to using the percentages calculated by discharges (see Fig. 8-5). This display of data was shared with the unit quality assurance councils for their professional evaluation.

Unit-Based QA Council Involvement

The Three West unit-based quality assurance council consisted of six members: the clinical nurse manager and five staff registered nurses, with representation from each shift. One additional staff RN was invited as a guest to each meeting. The council identified its role as twofold: to review nursing practice to determine compliance to professional standards, and to monitor clinical nursing practice to continuously improve the quality of care.

The council defined the scope of the unit as "a 36-bed medical surgical unit which focuses on a high percentage of chronic medical disorders of the geriatric patient." The scope included geriatric patients with alteration in mobility, altered nutritional status, alteration in elimination related to incontinence, and fluid-volume deficit. The unit-based council agreed that the departmentwide important aspect of care of skin integrity was of primary concern and in need of immediate action.

At the time discussions were beginning about the action to be taken, the trending done by the Hospital QI director was being presented to the unit council.

The trends validated the council's belief that action needed to be taken regarding the occurrence of nosocomial decubiti on the unit.

When the Three West QA council was given the task of professionally evaluating the patient care record for data on nosocomial decubiti, it was immediately apparent that an evaluation tool was needed for reviewing these records. A literature search was conducted, and a very basic tool was developed based on available articles (Braden, 1990, Goldstone, 1982).

Documentation

Through the use of the professional evaluation tool, the council found that documentation of all aspects of skin integrity was highly inconsistent. There was no continuity in a patient's care record of descriptive terms, staging methods, accurate measurements, or documentation of interventions and evaluations. Again, a literature search was conducted by the council and many pressure-sore status tools and skin-management profiles were examined (Gries, 1989, Gosnell, 1973, Goldstone, 1982). The group tailored a documentation flow sheet to the specific needs of the hospital and presented it to the Nursing Documentation Task Force, a group called to revise the documentation of nursing process. The flow sheet included a figure outline to clarify site location, a staging key with definitions for Stage I to IV decubiti, and columns for recording of data such as site, stage, appearance, treatment, and evaluation (see Fig. 8-6). This flow sheet would be used on all patients when a nursing diagnosis of "actual alteration in skin integrity" was initiated. The form was titled the Skin Management Profile and was well received by staff

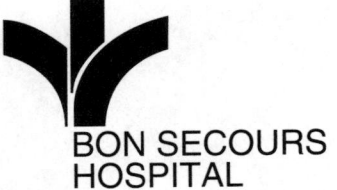

BON SECOURS
HOSPITAL
SKIN MANAGEMENT PROFILE

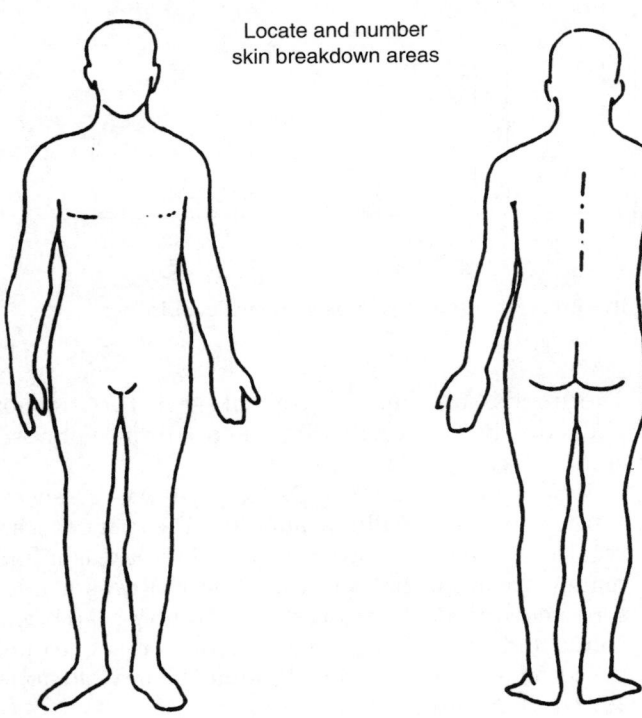

Locate and number
skin breakdown areas

STAGING KEY

STAGE I
Area is pink, red or mottled. Unbroken skin blanches on touch—lasts up to 15 minutes after pressure is released. Skin may be warm and firm.

STAGE II
Skin appears cracked, blistered and broken. Surrounding area is reddened.

STAGE III
Broken skin with deep pressure sore involving epidermis, dermis, and/or exposes muscle. May have necrotic tissue, infection, and/or drainage present.

STAGE IV
Broken skin, deep pressure sore with tissue, muscle and bone involvement. May have necrotic tissue, infection, and/or drainage present.

WOUND
Alteration in skin integrity requiring intervention.

Cultured: site # _____
date _____

Date	Site #	Stage	Diameter/Depth IN CENTIMETERS	Appear *	Drainage *	Odor *	Treatment	Signature

*DOCUMENTATION CHART KEY
1. Appearance: G = Granulating, Sl = Slough, B = Blackened
2. Drainage: S = Serosanguineous, P = Purulent, O = None
3. Odor: O = None, M = Mild, F = Foul

Fig. 8-6 Skin management profile for documentation of decubitus assessment and treatment.

nurses, as it simplified their documentation of decubiti assessment and treatment.

Measurement. Staff had made comments that it was difficult to obtain accurate measurements of pressure sores, particularly in centimeters. This led to the development of a disposable, transparent measurement grid. The grid was made up by the print shop and is available to all the nursing units through their quality assurance councils.

Assessment. After approving the Skin Management Profile, the Documentation Task Force invited the Three West QA Council to assist with the task of revising the Nursing Admission Data Base. The council was asked to develop a risk-assessment guide that would be used at the time of admission to target patients "at risk" to develop pressure sores. Many risk-assessment tools were reviewed, with special attention given to the Norton score and other numerical scales (Goldstone, 1982, Braden, 1990, Gosnell, 1973). In addition, valuable input was received from a staff physician who was actively developing a risk-assessment scale as well as an evaluation and follow-up form for a nearby extended-care facility.

The risk assessment tool that resulted is included as part of the initial assessment of the patient on admission. It provides eight risk categories for scoring the patient. A total score of 11 or above targets the patient at risk for skin breakdown. For those patients, a nursing diagnosis of "potential alteration in skin integrity" must be initiated, with interventions performed as outlined in the prevention portion of the decubitus protocol.

Decubitus Protocol

In referring nurses to the Nursing Protocol for Decubitus, the Three West QA Council felt it would be appropriate at this time to review and update the existing protocol. Use of current resources (Van Etten, Sexton, and Smith, 1990, Maklebust, 1991, Willey, 1989) provided a sound base for an updated protocol. A protocol that deals with nursing standards for review and approval was taken to the council. This updating of the protocol gave the Three West council the opportunity to meet with members of the purchasing department to discuss use of certain skin-cleansing agents, transparent and hydrocolloid dressings, and pressure-reduction devices. As a result of these discussions, several new products were brought into the hospital for trial and use. Members of the council also prepared a large teaching poster to complement the updated protocol. The poster was made available for circulation throughout the hospital units.

All the actions outlined here took place over several months. During this time, the Three West council was enthusiastically supported by its clinical nurse manager, the nursing quality, standards, and research specialist, various practice councils, and individual physicians and members of the nursing staff. Two registered nurse members of the Three West council have developed a much greater interest in skin integrity. They have attended seminars, workshops, and product fairs and were inspired to pursue an in-depth study of principles of skin healing and wound care. Three West has gained recognition throughout the hospital as a unit where skin integrity is a real quality issue.

Skin Integrity Task Force

Translating the progress made by the Three West council to the nursing department as a whole required a group with a broader scope than a unit-based council could provide. This need was met by the development of the Medical/Surgical Skin Integrity Task Force. This group is co-chaired by the nursing quality, standards, and research specialist and a registered nurse from the Three West council. Its other members are staff nurse representatives from the quality assurance councils of four medical/surgical units.

The main purpose of the task force is to evaluate professionally all nosocomial decubiti. This action was begun immediately with a review of the professional evaluation tool originally designed by the Three West council. Changes were made in the tool to facilitate good analysis of the variables in nosocomial decubiti (see Fig. 8-7). This tool is sent to each unit along with a listing of patients who developed nosocomial decubiti on that unit. A retrospective chart review is then done on each patient by the specific unit council, and completed tools are returned to the Skin Integrity Task Force.

The tool provides the Skin Integrity Task Force with valuable data such as whether the patient scored "at risk" on admission and how well the prevention portion of the decubitus protocol was implemented. It also enables the Task Force to determine if other problems associated with skin integrity, such as venous stasis ulcers or community-acquired pressure sores, are being reported as nosocomial decubiti. The tool gives the nurses on the unit where the decubiti developed the opportunity to contribute their professional evaluation of the variables contributing to the decubiti.

With the help of this tool, the task force will be able to chart trends for many of the variables using QI methodology. The task force hopes that this will lead to additional improvements in the assessment, prevention, and treatment of decubiti. This information will also provide a continuing check on how the revised nursing protocol is being implemented.

Routing/Reporting. The Skin Integrity Task Force decided to use one of the tools of QI to design the pro-

INITIAL DATA

Patient diagnosis and/or surgery: _____

Patient age:_____ Patient chart number (both #s): _____

_____

☐ Unable to locate incidence of decubiti (DO NOT FILL OUT THE REST OF THIS FORM)

☐ This was not an actual decubiti. It was _____.
(DO NOT FILL OUT THE REST OF THIS FORM)

1. Refer to the initial admitting assessment. Using the Nursing Admission Data
Base pressure sore risk scale, what was the patient's score?

SCORE: _____   NO SCORE OBTAINED: _____

2. a. If a score of 11 or above, was a problem of actual or potential skin
integrity alteration on the problem list?   YES   NO

b. If a score of 11 or above on admission, were any preventitive measures
instituted within 24 hours of admission?   YES   NO

3. a. On what day was it noted that a pressure sore had developed?

_____

b. What was the site of the pressure sore(s)?

_____

4. What stage was the pressure sore when discovered?

STAGE: I   II   III   IV

5. Did it progress to a more severe stage?

NO   YES to STAGE: I   II   III   IV

6. Was the patient consistently incontinent of urine?   YES   NO

7. Was the patient consistently incontinent of feces?   YES   NO

8. How was the nutritional status during hospital stay?

GOOD   FAIR   POOR   NPO   TPN   Tube Feedings

9. *Mobility*
☐ Full movement
☐ Limited assistance
☐ Moves only with assistance
☐ Immobile

LIST TREATMENT MEASURES HERE

Check all that were used:
☐ Egg crate
☐ Sheepskin
☐ Heel protectors
☐ Special beds
☐ Patient turned q 2°
☐ Other (mattresses, etc.)

Treatments
☐ Cara-Klenz spray
☐ Carrington wound gel
☐ Carrington moisture barrier
☐ Desiten
☐ Other (Granulex, etc.)

Dressings
☐ Tegaderm
☐ Tegasorb
☐ Other

List other wound treatments:

_____

_____

_____

Fig. 8-7 Decubiti professional evaluation tool.

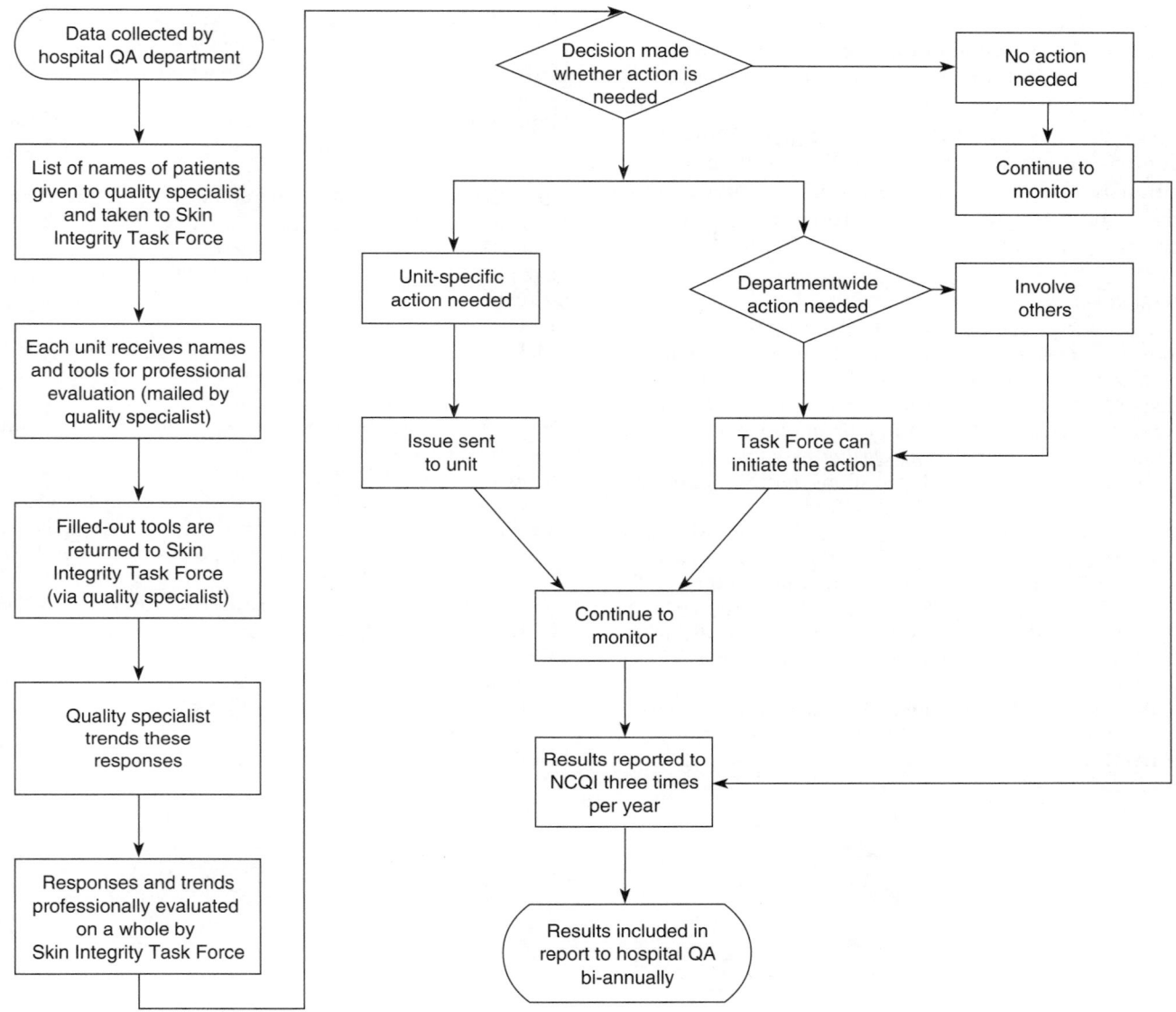

Fig. 8-8 Flowchart of the routing and reporting of nosocomial decubiti information.

cess to be used to route the decubiti information. A flowchart was developed to show how the decubiti information would be collected, routed, evaluated, acted upon, and reported (see Fig. 8-8). Often a flowchart is used to design a process as well as to examine an existing process.

Education

Because many of the innovations taken to improve maintenance of skin integrity were new to the nursing department, it was apparent that education for these was needed. The Skin Integrity Task Force members were urged to begin a review of the skin integrity program on their units. On a department level, it was felt that the program needed to be presented to new nursing employees during orientation and to nursing staff attending the annual nursing education day. A video format was suggested so that

the whole skin integrity program could be visible and "on the road" to each unit.

CONCLUSION

The response to the QI methodology has been very positive. The Skin Integrity Task Force is looking forward to using the QI tools to trend each variable as they continue to collect data from the professional evaluation tool. They will be looking for opportunities to improve the processes involved in the maintenance of skin integrity. The improved documentation forms for assessment and treatment of skin integrity were implemented in January 1992. The run chart shows a decrease in nosocomial decubiti for two months since that implementation. The task force looks forward to continued trend reporting in order to see whether actions have really resulted in improved patient outcome. The task force realizes the need for a long-term commitment to the issue of skin integrity and adopts the philosophy expressed by Roberta Abruzzese (1992): "The real success story involves months and years of caring, of monitoring progress, of paying attention to the problem, of continuously updating prevention and treatment strategies." The ultimate goal is to promote a quality skin care program as "the way we do it here."

REFERENCES

Abruzzese R (1992): Editorial, *Decubitus* 15(2): 6.

Andrews S (1990): QA vs. QI: The changing role of quality in health care, *Journal of Quality Assurance,* 13(1): 14.

Arikian V, C Kingery, K Beall, R Abbott (1990): Education and QA: a model for continuous improvement in skin integrity, *Journal of Nursing Quality Assurance* 5(1): 2.

Braden B, R Bryant (1990): Innovations to prevent pressure ulcers, *Geriatric Nursing* 11(2): 182-186.

Brassard M (1989): *The memory jogger plus+ ,* Methuen, Mass, Goal/OPC.

Casalou RF: Total duality management in healthcare. *The University of Michigan Department of Health Services Management and Policy,* Ann Arbor, University of Michigan.

Fifer WR (1990): Quality in moving upstairs. *Journal of Quality Assurance* 12(4): 17.

Goldstone L, J Goldstone (1982): The Norton score: an early warning of pressure sores? *Journal of Advanced Nursing* 7: 419-426.

Gosnell D (1973): An assessment tool to identify pressure sores, *Nursing Research* 22(1): 55-59.

Gries M, K Gladfelter (1989): Nursing practice briefs, *Nursing '89* 19(3): 81.

Joint Commission on Accreditation of Healthcare Organizations (1991): *Accreditation manual for hospitals,* Chicago, JCAHO.

Joint Commission on Accreditation of Health Care Organizations (1991): *Transitions: from QA to CQI.* Chicago, JCAHO.

Labovitz G (1990): From little "q" to big "d": an interview with George Labovitz, *Journal of Quality Assurance* 12(4): 11.

Maklebust J (1991): Pressure ulcer update, *RN* 54(11): 56-63.

Marek K (1989): Outcome measurement in nursing, *Journal of Nursing Quality Assurance* 4(1): 4.

Scholtes P (1989): *The team handbook,* Madison, Wisc, Joiner and Associates.

Schroeder P, J Katz (1992): Seeking consensus on important aspects of nursing care. *Quality Review Bulletin.* 65.

VanEtten N, P Sexton, R Smith (1990): Development and implementation of a skin care program, *Ostomy Wound Management* 27: 40-54.

Walton M (1986): *The Deming management method,* New York, Dodd, Mead & Co.

Willey T (1989): *A dressing application guide for the care of wounds, using moist wound healing principles* (Available from Smith and Nephew, 11775 Starkey Rd., P.O. Box 1970, Largo, FL 34649-1970).

CHAPTER NINE
PATIENT IDENTIFICATION
A Quality Imperative

Rhonda R. Stockard
Barbara Dianda-Martin

The evening nurse arrives on duty and receives reports on the four patients she is to care for during her shift. One patient under her care is Mrs. Smith, a 70-year-old woman in room 710, bed number two. Mrs. Smith is scheduled to receive cardiac medication at 6 p.m. The nurse carefully compares Mrs. Smith's medication record with her kardex. While at the medication cart, she also double-checks the pill name, dosage, and the scheduled time in the medication record for accuracy. Finally, she places the medication in a cup and goes to Mrs. Smith's room.

Upon entering the room, she approaches the silver-haired woman sitting in the chair next to bed number two. She states, "Mrs. Smith, I have your medication." The woman smiles and takes the medication with a sip of water. At this moment a patient transporter enters the room and announces that Mrs. Smith has just returned from Radiology. Unfortunately, the silver-haired woman in the chair was not Mrs. Smith, but her roommate, who is deaf and unable to speak. She was sitting in that chair because she enjoys looking out of the window.

What happened? This nurse had meticulously performed four of the five rights of medication administration (Smith and Duell, 1985). She was confident that she was giving the right medication, at the right time, in the right dose, via the route that was ordered. What she failed to determine was that she was giving it to the right patient; she did not check the patient's identification (ID) bracelet.

THE IMPORTANCE OF PATIENT IDENTIFICATION

Aitken (1973) believes personnel in nursing units become overconfident because they work with patients daily. They know a patient and therefore assume that everyone else does. Health care providers need to approach patients each day as if it were the first time the patient was encountered. All too often patients are identified by a room number, bed number, diagnosis, physical or behavioral description, or the fact they respond to a name when it is called. Nurses are often reluctant to check a patient's identification band because it is impersonal. According to the American

Hospital Association (AHA), verbal identification should not be used because patients may be indifferent or inattentive, sedated, or otherwise unable to respond. Patients may also have language barriers or speech and hearing defects or may be too young or too confused to comprehend (AHA, 1992).

In view of the risk and quality issues associated with failure to identify patients appropriately, adequate systems or processes are essential. To address this issue, it is important first to consider at what point a patient is formally identified following admission. At St. Vincent Medical Center, a 588-bed acute care facility in Ohio, adverse outcomes have not been documented related to an employee neglecting to check a patient identification band or patients not wearing an identification bracelet; however, the potential for this problem exists. The emphasis on cost containment in health care has resulted in patients being admitted through departments other than admitting. These departments may not have an admissions process in place, or the process may not be consistent with that of the admissions department. The AHA states that the patient identification band

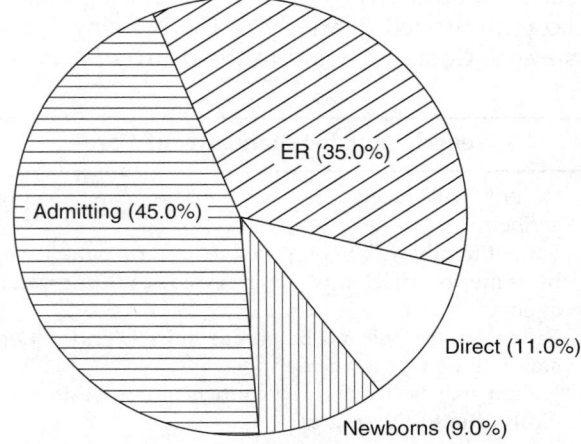

1991-1992
Routes of Admissions

Admitting (45.0%)
ER (35.0%)
Direct (11.0%)
Newborns (9.0%)

Fig. 9-1 Pie chart representing routes of 1991-1992 admissions to St. Vincent Medical Center.

should be prepared and affixed while the patient is still in the admitting department (1992, p. 1). However, nearly 50 percent of the patients admitted to St. Vincent are admitted through routes other than the admitting department (see Fig. 9-1). The implications of treating formally unidentified patients, coupled with a change in the system for banding patients, motivated the medical center to examine this quality issue. The ability to improve care and service by examining this issue became an operational imperative and an excellent opportunity to utilize quality improvement principles.

Approach to Quality

The Nursing Quality Assurance Program at St. Vincent Medical Center is decentralized and has been in place for three years. This approach to quality is consistent with the nursing management philosophy and goals and objectives. The framework that best supports this approach is unit-based. At St. Vincent, the belief is that:

- This approach enables each unit/department to define as well as measure the quality of care rendered and improved.
- Monitoring and evaluation should be at the level of the practitioner providing care or service.
- Nursing staff should be involved in all facets of the quality assessment and improvement process.

These beliefs validate the conviction that quality is everyone's business. Although the vice president of nursing is responsible for the quality of care delivered throughout the nursing division, each practitioner is responsible for his or her practice and the quality of care delivered. Four generic nursing standards guide the quality process (see the box below). Each unit develops and monitors department-specific indicators based on defined important aspects of care or service. The monitoring activities must support the generic standards. The results of monitoring activities are communicated quarterly to the Nursing Quality Assurance Committee and to the board of trustees.

Generic Nursing Standards of Care

1. Patient will receive medical/nursing care as prescribed.
2. Patient/family will be prepared to assume patient care by time of discharge or referred to appropriate agency.
3. Patient safety will not be compromised, and patient stay will be free of incident.
4. Patient will be discharged with no increase in morbidity due to nursing care.

Used with permission of St. Vincent Medical Center, Toledo, Ohio.

The quality programs in ancillary departments are also decentralized. Quality Assurance department findings are reported to the Support Services Committee and ultimately to the board of trustees. This committee is composed of representatives from ancillary departments supporting the provision of nursing care and the chairman of the Nursing Quality Assurance Committee.

Although successful, this decentralized approach to quality monitoring has not been without shortcomings. Opportunities to collaborate or to conduct multidisciplinary studies were limited. In addition, this approach often focused on identifying problems, reporting the negatives, and placing blame.

Early Concerns

The focus on patient identification at St. Vincent Medical Center began two years ago. Laboratory staff members perceived an increase in the number of patients without identification bands when they arrived on nursing units to collect blood specimens for testing. A phlebotomist reported this increase in unbanded patients approximately one month after the admitting department discontinued providing identification bands for patients during the admission process. The decision to purchase and apply patient identification bracelets was shifted from the admitting department to the individual nursing units.

An early assumption made by laboratory personnel was that the change in the accountability to the nursing unit led to an increase in unbanded patients encountered by the phlebotomist. It was necessary to confirm this assumption because the admitting department did not band all patients and this policy was not noted to be a problem prior to the system change. Laboratory personnel developed an indicator and began to monitor the frequency of occurrence. The monthly monitors revealed 1 to 12 percent of patients encountered were not wearing an identification band (see Fig. 9-2).

Working with patients without identification bracelets poses quality, risk, and productivity problems for all personnel. The complications caused by a lack of appropriate patient identification can result in potential injury when procedures are performed on erroneously identified patients. The incident that led to *Scribner* vs. *Hillcrest Medical Center* occurred when a hospital employee neglected to check the wristband of patient Rhonda Scribner. Ms. Scribner had correctly undergone a hysterectomy and then was taken by mistake to radiology for an ultrasound. She alleged in her lawsuit that the preparation for the procedure, which was not completed, tore her sutures. She had to undergo subsequent surgery to repair the site. Scribner was awarded 10 million dollars in punitive damages (Hudson, 1990).

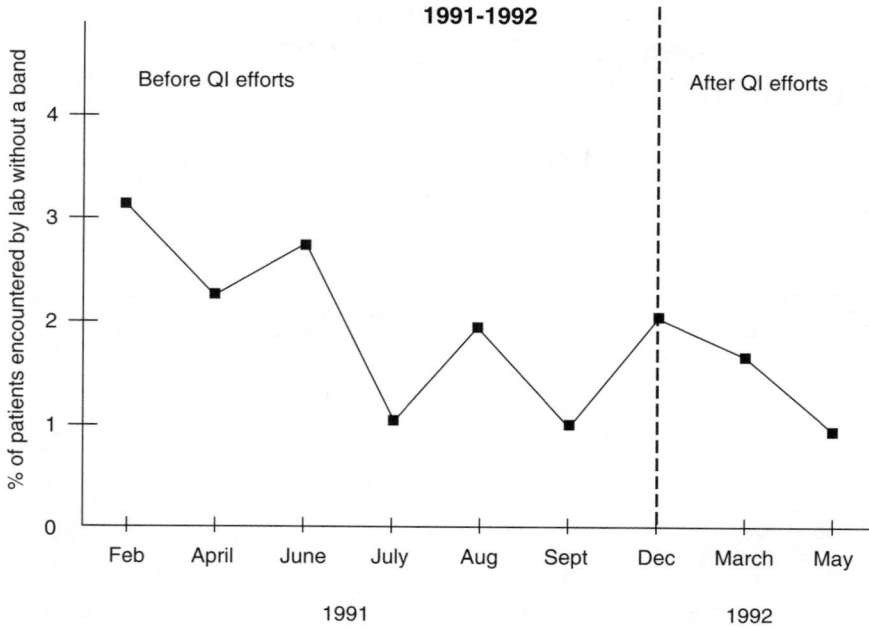

Fig. 9-2 Chart representing monthly percentages of patients encountered not wearing an identification bracelet by laboratory personnel.

According to Rakes, "Quality assurance has had a major role in recent years in the control of patient risk. Through the monitoring and evaluation of patient care activities, risk exposures in clinical areas that create a professional liability have been identified more expediently" (1991 p. 61).

Deming's philosophy also emphasizes improvements in productivity with the goal of achieving a fundamentally stable or predictable system (Duncan, Fleming, and Gallati, 1991). By having a stable and predictable system in place in an area such as patient identification, we gain efficiency and dependability.

Nursing Perspective

After the results of the laboratory studies were reported to the Support Services Quality Assurance Committee at St. Vincent the nursing division became involved in this project.

The Nursing Quality Assurance Committee chairman presented the information that was compiled to the committee members. The committee reviewed the laboratory's findings and the patient admission policies and procedures and discussed possible causes with laboratory personnel. The following was determined:

- The total cases reviewed only reflected patients that were having blood drawn.
- The compliance rates reported did not compare the number of patients encountered without identification bands with the total number of patients encountered.
- Many patients encountered were new admissions (see Fig. 9-3).

- The policies and procedures did not address banding patients on admission to the hospital.
- There was a need to look at all patients.
- The admitting department was critical to the process, yet was not involved.
- Nursing staff was not aware of the risk and potential quality issues associated with identification of patients.

A housewide study was needed to take a comprehensive look at the issues and to identify trends and possible causes.

The Study Process

The NQA Committee developed an indicator and a monitor for the generic standard: Patient safety will not be compromised and patient stay will be free of incidents. For a three-week period, personnel on all inpatient nursing units assessed every patient daily to determine if he or she was wearing an identification band. Numbers of patients with ID bands varied from unit to unit. An average of 3.5 percent of patients were encountered without proper identification. The reasons cited for patients not wearing an identification band were the following:

- Band was cut off by nursing/medical personnel to start or restart intravenous therapy.
- Band placement was delayed until admission numbers were available.
- Patient was admitted to nursing unit from another area without a band.
- Patient preferred not to wear a band.
- Patient admission status was outpatient or short stay.

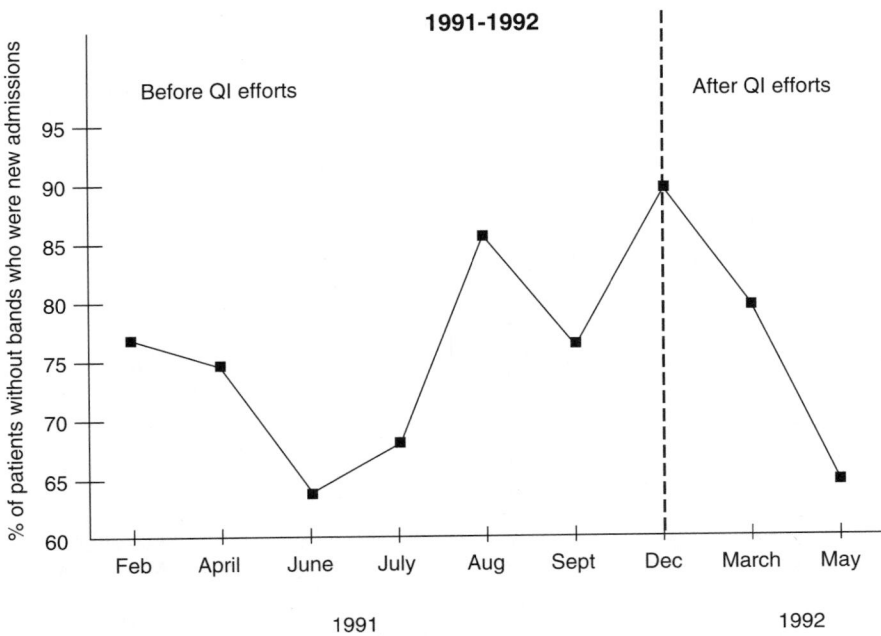

Fig. 9-3 Chart representing the percentage of patients encountered without bands who were new admissions to the hospital.

- Patient's physical condition contradicted use of an extremity.
- Considered a low priority upon admission.

THE TRANSITION TO QUALITY IMPROVEMENT

The findings of both the laboratory and nursing studies were reviewed and reported through the institutional channels. The studies gained the attention of the Quality Assurance Committee of the board of trustees. The leadership support to study alternatives to improve care provided the impetus to form a multidisciplinary committee and begin to introduce principles of quality improvement.

Through the formation of an interdisciplinary group, St. Vincent was able to eliminate departmental barriers and collaborate for a single purpose. The interdisciplinary group included representatives from nursing, the laboratory, and the admitting department. This group's charge was to examine the processes and develop a plan to improve current practice. The goal was to improve care without assigning blame. Quality management, write Katz and Green (1992, p. 28),

dictates that a practice guideline for patient safety be implemented that encompasses an organized plan for total patient safety. In the past, patient safety has been a singular ''nursing'' function. Realistically no one nurse is capable of observing every patient every minute. Together, however, the total health care team is able to ensure patient safety.

The group used brainstorming and a cause and effect (fishbone) diagram to identify possible reasons for lack of patient identification (see Fig. 9-4). This analysis suggested two strategies for action. The first strategy was to reinstitute the ongoing monitoring of patients on the inpatient nursing units. Daily monitoring could be an inherent component in care and would also serve to heighten the awareness of health care providers. The second strategy involved both nursing and laboratory personnel. Use of a data collection card was initiated for instances when a phlebotomist encountered a patient without an ID band (see Fig. 9-5). The card system provided nurses with an opportunity to follow up potential quality issues related to a lack of patient identification, misidentification, and treatment delays within a 24-hour period. The phlebotomist is responsible for completing the left side of the bright pink card and placing it in a designated area on each nursing unit. Nursing personnel are responsible for completing the right side of the card. In the spirit of continuous quality improvement, the card is not intended to be used punitively or to place blame.

Following a four-week monitoring period, the committee reconvened to check the results of the system changes and discuss the findings and problems associated with the study process. The measures proved to be successful; patient identification increased to 99.1 percent. Of those patients not wearing an identification band, 63.8 percent were new admissions. This percentage, though improved, was not acceptable to the committee, and a plan for improvement was developed. The committee agreed to continue ongoing monitoring and evaluation, to seek alternatives to use of an identification band, and to determine how other departments identified patients prior

Reasons Patients Are Not Identified

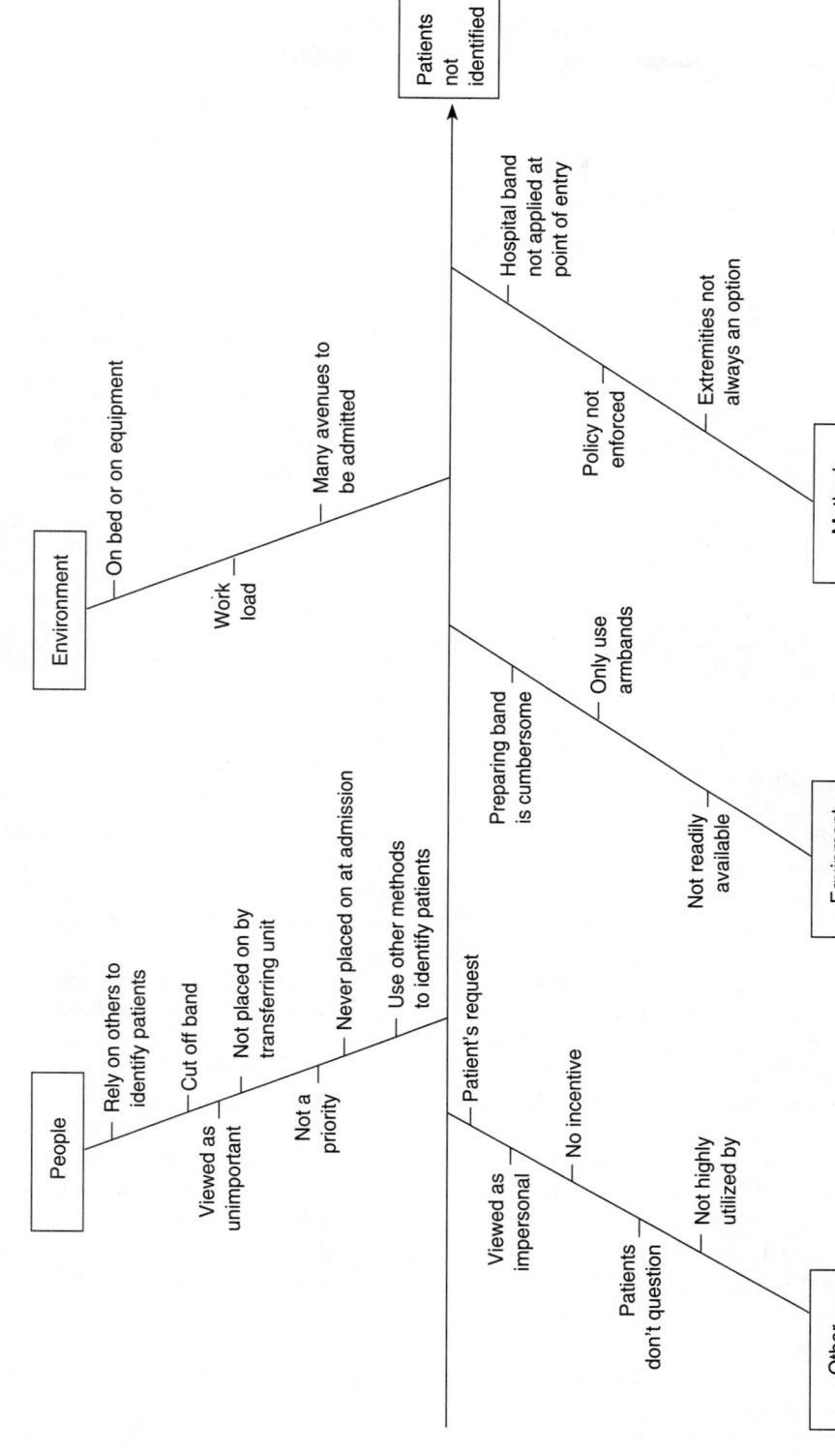

Fig. 9-4 Fishbone diagram showing the possible reasons patients are not wearing an identification band.

Patient Identification Band Alert

Important Aspect of Care: Patient Safety.　　　　Indicator: Patients Will Wear an ID Band during Hospitalization.

Lab Section

Date/time _____

Patient name _____

Patient room #_____

or

Place lab label

Nursing Unit Section

Admit date _____

Day of week _____

Admit time _____

Admit/transfer from _____

Reason not banded; if uncertain, note possible cause(s):

_____ New admit within one hour from
_____

_____ Transfer in within one hour from
_____

_____ Band cut off; reason:_____
_____
_____

Possible causes _____
_____
_____

Fig. 9-5 Revised patient identification band alert. *Reprinted with permission from St. Vincent Medical Center Nursing Quality Assurance Department, Toledo, Ohio, © 1992.*

to rendering care or treatment. Placing a permanent identification band on a patient at the point of admission was again considered.

Several problems were identified in the study process. First, phlebotomists were not consistently initiating a card when they encountered a patient not wearing an identification band. This was discovered when the laboratory log sheets were compared with the number of pink cards compiled. Causes cited included lack of phlebotomist education, and phlebotomists forgetting to leave a card on the unit or not wanting to get someone "in trouble." In some instances a band was immediately placed on the patient and the phlebotomist did not identify this person as a patient without an ID band. In other cases, cards were submitted with incomplete or inconclusive responses. This limited the ability to draw conclusions and develop appropriate plans.

Lessons Learned

1. Begin to collaborate early in process.
2. Select a mutual goal or outcome.
3. Provide regular ongoing reinforcement.
4. Keep board members informed of progress.
5. Celebrate victories with everyone involved in the process.
6. Don't allow finger pointing to enter the process.
7. Focus on the positives, not just the negatives.

The Action Plan

The committee reconvened to develop an action plan based on the data collected. Monitoring would continue, and the card to collect and track results would be revised. Nursing and laboratory personnel were reeducated about the process for and utilization of the data collection card.

A discussion with the administrative director for the admitting department led to brainstorming about alternatives to an identification bracelet for identifying patients. Potential methods included badges, credit-card-like stamps, or stickers. Also discussed was when the identification process should occur, as well as the need to determine a profile that delineates patients at risk for misidentification. The goal of the committee is to develop alternatives that prompt care providers to check a patient's identity, not just the presence of an identification band, prior to rendering treatment.

CONCLUSION

This experience is one hospital's pursuit to ensure that each patient is wearing an identification band. The committee has realized several accomplishments. The awareness of all staff has been heightened, increases in compliance have been noted, collaborative relationships have developed, and administrative and board support is evident. Lessons learned in the process are highlighted in the box on this page. The committee also recognizes, however, that patient safety is not ensured by simply placing an identification band on their wrists. "When a task is monitored, the evaluator still could not prove patient safety was adequate, for safety was and is a much broader issue than can be measured in isolated tasks," say Katz and Green (1992, p. 28). It is of paramount importance to go beyond simply making sure that each patient is wearing an identification bracelet, and instead to ensure that a reasonable approach to identifying patients is followed prior to delivering care. The ultimate patient care goal at St. Vincent Medical Center is to establish processes that support and facilitate a health care provider's ability to validate that Mrs. Smith in room 710, bed number two, is indeed Mrs. Smith.

REFERENCES

American Hospital Association (1992): *Quality management* (Management Advisory Catalog No. 049735), Chicago, AHA.

Aitken GJ (1973): Patient identification, *Medical Trial Technique Quarterly* 19(4): 439-49.

Cohen MR (1984): Check the patient's band before giving a medication, *Nursing 84* 47(10): 70.

Duncan RP, EC Fleming, TG Gallati (1991): Implementing a continuous quality improvement program in a community hospital, *QRB* 17(4): 106-112.

Hudson T (1990): Punitive damage awards create hospital problems, *Hospitals* 64 (24): 50-53.

Joint Commission on Accreditation of Healthcare Organizations (1991): *An introduction to quality improvement in healthcare*, Oakbrook Terrace, Ill, JCAHO.

Katz J, E Green (1992): *Managing quality*, St Louis, Mosby.

Rakes GM (1991): Risk management, safety management and quality assurance, *Topics in Health Records Management* 12(2): 59-66.

Renner SW, P Howanitz (1991): College of American Pathologists Quality Assurance Services. Q-Probes. Wristband identification error reporting. Data analysis and critique, *College of American Pathologists,* (No. 91-01A): 1-13.

Wenz B, ER Burns (1991): Improvement in transfusion safety using a new blood unit and patient identification system as part of transfusion practice, *Transfusion* 31(5): 401-403.

CHAPTER TEN

PATIENT SATISFACTION

A QI Pilot Project

Sharon J. Coulter   Mary Ellen Blatt
P. Mardeen Atkins   Lori Blashford
Dawn Bailey   Sandra Shumway

The changes in health care reimbursement systems have created a more competitive health care environment (Ellis, 1989). This competition has resulted in many community hospitals providing the same specialized clinical services that once were available only in university or medical center settings. Yet the one area of competitiveness that cannot be easily duplicated is patient satisfaction. For this reason, patient satisfaction has become an important quality indicator. Institutions are devoting more time and resources towards improving their patient / client services.

Health care institutions are embracing the quality improvement methodology to effectively and efficiently identify and resolve problems in systems and clinical areas that impact the quality of care or the patient's satisfaction with services or care. Using the QI methodology for a pilot project to improve patient satisfaction scores seemed ideal in a large tertiary-care group practice.

THE ORGANIZATION

The Cleveland Clinic Foundation is a large tertiary-care group practice with a 1000-bed hospital. Annually, there are more than 30,000 admissions and 600,000 outpatient visits. The Division of Nursing has more than 2000 staff members consisting of registered nurses (RNs), licensed practical nurses (LPNs), nursing unit assistants (NUAs), patient care technicians (PCTs), and clerical staff. Patient services within the Division of Nursing are provided on 21 medical surgical units, 10 intensive care units, 4 psychiatric units, the Children's Hospital, 50 operating rooms, PACU, and an emergency department.

The chairman of the Division of Nursing has responsibility for the overall management of the division. The chairman is assisted by an administrative team composed of an assistant to the chairman, directors for five clinical departments (Medical, Surgical/Oncology, Cardio-Thoracic, Critical Care, and Operating Room), the Center for Nursing (Quality Management, Infection Control, Nursing Education, Recruitment and Retention, Staffing and Scheduling,

Nursing Operations, and Information Systems), the Department of Nursing Research, a financial manager, and a project director for case management (see Fig. 10-1).

The head nurses on the specialty-oriented units have the autonomy to implement the patient care-delivery system that would best meet the nursing care needs of their patient population. On most units, case management and managed care, both involving a multidisciplinary approach to patient care, have been identified as the most effective care-delivery systems and are in the process of being implemented.

The structure of the Division of Nursing's quality management (QM) program supports both centralized and unit-based components. Each unit has a staff nurse serving as the unit QM coordinator. This staff nurse, working in conjunction with the unit management staff, is responsible for coordinating the monitoring and evaluation activities on the unit and assisting with staff education related to quality methodologies. The unit-based activities focus on the high-volume or high-risk nursing diagnoses or nursing care functions.

The data-collection system's centralized and unit-based components are based on the 10-step monitoring and evaluation process. The centralized process involves the use of a screening questionnaire with indicators for each of the identified aspects of care. Indicators that can be applied to the majority of the patient populations are developed / revised annually with input from the unit QM coordinators (see Table 10-1). On an annual basis, the coordinators, in conjunction with the unit management staff, select from these indicators or develop indicators specific to their unit for monitoring and evaluation. Data are collected on each inpatient area continuously throughout the month. Units receive immediate patient-specific information as well as aggregated reports for the unit, department, and division on a monthly basis.

The Nursing QM Department has initiated steps to familiarize the nursing staff with the QI language. The Joint Commission on Accreditation of Healthcare Organizations (JCAHO) has converted the 10-step

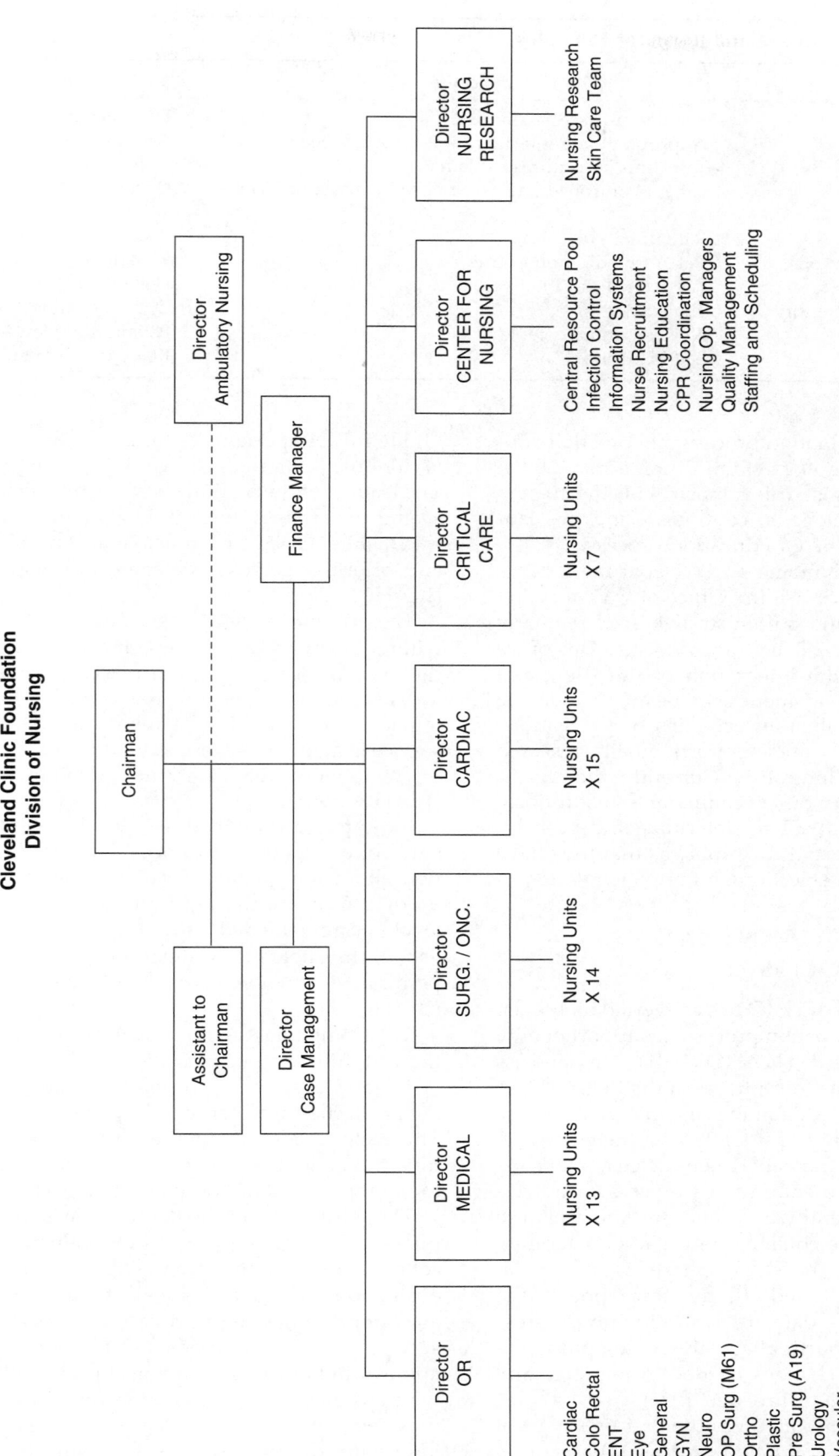

**Cleveland Clinic Foundation
Division of Nursing**

Fig. 10-1 Cleveland Clinic Foundation Division of Nursing table of organization.

TABLE 10-1 Aspects of Care and Indicator Examples

Aspect of Care	Indicator	Data Source
Nursing Process	Admission Assessment in 24 hours	Documentation
Discharge Planning	Appropriate identification of discharge needs	Documentation
Patient Education	Tests and procedures explained	Patient interview
Comfort	Patient-controlled analgesia: dose increased if level > five	Documentation
Patient Safety: Falls	Rate of falls	Risk-management system
Patient Safety: Medications	Rate of medication events	Risk-management system
Patient Safety: IV Therapy	IVs rotated at 72 hours	Documentation / observation
Patient Safety: Skin Integrity	Skin intact	Documentation / observation
Patient Satisfaction	Noise at an acceptable level	Patient interview
Respiratory Care	Self-extubation	Risk-management system

monitoring and evaluation process into one that supports the QI methodology (Joint Commission, 1991). Because the nursing staff is familiar with the 10-step process, it was decided to continue using this language throughout the QI education process.

The Division of Nursing's QM Department has a collegial relationship with the Office of QM, meeting with the director and administrative staff regularly and participating in collaborative projects. This office is responsible for the integration of the Cleveland Clinic's quality management activities, assists in the monitoring and evaluation activities of the various clinical departments, and supports quality research projects for clinical indicators. Currently, the organization is researching other, comparable institutions' efforts to implement QI to determine the best approach in order to avoid the problems that they have had to overcome in selection and implementation.

QUALITY IMPROVEMENT AND THE 10-STEP PROCESS

As stated earlier, the JCAHO has converted its 10-step monitoring and evaluation process to support quality improvement concepts (JCAHO, 1991). This process can be adapted to the four phases of the PDCA (Plan, Do, Check, Act) cycle. Planning, the first phase, is the process of identifying customers and their expectations. Then a comparison between the customer's expectations and the organization's processes and services is made to identify and then develop a plan to ensure that they are equal or similar to one another. The second phase, the Doing phase, is the one in which data are collected. In the third phase, the Checking phase, the data are analyzed and progress is monitored. The fourth phase, the Acting phase, involves making the changes needed to reinforce and continue to improve (Schroeder, 1992).

The Planning phase involves the first five steps of the monitoring and evaluation process: (1) assign responsibility, (2) delineate the scope of care or service, (3) identify important aspects of care or service, (4) identify indicators, and (5) establish thresholds. The leaders of the institution are responsible for overseeing the strategy to continuously improve quality, establishing specific responsibilities for improvement and prioritizing these strategies and responsibilities (JCAHO, 1991).

The scope of service is defined as a key function within the organization. Key functions are defined as the organization's key governance, managerial, clinical, and support functions that can have the greatest impact on the quality of patient care. The aspect of service is defined as those key functions, procedures, or treatments that warrant ongoing monitoring (JCAHO, 1991).

Indicators are defined as specific, objective measures of events or occurrences that provide information about the quality of care. These indicators are used to measure the level and improvement in the level of care delivered. After the indicators are established, thresholds for evaluation are set; they are the points at which more intensive evaluation is triggered (JCAHO, 1991).

The Doing phase of the PDCA cycle corresponds to the collection and organization of data in the monitoring and evaluation process. The methodology for data collection is determined by the teams involved. This includes identifying the sources, the data collectors, the patient population, the frequency, and how to organize the data for analysis (JCAHO, 1991).

The third phase of the PDCA cycle is the Checking phase, which is the process of evaluating the data collected against the preestablished thresholds for evaluations. The analysis seeks to determine if there are opportunities to improve the process of care or service. It is not the process of identifying the "bad apples," but one of identifying chronic problem areas with systems, staff preparation, or technology. Addressing these issues can have a greater impact on improving the process than removing the "bad apple" (JCAHO, 1991).

The Action phase, the final phase of the PDCA cycle, includes the process of taking action, the eighth step in the monitoring and evaluation process, when opportunities to improve care or service were identified. Actions should be determined by the team evaluating the aspect of care. After the actions have been implemented, a reassessment should occur to determine the impact of the actions on improving the care. The final step in this phase is reporting conclusions, recommendations, actions, and follow-up to the appropriate groups or committees within the organization (JCAHO, 1991).

PATIENT SATISFACTION: AN INDICATOR OF QUALITY

A new paradigm shift that is occurring in health care is the recognition that patient satisfaction is as important as customer service is in retail business. Despite abundant literature about successful companies valuing and responding to their customers' concerns, most health care providers and organizations have given only lip service to ensuring patients' satisfaction.

Health care professionals have retained a parochial and paternalistic definition of quality care. Until now, they have successfully argued that they, not the lay public, have the qualifications to establish appropriate standards of care. Some in health care question the value of measuring patient satisfaction, arguing that it only measures the perception of care rather than the actual medical outcome.

In these uncertain times of fierce competition, consumerism, shrinking reimbursement, managed care, and general dissatisfaction with the health care system, many providers now acknowledge that it is necessary to furnish the services that *patients* define as important. Respecting the patients' perspective is bringing about new and refreshing changes in the delivery of care.

Increased patient satisfaction has been linked not only to higher quality of care but to sound business practice. Satisfied patients are more likely to return and also are more likely, through word of mouth, to tell their friends and neighbors about their positive experiences (Press, Ganey, and Maloney, 1991). Content no longer to be the passive receivers of care, patients now expect to be decision makers in their care—to choose the standards by which that care is delivered, by whom it is delivered, when and where, and at a price acceptable to them. Unable to evaluate the quality of medical diagnoses and treatment, patients make judgments about their care based on the human interactions through which that care was given.

It has been recognized that patients value care far more when it is delivered by a thoughtful, concerned, and respectful individual rather than by someone who is abrupt and concerned only with meeting narrowly defined professional standards of care (Shapiro, 1991). A review of patients' letters of commendation or criticism shows that patients value the human interactions by which their care was delivered as much as the medical care they received. They write to say how much they appreciate our understanding of their unique needs, that we take the time to talk to them, give them explanations about procedures or routines of care, are willing to bend the rules when necessary, and make provisions for their families when appropriate. Rarely, if ever, do they write expressing how much they valued the new CAT scanner, balloon pump, or modern facilities. Modern miracles have given people faith in medical technology so that people seldom question its effectiveness, but human behavior and interactions are continually evaluated.

Each patient encounter with any employee leaves a lasting impression and defines quality for the patient. We make a choice to be rushed and curt, or to be courteous and accommodating; to make patients feel welcome, or feel like an intrusion in our already hectic day; to deliver impeccable service, or just good-enough service. Hundreds of good or bad seemingly unimportant little decisions each day have a huge impact upon a company's ability to act in congruence with the strategic message (Shapiro, 1991).

The first step toward improving patient satisfaction is identifying barriers. Patient satisfaction cannot be achieved when necessary work guidelines are unclear and policies are inefficient and too rigid. Standard operating procedures don't always support the goal of achieving patient satisfaction. People on the front lines need to make judgment calls; rules and regulations need to be bent if they get in the way of patient care and satisfaction. It takes courage to stand up for the patient instead of defending rules. "That's our policy" is not an appropriate answer to someone with a justified need. Legends are made of stories recounting how one employee singlehandedly overcame multiple obstacles to providing good care and service (Pritchett, 1989).

The presence of poorly prepared staff is another barrier to patient satisfaction. Good intentions and a pleasant manner will never compensate for a knowledge deficit. Everyone must take personal responsibility for acquiring job knowledge. "No one told me how to do that" will never satisfy patients' wants or needs. When co-workers do not meet their responsibilities, their failing places a burden upon others. Those at the forefront of patient care often know that their success in delivering superior patient care rests upon their team members and support departments.

Mediocre or flawed cultures also block patient satisfaction. The standards of performance an organization sets for itself sometimes leave a great deal to be desired. If organizational pride is lacking, it is almost impossible to consistently deliver high quality service and care. Only a genuine desire to achieve excellence can overcome such a cultural obstacle.

Leaders need to be mindful that the attitude of "good enough" does not support superior patient care. The most difficult time to deliver excellent patient care and service is when your co-workers have failed, the systems are down, and your workload is high. It is then that we ask ourselves why we bother, and that still, quiet voice within us should say, "because it's my responsibility—it's my job" (Pritchett, 1989).

Patient Satisfaction Project

Approximately three years ago, a coalition of Cleveland business leaders, hospital administrators, and physicians created a new program that was directed toward lowering cost while assuring the highest quality. That initiative became known as the Greater Cleveland Health Quality Choice Project (GCHQCP). This project comprises three measuring tools: (1) a risk-adjusted outcome tool for specific DRGs; (2) Acute Physiological and Chronic Health Evaluation (APACHE III) for the ICUs; and (3) the Nashville Consulting Group's patient satisfaction instrument, which measures all aspects of the patient's hospitalization.

Knowing that large, urban, teaching hospitals frequently fare less well in patient satisfaction surveys than smaller, rural hospitals, the Cleveland Clinic decided to focus efforts on the key issue of patient satisfaction to enhance ratings. The chairman of the Division of Nursing viewed this project as an opportunity to make patient satisfaction a priority issue. While the nursing staff plays a major role in influencing the patient's perception and satisfaction with the care he or she receives, other members of the health care team also have a role. The chief executive officer and the chairman of nursing felt strongly that the effort to improve patient satisfaction would have to be a collaborative effort. To accomplish the improved ratings, Nursing, the Division of Operations (which includes areas such as Building Services, Dietary, Admitting, and Patient Transportation), and the Department of Marketing undertook a one-year pilot program to increase patient satisfaction. Program success was to be measured by an increase in the scores of the patient satisfaction instrument. Administration viewed this pilot program as an excellent introduction to the concept of quality improvement methodology.

To achieve an increase in the scores, five principles to stimulate the necessary employee behavior change and improvements were set forth by the Board of Governors and expressed as follows:

First, we are measuring patient satisfaction data every quarter to provide timely feedback to our nurses, physicians, and other staff.

Second, we are using peer pressure to motivate actions. Each unit's data and scores are shared with the other units so that comparisons can be made.

Third, we are letting the employees closest to the patient generate the ideas. We know without employee involvement, there is no commitment to the program.

Fourth, we are using incentives and rewards to show management's interest in the project. Every quarter, the units and support departments (Patient Transportation, Billing, etc.) showing the greatest improvement are recognized in front of their directors and peers.

Fifth, we are using the success of the previous measurement period to motivate and inspire the nurses, physicians, and support departments to continue to improve.

At the conclusion of the pilot, the program may be expanded to all units.

Program Objective

The objective of the program was to continuously increase patient satisfaction on inpatient nursing units. During the pilot, a generic process was being mapped for use when the program was expanded to the remaining nursing units.

Planning Phase. The responsibility for managing the Patient Satisfaction Improvement Program was given to the Patient Satisfaction Improvement Steering Team. This team was composed of the chairman of nursing and members of the nursing administrative staff, the director of marketing, who had used the process in another institution, and administrative representatives from the Division of Operations. The team's charge was to devise the plan for the program, from unit planning to implementation hospitalwide. The steering team perceived that their responsibilities would include the following:
- Educate unit teams to the process
- Coordinate data collection through the mailing of the satisfaction survey at the specified intervals
- Respond to reasonable budget needs
- Address hospitalwide issues
- Communicate unit needs to management, clinical areas, and operational areas
- Generate internal awareness among Foundation employees
- Provide quarterly satisfaction results to units.

The steering team would work with the units in identifying unit-team members, implementing their plans for improvement, and coordinating the overall process.

First, the steering team needed an introductory education to the QI process. Because the organization had not begun its overall implementation of QI, the education was under the auspices of the director of marketing. The education was directed to providing the team with a basic understanding of the QI process particularly as it related to the patient-satisfaction pilot and the patient-satisfaction measurement tool.

The scope of service was defined as customer satisfaction, a key function performed by all employees whether their customers are patients and families or other employees. The customers during this pilot would be any hospitalized patient or family of a patient. The essential aspect of service was defined as inpatient satisfaction. The perceived benefits of meeting the patient's and family's expectations would include a more satisfying hospital experience, increased patient compliance with treatment regimens, resulting in higher quality, and improved market preference for the Cleveland Clinic Foundation through positive word-of-mouth commentary and referrals. It was hoped that the improvement would result in an increase in patient loyalty and an improved revenue stream and increased net income.

The indicators for the Patient Satisfaction Improvement Program would be obtained through the Nashville Consulting Group patient satisfaction survey tool (NCG instrument). This mail-based survey focuses on the experiences reported by discharged patients during all phases of the hospitalization. It was developed in collaboration with the Hospital Corporation of America, The Rand Corporation, the New England Medical Center, UCLA, and the Harvard Community Health Plan. It is being used in 100 acute care hospitals in the United States (Greater Cleveland Hospital Association, 1990). Patient demographic information is obtained as well as the patient's previous hospital experiences. The data can be aggregated at the unit level, department level, and the hospital level. In the Cleveland program the unit teams would be able to select from the instrument those indicators that would have the most impact on their patient population. Fig. 10-2 provides examples of questions included in the survey. The thresholds would be set above the initial survey results to provide the team with a goal.

The chairman of nursing and the director of marketing sought volunteers for participation in the pilot from among the head nurses. The chairman of nursing felt it was important that participation be voluntary, because it provided the foundation for improvement to occur, as members of the nursing unit would perceive this as their work and accomplishments. Because this program was considered a learning experience for all levels of staff, participation was limited to six pilot areas. This small number allowed an appropriate level of support for the nursing units.

The initial set of instructions given to the nursing units were:

- To identify teams from nursing and ancillary departments (transportation, dietary, and building services, etc.)

- To select the indicators from the NCG tool they believed would have the greatest impact on patient satisfaction
- To solicit ideas for improving satisfaction from all staff members
- To generate two-way communication with unit members to discuss goals, solicit ideas, build enthusiasm, and monitor results

Unit Team Responsibilities

The nursing unit teams included RNs, LPNs, NUAs, unit secretaries, and physician staff. Also included were personnel from the support departments providing direct service to each unit—dietary staff, housekeeping, and transportation. Personnel from radiology, billing, parking, facilities engineering, admissions, laboratory, and physical therapy were included to solve specific problems arising on a unit. Each unit team consisted of 10 to 14 people.

Rationale for involvement of all staff, both unit and support departments, was influenced by two considerations: employee involvement at every level enhances generation of ideas and commitment; and staff action is motivated through the peer pressure generated by the sharing of unit scores. It was important that the units develop their own strategies and implement and evaluate their effectiveness to impress upon them that they can make a difference in patient care. The steering team provided oversight of the program and served as an avenue for the units to bring systems problems to generate organizationwide problem solving.

The steering team working with each unit met initially with each unit's head nurse, a unit coordinator for the project selected by the head nurse, and the director of nursing responsible for the clinical area. This meeting consisted of a discussion of the project's goals, a review of the indicators that would be used to evaluate progress, and a review of the incentives that would be given when specific patient satisfaction goals were achieved.

Education of the unit team members regarding the objectives, goals, and benefits of the pilot was the responsibility of the head nurse and steering team members. Methods used were handouts, explanation of the process, and the NCG Survey Instrument. Information about the incentives and rewards was also shared. An effective strategy was to review with the unit team members previous scores from the initial survey and specific patient comments from unit scores. The same process was used to educate unit and support departmental staff.

Doing Phase

In the first phase of the project, the data collection would be a function of the steering team. The surveys were mailed to all patients discharged from the par-

Your Hospital Stay: The Patient's Viewpoint	Excellent	Very Good	Good	Fair	Poor	Doesn't Apply
ADMISSION: ENTERING THE HOSPITAL						
12. EFFICIENCY OF THE ADMITTING PROCEDURE: Ease of getting admitted, including the amount of time it took	1	2	3	4	5	6
YOUR DAILY CARE IN THE HOSPITAL						
15. CONSIDERATION OF YOUR NEEDS: Willingness of hospital staff to meet your needs	1	2	3	4	5	6
KEEPING YOU INFORMED						
21. INFORMING FAMILY OR FRIENDS: How well they were kept informed about your condition and needs	1	2	3	4	5	6
YOUR NURSES						
22. SKILL OF NURSES: How well things were done, like giving medicine and handling IVs	1	2	3	4	5	6
23. NURSING STAFF RESPONSE TO YOUR CALLS: How quick they were to help	1	2	3	4	5	6
YOUR DOCTOR						
27. ATTENTION OF DOCTOR TO YOUR CONDITION: How often doctors checked on you to keep track of how you were doing	1	2	3	4	5	6
OTHER HOSPITAL STAFF						
33. HOUSEKEEPING STAFF: How well they did their jobs and how they acted toward you	1	2	3	4	5	6
LIVING ARRANGEMENTS						
39. PRIVACY: Provisions for your privacy	1	2	3	4	5	6
DISCHARGE: LEAVING THE HOSPITAL						
48. DISCHARGE PROCEDURES: Time it took to be discharged from the hospital and how efficiently it was handled	1	2	3	4	5	6
BILLING BY HOSPITAL						
51. EXPLANATIONS ABOUT COSTS AND HOW TO HANDLE YOUR HOSPITAL BILLS: The completeness and accuracy of information and the willingness of hospital staff to answer your questions about finances	1	2	3	4	5	6
LOOKING BACK ON YOUR CARE						
53. HOSPITAL QUALITY: Overall quality of care and services you received from the hospital	1	2	3	4	5	6

OVERALL SATISFACTION WITH HOSPITAL	Strongly Agree	Somewhat Agree	Somewhat Disagree	Strongly Disagree
56. The care I received at the hospital was so good that I have bragged about it to family and friends.	1	2	3	4

Fig. 10-2 NCG Patient Satisfaction Instrument sample questions.

TABLE 10-2 Internal Medicine / Gerontology Unit Patient Satisfaction Survey Scores

Select Questions	Scores		
	First Wave Scores	Second Wave Scores	Third Wave Scores
How quickly nursing staff responded to your call	70	74	77
Courtesy and respect you were given by nurses	81	79	84
How well nurses communicated with you and your families	72	79	81
How well housekeeping staff did their jobs and acted toward you	73	74	74
Quality of food	50	52	54
Amount of peace and quiet	60	64	70
Nurses	76	77	80
Hospital quality	75	76	81
Admissions	65	70	72
Daily care	74	78	79
Overall satisfaction	84	86	89

ticipating units for one month during each quarter of the pilot. The Marketing department would be responsible for mailing the surveys and collating the data by unit. Prior to the beginning of the pilot, an initial survey, referred to as the "first wave," had been conducted to provide a base for setting the thresholds and to provide the units with initial data from which to develop their improvement plans.

Every quarter, units would be provided with satisfaction scores and with written comments from their patients. These data enabled staff to determine if their trial activities had affected satisfaction levels.

Checking Phase

The survey data would be analyzed at the unit level. Improvement plans were developed for the indicators with the lowest scores or for those that the team felt it could impact the most. In most cases, the plans were developed around groups of indicators that expressed a common theme. For example, if the indicators with the lowest scores were related to instruction or the quality of information provided, the plan would be focused on improving that process. Although some of the units selected the same indicators, their approach to the improvement plan and staff involvement varied.

Internal Medicine / Gerontology Unit

Reason for Volunteering. One unit participating in the Patient Satisfaction Improvement Program was a 37-bed Internal Medicine/Gerontology unit. Its members readily volunteered to take part in the project as they were eager to have a chance to have a positive affect on interdepartmental changes. Previous satisfaction-improvement efforts had been more limited in scope, able only to address areas directly within nursing's control. The new project, however, having received such tremendous support from all executive levels,

promised to make changes in support departments a reality. The nursing staff was empowered as the leaders in this endeavor. Nursing responded to an opportunity to lead a multidisciplinary team of hospital personnel and institute change across traditional departmental barriers.

Indicator Selection. To determine which areas of the hospital stay patients perceived as most problematic, the unit team reviewed the indicator scores. The team members analyzed the results of the survey generated by patients for whom they had *actually provided care.*

The areas of the care consistently cited by patients as important, or having made a difference, were identified as (1) the availability of the staff simply to spend time with the patient, (2) the attention and information provided to the patient and family at admission, (3) the provision of a quiet, restful atmosphere, (4) interaction with their physicians, and (5) the quality of the food served. A common theme that prevailed throughout the feedback was the desire for kindness and a personal touch. This concern would be the focus for the unit improvement plan (see Table 10-2).

The unit team decided to establish an overall theme for the program. They believed launching a patient satisfaction *campaign,* with a slogan and logo, would create more enthusiasm, energy, and motivation than the mere implementation of a "project." The team wanted a broad-based campaign idea that would encompass the multidisciplinary focus without emphasizing or highlighting the *nursing* unit or nursing work. The team also believed that the concepts of *kindness* and attention to *the patient as a person* were of great significance to patient satisfaction. They wanted the campaign, therefore, to reflect and emphasize kindness and the "personal approach" to patient care. With these criteria in mind, the project team developed the idea of the "S.W.A.K. Campaign": Service with Abundant Kindness.

Various plans and protocols were established to address the areas patients cited as key to a high degree of satisfaction.

1. To provide the personal touch and allow staff to spend more time with patients, an "HS Care" protocol was established. Hospital volunteers were enlisted to spend time reading to patients, writing letters, and simply dropping in to visit. An "admission" protocol was developed to ensure that patients and families were promptly welcomed to the unit, made comfortable, and provided with appropriate information to orient them to the unit and the hospital.

2. To provide sufficient information, a Patient Welcome letter was drafted, on S.W.A.K letterhead, and a hospital information booklet was made available to be included in each patient's admission packet.

3. To provide a quiet and restful atmosphere a "Quiet Time" and an "Intercom Etiquette" protocol (as shown in the box) were established.

4. To promote the physician-patient interaction, a physician information card was developed to ensure that patients would more easily know who their attending physician, senior resident, and intern staff would be.

5. To improve satisfaction with the dietary service, Dietary was able to provide a variety of herbal teas and snacks to patients and families. Other plans were enacted to improve the quality and appearance of the food. Dietary also provided the daily newspaper to the patients as an extra courtesy.

After six weeks of extensive planning and preparation, the project team was ready to mobilize the support and energy of all staff members and to implement their ideas. Gaining full staff support and commitment was clearly of great importance to the success of the campaign. Staff education and opportunity for input were considered key elements in gaining that support. Several techniques were employed to achieve this objective. In-depth in-service sessions were conducted by project team members to share the purpose, goals, and benefits of the program. Each staff member was provided with copies of the First Wave survey results, actual comments from patients on the unit, and protocols and action plans. Staff was given the opportunity to provide feedback and offer suggestions, and refinements and revisions were made in the plans and protocols, based on staff input. In addition, four former patients were interviewed, on videotape, regarding "satisfiers" during their hospital stay, as well as what areas that could improve. To see and listen to this evaluative feedback from their former patients was powerful and mean-

---

Intercom Etiquette Protocol

Purpose
To ensure considerate, professional use of the intercom for communication with patients and staff

Time
At all times when using intercom.

Responsible Person
All staff members who use the intercom.

Procedure
ALWAYS
1. Speak in a clear, courteous manner.
2. Speak in a normal tone of voice.
3. Let patient know that his or her request was heard, understood and that his or her nurse will be in within 5 minutes.
4. Make sure that both patients are addressed.
5. Follow up that patient request has been attended to via the "aid" system.
6. Be aware of patients who are hard of hearing or who have had a tracheostomy.

WHENEVER POSSIBLE
1. Address the patient by name.
2. Avoid the "all-call." If the nurse is assigned to patients in Rooms 30-38, "all call" these rooms only. If no response, then call into the other rooms.
3. Look for narcotics keys or Accu-Chek machines before calling over the intercom.

NEVER
1. Use the intercom between 11 p.m. and 7 a.m., unless it is an emergency situation.
2. Carry on a conversation over the intercom.
3. NEVER WALK PAST A RINGING CALL LIGHT!!!

---

ingful for staff members. The group was ready to make some changes!

Actual implementation of the campaign was enjoyable for staff and patients. A party was held on all shifts and weekends to kick off the campaign and to further perpetuate the staff's enthusiasm and energy. All current patients and families, and hospital departments and personnel were invited to attend. S.W.A.K. posters and balloons were placed in each patient room and around the unit; S.W.A.K. buttons were given to all staff. Inspirational and motivational bulletin boards and posters regarding patient satisfaction and the S.W.A.K. campaign were in place on the unit. The patients' videotape about their previous hospital experience was shown around-the-clock to educate and inform staff from all departments. Refreshments were served.

The kick-off sessions were exceptionally well attended. The excitement of the project team and staff was contagious. Patients truly enjoyed the activities and related well to the S.W.A.K. theme. Staff were enthusiastic and eager to implement the action plans.

The unit team began making inpatient visits immediately, to obtain early feedback. Patients had only positive comments for the staff, stating that they were enjoying the back rubs and the personal attention. Patients also remarked on how the unit was quieter, especially at night.

Acting Phase. Formal feedback came three months after the initial implementation, when the first group of patients participating in the campaign was surveyed. Much to the delight of all, the second wave scores showed significant improvement in nearly all areas (refer to Table 10-2). Patient comments also were particularly rewarding, as they cited the S.W.A.K. campaign by name. The action plans and protocols that had been successful in improving patient satisfaction were officially adopted as standard unit practice. Patient satisfaction scores in regard to several other hospital departments, however, showed no improvement or declined. These were areas that the project team decided to include in its efforts.

Survey results showed that patient transportation, laboratory medicine, parking, and billing could improve. Staff members from these departments were promptly invited to join the project team. The departments were eager to participate in the campaign.

Action plans were developed to include the new group members. Several patient transporters were consistently assigned to the unit, to ensure the timely transportation of patients to appointments, and to minimize patient waiting and delays. Several consistent phlebotomists were assigned to the unit, to establish better patient rapport and to coordinate and minimize the number of laboratory draws for each patient. Arrangements were made to provide free parking for patients and families on days of admission, discharge, surgery, and bereavement. Billing personnel agreed to contact all patients two weeks after discharge, to explain the bill, when necessary, and to address any questions or concerns. These changes were easily negotiated and accepted, as the survey data clearly demonstrated the departments' impact on patient satisfaction.

Other non-departmental-specific plans were implemented:
1. A TV/VCR was purchased by the unit, to provide free television services to patients who could not afford to purchase the service. Families also could now bring in VCR tapes for patients' enjoyment.
2. Patients were provided with a homegoing tote bag on discharge to pack their belongings. The tote bag also contains a preaddressed, stamped postcard that patients may use after discharge to let staff know their progress. About half the patients write back to the unit with positive comments as well as suggestions for further improving services.

Staff motivation and encouragement are also viewed as highly important for keeping the positive momentum of the campaign. Staff are kept abreast of changes and revisions in the campaign through a monthly S.W.A.K. newsletter. The newsletter, generated by members of the project team, is motivational as well as informational. Individual staff contributions to patient care and the satisfaction effort are recognized through the *patient-nominated* S.W.A.K. employee of the month award. Nominations are submitted to the project team for final review and selection. The chosen employee is featured in the newsletter, and the employee's picture is posted.

Overall, the group continues to look for ways to emphasize kindness and their "personal approach" to patient care.

Nephrology / Gastrointestinal Medicine Unit

Reason for Volunteering. During the six months before implementation of the hospitalwide Patient Satisfaction Improvement Program, the nephrologoy unit underwent several changes. The clinical specialty was changed to include gastrointestinal medicine. Nursing staff members found themselves caring for patients with very different needs, both physical and emotional, and working with an unfamiliar group of physicians and diagnostic procedures. Simultaneously, nursing case management was being implemented on the unit, and while this was perceived as positive, participants found adapting to the change to be stressful.

The unit management staff felt that participation in the Patient Satisfaction Improvement Program would be an outstanding opportunity to improve patient satisfaction and to involve the unit staff in learning effective methods to improve the quality of care. Patient satisfaction had decreased on the unit since the additional clinical specialty was added; therefore, the staff offered to participate in this pilot program.

Indicator Selection. The team critically reviewed the first wave survey results to compare this unit with the other units involved in the pilot and to identify the specific areas for improvement. After discussion and review of the survey results, it was decided to focus on two areas: (1) implementing basic comfort and caring strategies for patients; and (2) involving all staff members on the unit along with the staff from the ancillary departments as members of the team (see Table 10-3). The improvement plan focused on the indicators needing the most improvement and on those that nursing could affect with a positive outcome on patient comfort, efficiency, ease of implementation, and cost effectiveness.

A logo with the slogan "We Care for You" was developed. It was displayed on lapel buttons, on a unit introductory brochure given to every patient on

TABLE 10-3 Nephrology / Gastroenterology Unit Patient Satisfaction Survey Scores

	Scores		
Select Questions	**First Wave Scores**	**Second Wave Scores**	**Third Wave Scores**
How quick nursing staff responded to your call	64	73	65
Courtesy and respect you were given by nurses	73	80	77
How well nurses communicated with patients and families	70	76	71
How well housekeeping staff did their jobs and acted toward you	60	78	65
Overall, how good the food tasted; adequacy of serving temperature and variety available	44	55	41
How well transportation staff did their jobs and acted toward you	65	76	73
Amount of peace and quiet	58	68	61
Nurses	71	78	70
Physicians	77	81	73
Hospital quality	71	77	75
Overall	87	88	83

admission, and on a banner made for the unit hallway. The team then brainstormed and developed strategies that would reflect the "caring" theme. Cost effectiveness and efficiency were paramount considerations. The plan included actions to:

1. Decrease the response time to call lights
2. Provide back rubs to each patient at bedtime
3. Provide daily newspapers for each patient; feeling isolated from what was happening in the world was a frequent patient comment.
4. Promote a quiet and restful atmosphere; the intercom was not to be used from 11 pm to 7 am. Signs were posted in the report and conference rooms reminding staff that they were in a quiet zone once they departed from these employee areas.

Responsibility for the education of the staff members to the Patient Satisfaction Improvement Program was assumed by the unit team. The education process involved explanation of the program and results of the pilot project and unit survey. A copy of the written plan was given to each staff member. Through this process the unit team demonstrated ownership for the plan to peers.

A kick-off celebration involved all staff on the unit, staff from other departments, and patients and their families, all proudly wearing the neon pink logo buttons. The staff's enthusiasm for and diligence at making the project a success were evident.

One of the head nurse's personal goals for the unit was to demonstrate to staff that if patient comfort needs were met, the number of unexpected calls would decrease. This result would be accomplished through frequent checking with each patient to see if he or she needed anything, and in the evening, offering a backrub to each patient. The impact would be

fewer unanticipated interruptions and less noise on the unit from the intercom. Although there was initial resistance to this idea, after one week, all staff on the unit recognized something had changed. The unit was quieter and more organized, and staff was actually responding to fewer unanticipated patient requests because the patients felt they knew that "they would be coming to check on me or to give me a backrub." One nurse related her experience with a patient transferred from another hospital. Soon after his mid-evening arrival he was offered a backrub. With total surprise he responded that he hadn't been there long enough to have "earned" a backrub.

This unit is a teaching unit for the internal medicine residency program, so physician involvement was a major component of the plan. The head nurse and nursing case managers participate in their monthly orientation at the beginning of each new rotation. The Patient Satisfaction Improvement Program is described during this orientation, and interns and residents are expected to participate and to wear the unit logo button. Survey results and incentives are shared with the residents.

Acting Phase. Comparison of the scores of the first wave and the second wave surveys was done during a team meeting and resulted in minor additions to the plan. Positive comments from individual survey responses were reviewed and shared with the unit staff. The improvement plan was not changed; scores had improved as shown in Table 10-3. The analysis of the third wave of scores demonstrated a decrease from the second wave, but were still improved over the first wave scores. Revisions in the improvement plan were made to address the score decreases.

TABLE 10-4 Cardiology Stepdown Unit Patient Satisfaction Survey Scores

Select Questions	Scores		
	First Wave Scores	Second Wave Scores	Third Wave Scores
How quick nursing staff responded to your call	77	79	77
Courtesy and respect you were given by nurses	82	85	84
Information provided by nurses	80	82	79
Information provided by physicians	83	82	80
Discharge instructions	75	71	73
How well nurses communicated with patients and families	76	80	78
How well housekeeping staff did their jobs and acted toward you	74	77	73
How well transportation staff did their jobs and acted toward you	76	75	73
Overall, how good the food tasted; adequacy of serving temperature and variety available	53	58	53
Amount of peace and quiet	70	71	67
Nurses	80	83	80
Hospital quality	79	83	81
Overall satisfaction	87	88	84

The area of peace and quiet demonstrated a decrease in score and an increase in the number of negative patient comments. This regression was the focus of the changes in the improvement plan. The primary action was the elimination of the use of the intercom system expected during emergency situations. Patient lights would be answered in person within two minutes. This strategy was reluctantly accepted by staff, which believed that workload would increase. Two weeks after implementation the staff's perception had changed: there was a decrease in the noise level and there were fewer patient calls with requests.

An additional measure to increase the patient satisfaction scores is currently under way. The clinical instructor and the Department of Nursing Education will be conducting "people awareness" classes for all the staff. The idea is to increase the staff's understanding of patients' expectations and identify approaches for successfully meeting them. The impact of the classes will not be realized until the fourth wave of scores.

Staff members remain enthusiastic about the program and the gains they have made. They are confident that the latest changes in the improvement plan will improve the level of patient satisfaction.

Cardiology Stepdown Unit

Reason for Volunteering. The 36-bed cardiology stepdown unit volunteered for the Patient Satisfaction Improvement Program for two reasons. First, the unit wanted to be a part of the future, one that realizes that patients' expectations are rising and that patients *demand* high-quality care. Second, the unit accepted this program as a challenge to improve its capacity to provide high-quality care.

Indicator Selection. The team reviewed the results of the initial NCG survey and selected the indicators that it could primarily affect (see Table 10-4). The team then brainstormed ways to address these indicators. These ideas as well as the suggestions solicited from the staff were recorded and were considered in the improvement plan development.

In deciding on a theme, the team considered several factors. The first was the availability of materials needed to make the idea work. Would the materials be easy to obtain? The second was the practicality of the idea. Would it impact the patient enough to increase his or her satisfaction level? The third was to consider the group's cooperation and participation in the program. Would the members of the unit be willing to carry out a specific action or task for an indefinite period of time? And the fourth factor was cost effectiveness. Would the continual implementation of these ideas be too costly for the unit's budget? With these things in mind, the head nurse and the patient satisfaction coordinator formulated a plan that included elements for staff education changes in staff responsibilities and new services. Education of the staff was the next step.

The education of the unit staff was the responsibility of the coordinator and the head nurse. After the improvement plan was developed, staff meetings were held for all unit staff and support department personnel involved. At these meetings, the patient satisfaction coordinator and head nurse provided an overview of the Patient Satisfaction Improvement Program and shared the unit's patient satisfaction plan, purpose, and rationale.

The plan included the following elements:
1. To decrease the lack of familiarity with the process for addressing problems or questions, a memory

board (a dry marker board) displaying the name and phone extension of the patient's nurse and NUA for each shift, head nurse, dietitian, and housekeeping personnel was proposed for each room. Nurses were responsible for identifying themselves upon meeting their patients for the first time and for updating the board.

2. To address dietary concerns, a "Courtesy Cart" that included warm, wet wash cloths, coffee, tea, juices, and crackers was implemented. Before breakfast and in the evening, the cart was offered to patients, except those with dietary restrictions. The NUAs were responsible for clearing overbed tables for meal trays and offering wet wash cloths before all meals.

3. To improve the response time to patient calls, answering patient call lights within one to two minutes was a goal.

4. To provide a quiet and restful atmosphere, the staff was shown a video tape on noise reduction. Staff members were encouraged to give shift reports away from the nurses' station and away from patient rooms.

5. To keep patients informed about news of the world, newspapers were made available on the unit. A set number of newspapers was purchased each day.

The length of stay on this unit can range from 48 hours to 2 weeks. Most patients require extensive education for lifestyle changes related to their cardiac condition. To better organize the educational information and provide the patients with more information about the Cleveland Clinic Foundation and the unit, a brochure and folder were developed by the coordinator and head nurse. In the folder, patients find educational booklets, a unit brochure, puzzles, financial information about the hospital, the head nurse's professional card, and a pencil with the unit logo.

Acting Phase: Second Wave. The second wave of data collection came shortly after the plan was chosen and the staff was educated, but before most of the ideas were implemented. Yet the results (see Table 10-4) showed an increase in the ratings from the initial measurement. A possible reason for the increased scores was that the unit had, for the most part, "bought into" the program. Staff members might have been more conscious of their actions and their dealings with patients, thus affecting the patient satisfaction levels. Another possible reason was that the few ideas already implemented had been successful. Patients commented that the courtesy cart and warm cloths were "nice," but the newspapers seemed to be the bigger hit with the patients.

The relationship between the nursing staff and the dietary workers improved. The dietary workers stated that having a cleared bedside table on which to place meal trays helped them to do their job more efficiently.

The memory boards were well received by the patients. The patients appreciated having a reference when something was needed. The full impact of this action will not be known until the fourth wave data collection.

The third wave data scores also showed that noise continued to be a major complaint. The patient satisfaction coordinator interviewed patients and determined that the change of shift and the mid-morning hours were the times of most concern. The action plan was revised to focus resources to this area of concern.

Acting Phase: Steering Team

The steering team organized quarterly joint meetings, at which time the units would report the actions taken and their analysis of the impact of those actions on the patient satisfaction scores. These meetings also served as a forum to discuss problems experienced on the unit that were felt to be common to other units. The steering team was responsible for communicating these issues to the executive groups that could affect systems.

Several common issues have been identified, with two being actively addressed by the team currently and others being deferred to permit plans for revisions in departments to be fully implemented. For example, implementation of a new billing system has just been completed; the system should result in improved satisfaction with the billing process. The two issues being addressed by the team are:

1. The inability to have patient television service activated after 5 pm. This information was presented to the administrative committees, and arrangements were made for 24-hour television service throughout the hospital.

2. The noise on the units, whether from staff, visitors, or equipment. This is currently being addressed by the steering team. Additional data will be collected to identify the geographical problem areas and the problem times of day, and an action plan will be developed.

The steering team also sponsors periodic luncheon meetings to recognize achievements of the units and support departments and to provide a forum for discussion and networking. This is the time when unit head nurses, unit coordinators and directors of nursing responsible for a unit, and directors of the support departments are recognized for achieving significant improvements in satisfaction scores.

CONCLUSION

The pilot for the Patient Satisfaction Improvement Program has been a successful introduction to the concept of quality improvement. Use of a unit approach with central coordination has had many benefits. The nursing units have taken ownership of the program and have been assertive in pursuing the ideas that improve the scores. The nursing units involved in the program have each developed their own personality for approaching patient satisfaction. They have also gained a certain status among the other units. The program is in the third of the four measurement phases, and other units are requesting to be the first to participate in the program expansion. The units currently involved in the program will serve as mentors for additional units. They should be able to help the other units avoid the problems they encountered and provide them with improvement plans that worked. The expansion units also will be at an advantage because two of the issues expressed by patients as areas for improvement have been addressed.

The steering team's oversight function for coordination and for providing a forum for the discussion of common areas of concern has tied the program together. The team works closely with a unit to ensure the unit has the resources to pursue its intended actions. The team also informs the unit when its actions are outside budget limitations. The team has addressed the areas of concern that cross departments. The television-service issue was a longstanding problem that has finally been resolved. It is hoped the same will occur with the noise-level issue.

Unit scores for patient satisfaction have demonstrated a continued improvement in most areas. The units are still distinguishing between the actions that did and did not work. The action plans are being revised and implemented to achieve the desired results. The next task of the steering team will be to identify specific actions that influence patient satisfaction on all units to have available resources for the remaining inpatient units.

The lessons learned during this pilot are related to planning and education. Because of the feeling of urgency to begin the project, the education process for QI concepts and the overall and unit-level planning were abbreviated. This resulted in misunderstandings of what was to be accomplished. Most of the unit teams believed that their initial improvement plans should have resulted in a marked improvement in the second wave scores. They had missed the idea of continuous improvement. Much time was spent by the steering team with the unit teams to review the program objectives. Over the past year all managers have been encouraged to become familiar with QI terminology, which will be beneficial for the program expansion. A longer education and planning phase will be the standard as the program is expanded.

Another point realized was that there were more issues common to all units than at first realized. These issues are being addressed by the steering team and are being implemented on all units. The nursing units participating in the program can then focus on actions that would be oriented more toward the patient population, outcomes, and treatment-specific issues, or those that present opportunities for the staff to make behavior modifications related to customer service.

The process that was followed reinforces what was earlier stated: patients do not respond to amenities in the absence of human interactions that convey caring, understanding, and the realization that they are part of the treatment-planning process.

REFERENCES

Albrecht K, R Zemke (1985): *Service America!*, Homewood, Ill, Dow Jones-Irwin.

Crosby P B (1984): *Quality without tears*, New York, Penguin Books, USA.

Joint Commission on Accreditation of Healthcare Organizations (1991): *Transitions: from QA to CQI: using CQI approaches to monitor, evaluate, and improve quality*, Oakbrook Terrace, Ill, Joint Commission on Accreditation of Healthcare Organizations.

Pritchett P (1989): *Service excellence!* Dallas, Pritchett Publishing Company.

Press I, R Ganey, M Maloney (1991): Satisfied patients can spell financial well-being, *Health Care Financial Management* 45(2): 34-6, 38, 40-2.

Schroeder P (1992): Using the PDCA cycle, *Nursing Quality Connection* 2(1).

Shapiro E C (1991): *How corporate truths become competitive traps*, New York, John Wiley & Sons.

CHAPTER ELEVEN

CUTTING THE BLAME ROPE IN THE TRANSFER TUG OF WAR

A QI Project Team Approach

Janet E. Yskes
Cheryl Czech
Pete Knox

BELLIN HOSPITAL AND ITS QI STRUCTURE

Bellin Hospital of Green Bay serves as the regional medical center for northeast Wisconsin and Michigan's Upper Peninsula. It was established in 1907 by Dr. Julius J. Bellin, whose entrepreneurial spirit has guided Bellin Hospital's unique health care vision since that time.

Today, Bellin is an acute care 180-bed, multispecialty hospital, employing more than 1600 people. In addition to being a comprehensive cardiac center, Bellin also specializes in mental health and addictive services, as well as reference laboratory, surgery, pediatrics, obstetrics, general medicine, orthopedics, and neurology services.

The hospital, the 87-bed Bellin Psychiatric Center, and the Bellin College of Nursing constitute the total family of services offered by the nonprofit organization Northeast Wisconsin Health Care, Inc.

Continuing with a long history of being a leader in health care change and innovation, Bellin introduced the concepts and principles of total quality management (TQM) in 1988. Realizing the need for changes in the health care system in which it operated, Bellin embraced total quality management as a tool to improve overall performance at every level. Creating the culture in which this can occur has been and will continue to be the primary focus of quality efforts at Bellin.

Efforts related to total quality management at Bellin revolve around the three central values of the organization: superior service, continuous improvement, and people (Fig. 11-1). Understanding the core values has provided a foundation for specific action in each of the three areas to ensure the optimization of customer value, work processes and systems, and people. The specific activities for each of the three value areas are defined below:

Superior Service
1. Development of ongoing feedback and measurement systems
2. Policy deployment
3. Quality function deployment
4. Innovation

Continuous Improvement
1. Supplier partnerships
2. Quality in daily work
3. Design and improvement teams
4. Benchmarking

People
1. Clear roles and expectations
2. Effective learning systems
3. Recognition and reward systems
4. Supportive management systems

Each of the activities is carried to an action level through the quality planning process. The actions relate to both short-term and long-term initiatives that will drive the organization toward its overall vision.

IMPROVEMENT TEAM STORY

What follows is the story from an improvement team at Bellin.

The Rope

Silently, a struggle was unfolding. Amid the conflict ran a rope so heavy with blame no one person or nursing unit was able to pull the load any longer. The players who were grasping to this invisible tug-of-war rope included nurses from the Critical Care Unit (CCU), the Intermediate Care Unit (IMCU), and the Cardiac Floor (Two South). Over time, the blame rope had emerged because there was no smooth, consistent process for transferring patients between the units. The inconsistencies caused transfers to occur at inappropriate times of the day, resulting in secondary problems adding weight to the already burdened blame rope. Recognizing this struggle as being inconsistent with Bellin Hospital's basic value of continually striving for quality improvement made it easy to choose this process as a focus for improvement. It was clear the blame rope needed to be severed and

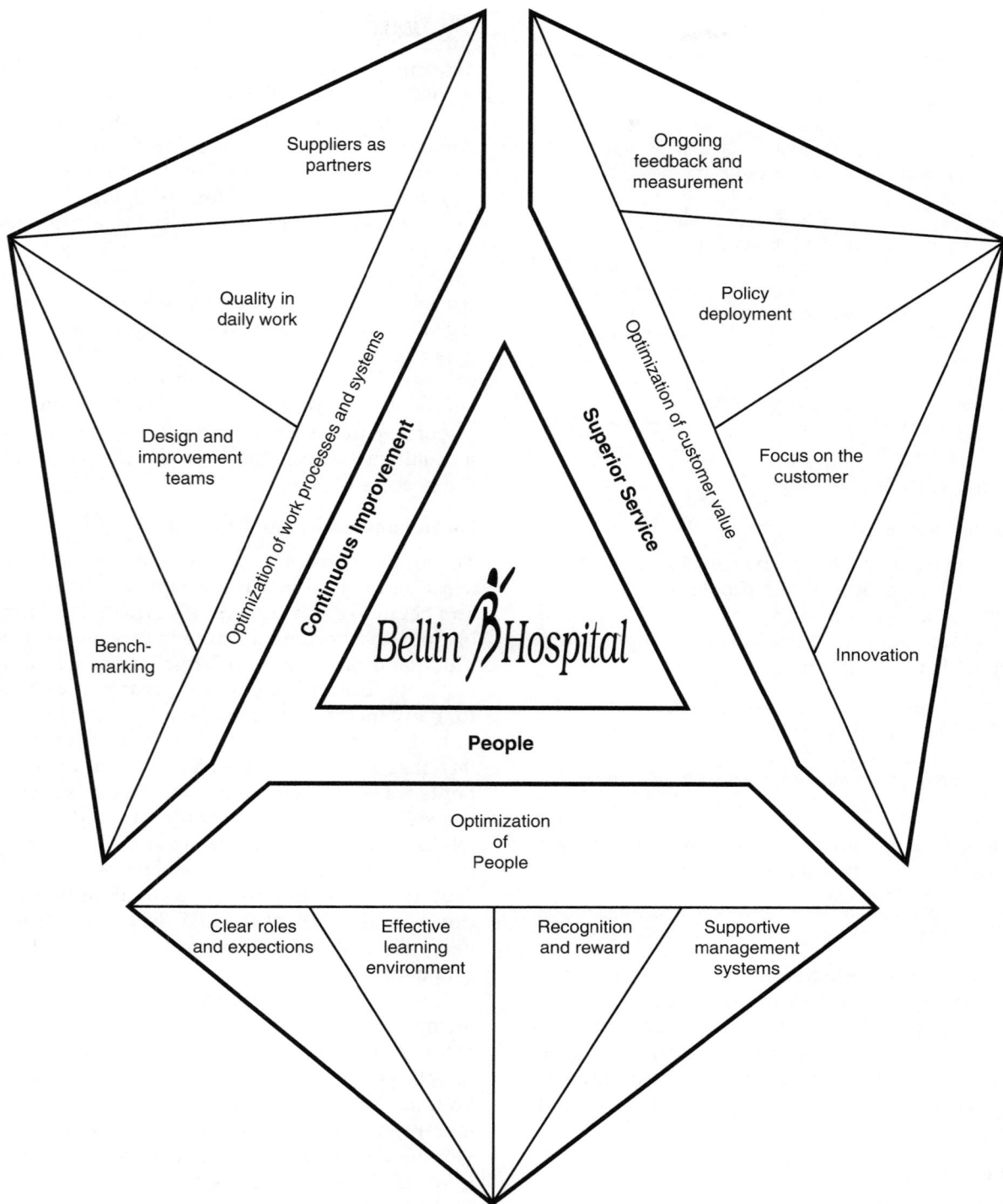

Fig. 11-1 Bellin total quality model.

shredded, allowing the negative, pulling energies to be converted into positive, problem-solving energies. Thus the journey began in the destruction of the strong, unyielding rope woven of blame.

The Problem-Solving Process

The Bellin VALUE PDCA+ model would be the tool used to cut the blame rope. Bellin employees devel-

oped this tool to facilitate quality improvement activities throughout the institution. VALUE PDCA+ is an acronym (see the box on p. 118) that describes the steps in the problem-solving process at Bellin. It uses a scientific approach and requires statistical thinking. What follows is a step-by-step description of how the process progressed, including the achievements and hardships faced along the way.

```
┌─────────────────────────────────────────┐
│         Value PDCA + Model                │
├─────────────────────────────────────────┤
│ Verify a problem exists.                  │
│ Assemble a team.                          │
│ Locate and isolate the problem.           │
│ Understand the cause of variation.        │
│ Establish the real causes of the problem. │
│ Plan—Plan the change.                     │
│ Do—Implement the change on a pilot basis. │
│ Check—Determine if it met intended need.  │
│ Act—Determine the effectiveness of the    │
│    change and make appropriate decisions; │
│    implement fully and develop a          │
│    measurement to hold the gain; repeat   │
│    the cycle.                             │
│ +—Recognize and celebrate.                │
├─────────────────────────────────────────┤
│ Courtesy Bellin Hospital. Copyright 1992. │
└─────────────────────────────────────────┘
```

STEPS IN THE PROCESS

Verify a Problem Exists

It was clear from the heavy burden of blame being carried by all three units that a problem existed. Clarifying the problem in a written statement would allow all to understand and provide a starting point for resolution. This statement read:

The current process of transferring patients from CCU and IMCU to Two South is occurring at inappropriate times of the day, which causes staffing issues, backlog of patients, delays in patient transfers, staff frustration, stress, and overtime.

The action to be taken to combat this problem was then clarified in the mission statement, which read:

Develop a process to facilitate timely and efficient patient transfers between the units.

At times the team working on the issue would get off track and have to refer back to the mission statement to stay focused. Hence, the mission statement was vitally important because it prevented the team from losing precious time and energy trying to solve ostensibly related, but actually separate and nonurgent, problems.

Assemble a Team

The destruction of the blame rope began with the development of a team whose mission was to devise an efficient process for transferring patients from unit to unit. Persons were selected to be team members based on their working proximity to the process. No one was coerced to participate; instead, persons were asked to volunteer their individual expertise. It was vitally important to select team members close to the problem because these individuals understood the process and were the best candidates to aid in its improvement. This team was composed of charge and staff nurses from each area. There were four nurses from Two South, two nurses from CCU, and two nurses from IMCU. The team also included a facilitator whose role was vital in leading the team through the quality improvement journey. Two additional members were incorporated into the team midway through the process. One represented Transport and the other was from Housekeeping. The multidisciplinary aspect proved to be quite advantageous as the process progressed. And although managers were not actively involved on the team, their role was crucial to the success of the mission. The team had the support from each unit manager to make any necessary changes resulting from the problem-solving process. The managers' absence from team meetings, yet their ever present support, led team members on a journey that started with blame and ended with mutual trust and respect for the people involved in the process.

Locate and Isolate the Problem

The initial battle the project team would face was learning to lay down the weapons of condemnation and begin to cultivate a spirit of trust. Over time, lack of trust had become a learned response between the units, and breaking down this barrier was a difficult task. The concept of people versus process was new to many members of the team. Much time was spent during the initial meeting sessions emphasizing the fact that the current problem with transferring patients was not originating from the people behind the transfer, people who inherently wanted to do a good job, but rather from the process itself. Even with repeated emphasis on this people-versus-process concept, it was not until the phase of identifying the true causes of the patient transfer delays that team members fully realized the absurdity in calling it a people problem.

Locating the problem areas in the process of transferring patients could only be fully identified through a flowchart (Fig. 11-2). The flowchart revealed several directional branches that led to many, unneeded, built-in delays and rework in the process. A delay loop representing a particularly problematic area was identified in the flow diagram. This would be the area to which the team would give particular attention and focus on improving.

It was noted by simply looking at the flow diagram that the transfer process was overly complex. There were too many ways of doing the same thing: transfer a patient from one unit to the next. Some ways were more efficient at carrying out the process than others. The team needed to find the most efficient way of transferring a patient and make it universal for all.

Another problem identified was inefficient use of resources. RNs were doing nonnursing activities—for example, spending up to 20 minutes looking for a

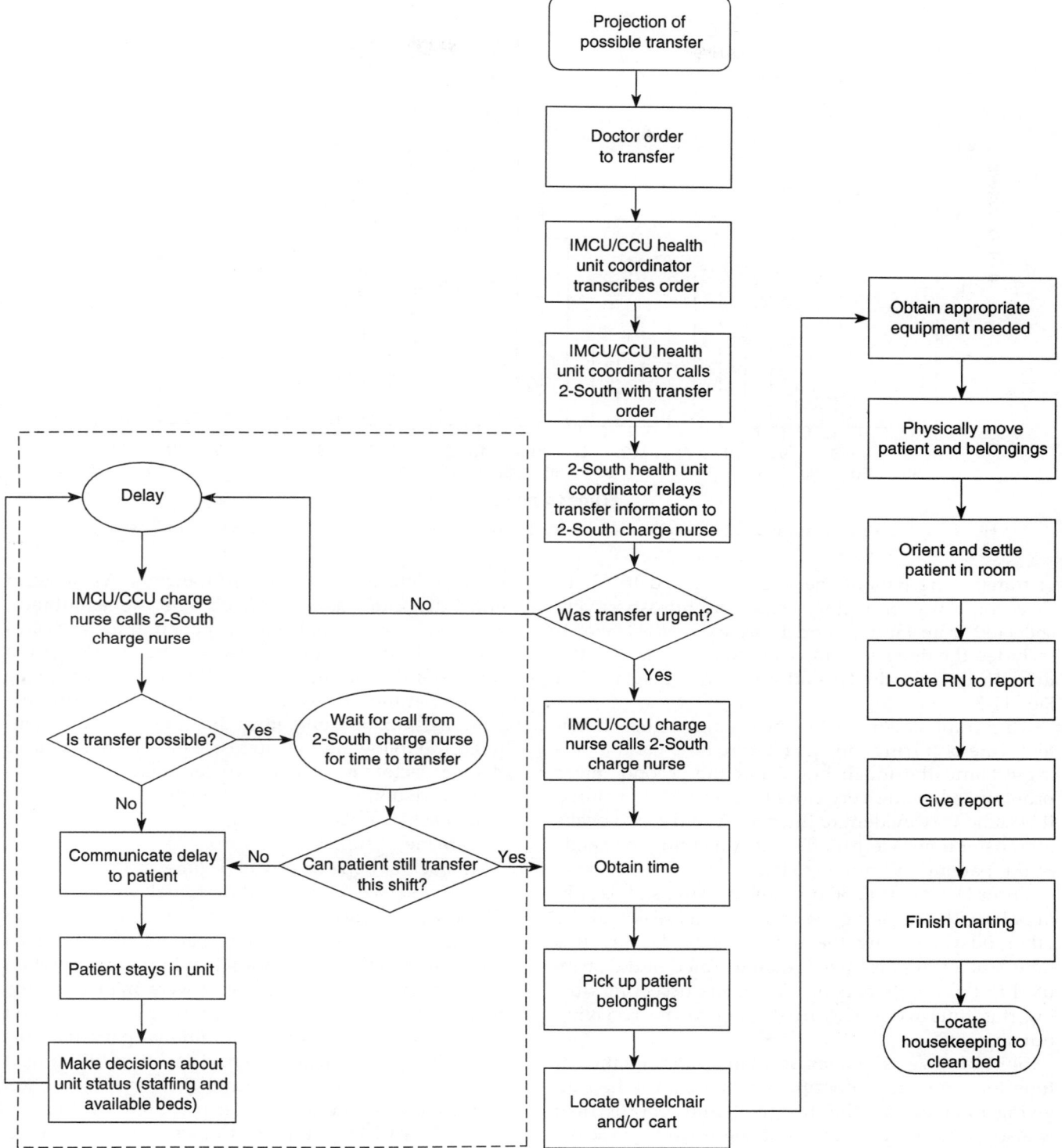

Fig. 11-2 Old process of transferring patients from CCU/IMCU to Two South. The area delineated with the dotted line represents the delay loop the team focused on for improvements.

wheelchair or cart to transfer a patient. This activity could be delegated to nonnursing personnel, allowing the nurse to carry out assigned activities.

All identifiable problems eventually led to postponed transfers. Each delayed transfer, one might say, represented another brick in a wall of blame that would grow so high that effective communication between the units was almost an impossibility.

After reviewing the flow diagram, the team needed to better understand how the current process

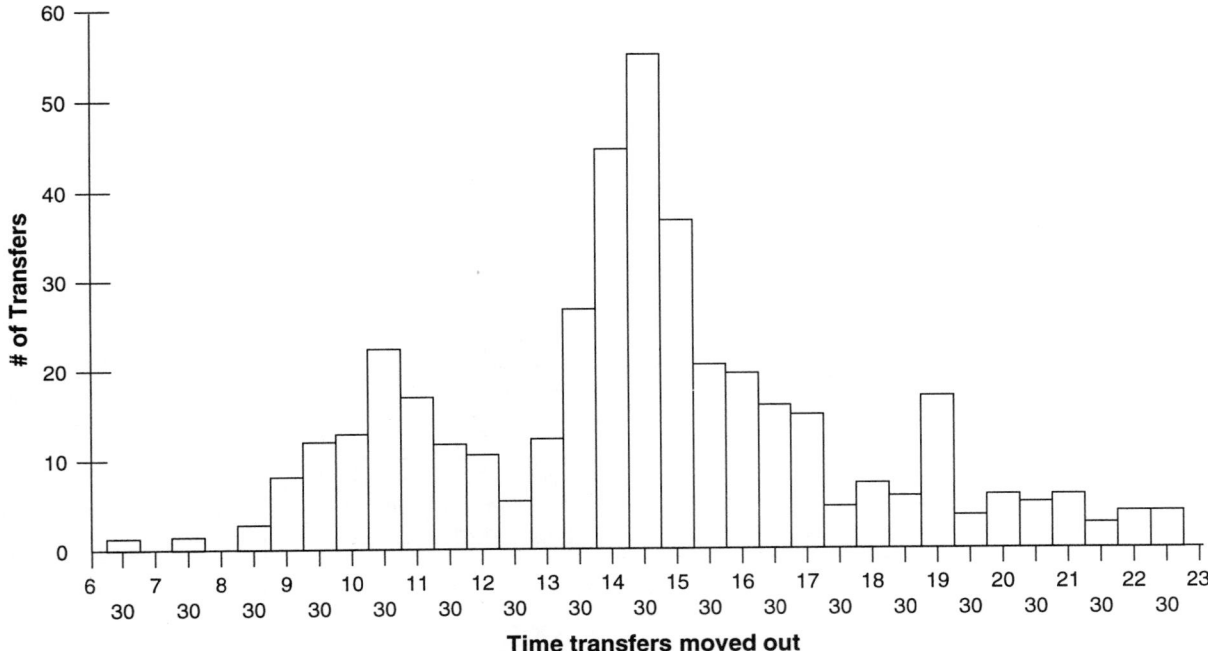

Fig. 11-3 CCU/IMCU transfers to Two South January 1 through February 28, 1990 (59 days, 414 transfers).

of transferring patients between CCU and IMCU to Two South was occurring. Data were retrospectively collected from January and February of 1990, which included the times patients were transferred from the units to Two South. This information is displayed in Fig. 11-3.

This graph illustrates two peaks in the times transfers were occurring, one just before lunch and tapering off into the lunch hour, and the second, more pronounced, being very close to the change of shifts. It became very evident to the team that the two peaks in transfer times were inefficient in meeting the needs of the patient and nursing staff.

From 11 a.m. to 12:30 p.m. the nursing staff is split in half, with one half gone on its lunch break and the other busy covering the unit's needs. During this time lunch trays also need to be warmed and distributed to the floor's patients. Transfers occurring during this time were very frustrating to the receiving nursing staff.

Shift change is the most chaotic and inefficient time for a transfer to occur. Nursing staff is tied up giving and receiving the change-of-shift report. There is also increased congestion at the nursing desk because of the presence of the oncoming shift. A patient transferred during this time frequently wasn't seen until the staff was out of report.

Understand the Cause of Variation

The flow diagram and data collection now gave the team a better understanding of the process and what was actually occurring. The next step was to determine why delays were occurring, leading to the focus

on the inefficient times of most transfers. A cause and effect diagram was constructed, and the team brainstormed reasons that led to the patient transfer delays (Fig. 11-4). It was at this time that the team began to understand that the focus of blame needed to be pointed at the process and not at the staff. After examining the cause and effect diagram, the team identified the following four items, which were felt to be the key factors in patient transfer delays:

1. Variation in number of transfers
2. Lack of RNs
3. Time of transfer
4. Lack of beds or private rooms

The first two factors leading to delays are related. There was no mechanism in place to predict or plan for the transfers that would be made floor status each day. The transfers were not taken into account when staffing levels and assignments were made on Two South, and as a result there frequently weren't enough RNs to take on the additional patients. This meant that the transfers were delayed until the next shift, or sometimes even until the next day, when staffing levels would be better prepared for them.

The third factor, time of transfer, was uncovered when the team again reviewed the times that transfers had been occurring. There weren't any designated times for patient transfers to occur. Two South was notified when a patient was made floor status. When a bed and RN became available to receive the patient, Two South would then notify the transferring unit. The time span could be as short as minutes to as long as hours. The patient could then transfer to Two South any time after that. Sometimes the trans-

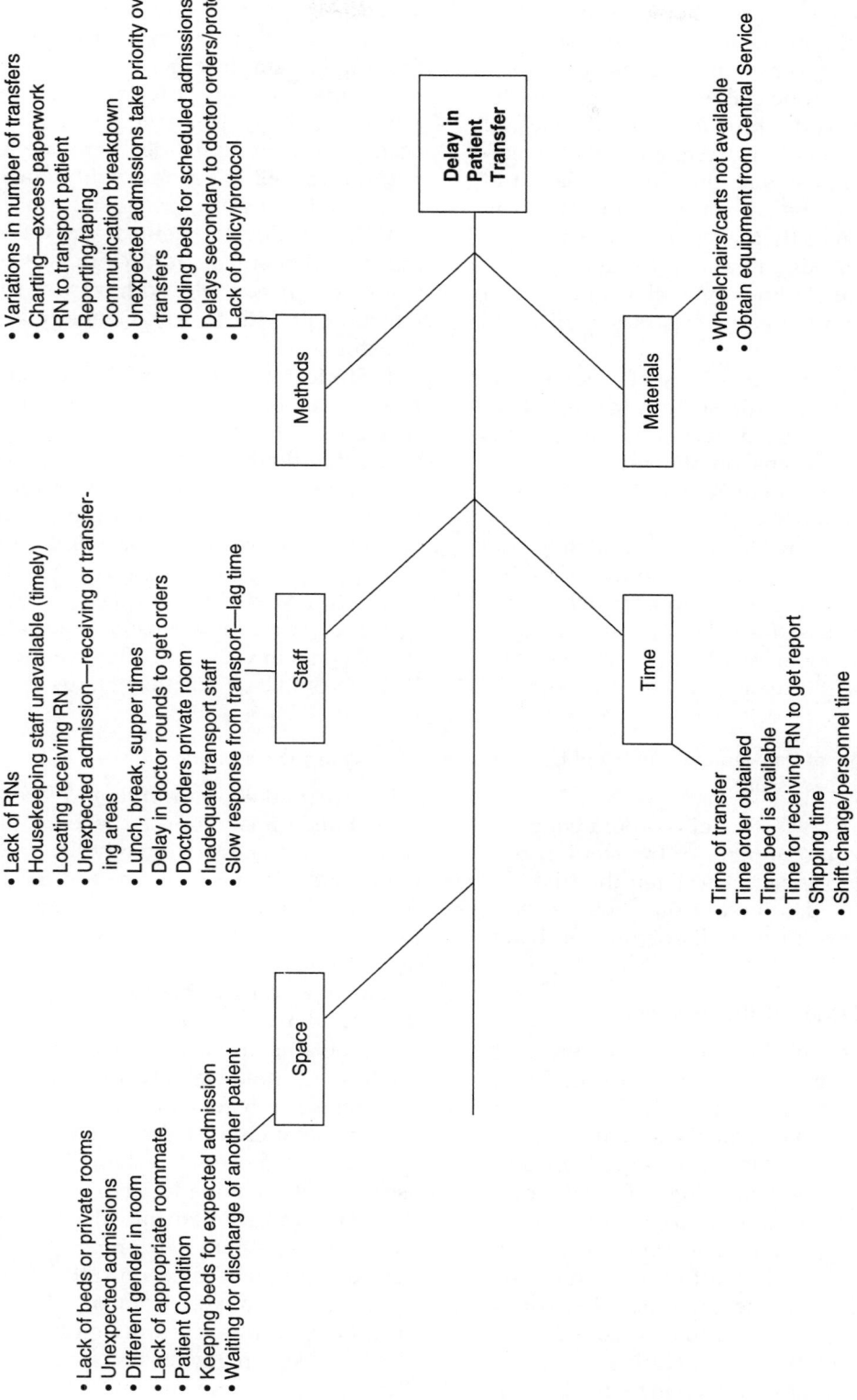

Fig. 11-4 Cause and effect diagram.

fer would not occur until after the next shift began. The receiving RN and the patient had no way of planning their day, not knowing when the transfer was going to occur. Lack of communication played a large role in this factor. A phone call was requested by the receiving unit prior to the transfer to notify the RN that the patient would be transferred shortly thereafter. In the midst of a busy day, this phone call would often be forgotten by the transferring unit. If a call was placed, many times there were other unexpected things that the RN needed to attend to, delaying the transfer. These untimely and somewhat unexpected transfers added to the already frustrating dilemma that was evolving.

The last factor, lack of beds or private rooms, was something the team was unable to address. There will always be times when there aren't enough beds or requested private rooms on the receiving floor, with the result of the patient remaining in the unit until one becomes available.

Recently Two South underwent remodeling and increased its number of private rooms. This has served to further reduce patient transfer delays that were caused by the need for more private rooms.

In reviewing the key areas identified in the cause and effect diagram, the team uncovered a potential theory:

Predictability in time of transfer and number of transfers will improve staff and bed issues.

The theory contains two elements—predicting the time of transfer and the number of transfers. If both of these could be addressed, it was felt that the staff and bed weaknesses identified in the problem statement would improve, further dissolving the blame rope.

Establish the Real Causes of the Problem

The first step to identify the real cause of the problem was to determine the best time to transfer patients from unit to unit. These times would take into account the needs of the patients and the nursing staff. Two time frames were mutually agreed upon by the three units as best meeting the needs of all those involved. The two time frames were 9:30 a.m. to 10:30 a.m. and 1 p.m. to 2:30 p.m. These were referred to as morning and afternoon time slots. These were identified as times in which the work of the nursing staff and the schedules of the patients would be least interrupted or disturbed. The time slots avoided meal times and change of shift. By preparing for the designated time slots, the RNs involved could be able to better plan their activities, knowing approximately when a patient would be transferred. Likewise, the patient and the family had a more definitive idea of when the patient would be moved to a different bed.

In reviewing the data that had already been collected from January and February of 1990, the team transposed the newly made transfer time slots onto the original graph to get a better idea of whether or not transfers were occurring during appropriate times (Fig. 11-5). There were many transfers that had occurred outside the "ideal" transfer time slots. This pattern was felt to be inefficient in meeting the needs of the patients and nursing staff.

With the development of the transfer time slots, the first element of the theory was addressed. The team now needed to address the second element, which dealt with the predictability in the number of transfers.

Historical data that had been collected showed a relationship between transfers out of CCU and IMCU and the units' respective censuses. The team also noted that there was a consistent pattern of transfers that occurred during each day of the week and that this pattern correlated with the census in the units. From this information a formula for predicting transfers to Two South was devised (Table 11-1). For example, on Monday morning Two South can, based on Sunday evening's census, predict that 5 percent of the patients in CCU and 20 percent of the patients in IMCU would be made floor status and would transfer that day.

Plan—Plan the Change

With the prediction formula in place, along with the designated transfer times, the team was now ready to plan a new process to remedy the problem. The team made a flowchart of a process for patient transfer from CCU and IMCU to Two South utilizing the two new additions: transfer time slots and the predictability formula (Fig. 11-6).

The new transfer process originates at 7 p.m. each day. At that time the PM charge nurse from Two South obtains the current CCU and IMCU census and applies the predictability formula to determine the number of transfers to expect the next day. These predicted patients are then figured into staffing levels for the next morning. When Two South's morning assignments are made, the predicted transfers for that day are included into the RN's normal patient load. Transfers are no longer dealt with as unexpected patients who add further stress to the RN.

The charge nurses from the three units involved meet every day at 8:30 a.m. to discuss which patients are most likely ready for transfer. The number of predicted transfers and the time slots that are most appropriate are also discussed, along with any special circumstances or needs that may affect that day. This meeting has served to keep the lines of communication open among the units and has reinforced the interdepartmental teamwork and growth that had developed.

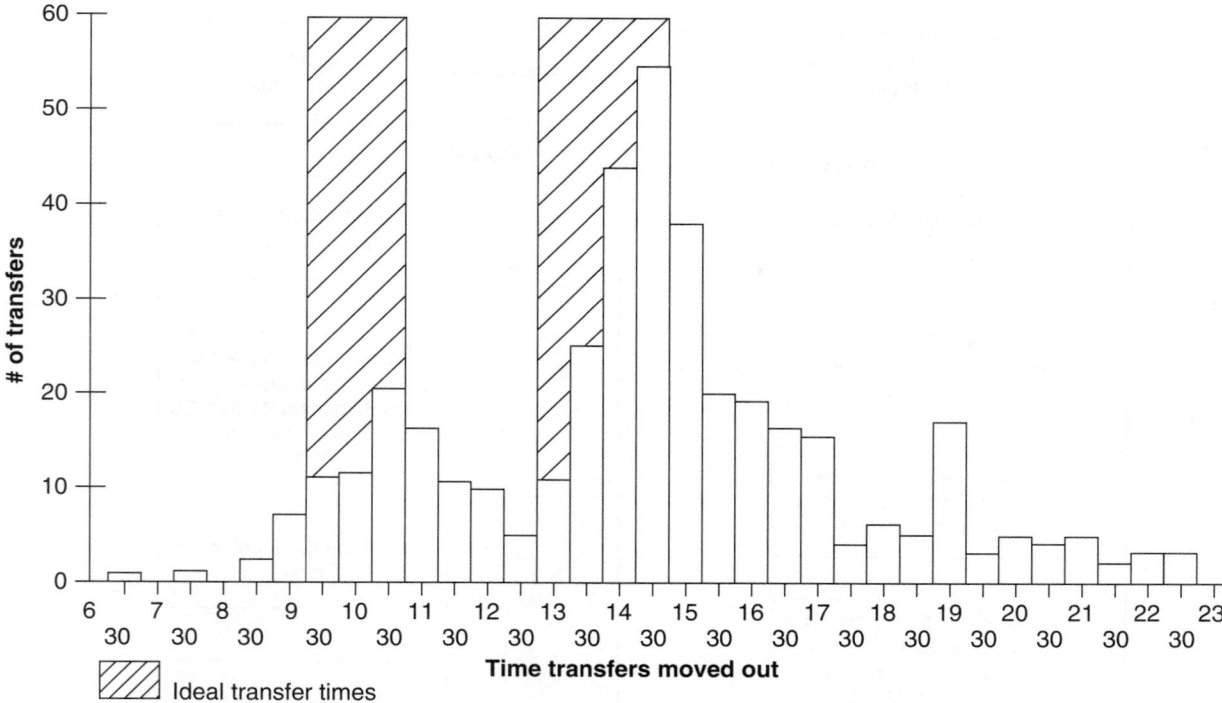

Fig. 11-5 CCU/IMCU transfers to Two South January 1 through February 28, 1990, with ideal transfer time slots highlighted.

The new process required the assistance of two other departments. The first was of the Transport Department to help in locating enough wheelchairs and carts in the morning for CCU and IMCU to use during the transfer of the predicted amount of patients between units. The request for them is entered into the computer system in the morning and the Transport Department delivers the requested wheelchairs and carts shortly thereafter. This procedure relieved the RN from spending up to 20 minutes in locating the necessary equipment to transfer the patient.

The Housekeeping Department routinely took a break during the designated morning transfer time slot. In order to facilitate a smooth flow of transfers between units, the Housekeeping Department adjusted its schedule to make its staff available to clean vacated rooms immediately. Thus, clean rooms were available for new patients at a moment's notice.

When a patient was made floor status, the charge nurse from that unit contacted Two South. At that time a room number, transfer time slot, and the RN's name expecting that transfer was given. This new process was more systematic, shorter, predictable, and would prove to reduce patient transfer delays.

Do: Implement the Change on a Pilot Basis

The new process was piloted and studied to determine its effectiveness. Fig. 11-7 represents the transfers that occurred during July of 1990. There had been a definite shift of transfers occurring during the designated transfer times. During each of the studies the team also tracked the predicted number of transfers and the actual number of patients that were transferred to check the reliability of the prediction formula (Fig. 11-8). It proved to be highly reliable throughout this and further studies and hasn't required any adjustments.

One thing that was noticed on all data reviews was that significant numbers of transfers were occurring from 3 p.m. or change of shift on into the evening. An investigation into the reasons disclosed that these late transfers were related to a procedure that required the patient to remain in the unit for approximately six to eight hours after being made floor status before the transfer could occur. After reviewing the data, a further adjustment was made to the process. An additional transfer time slot, from 6 p.m. to 7:30 p.m., was added to accommodate any patient transfer that didn't occur in the afternoon (Fig. 11-9). The

TABLE 11-1 Predicted Percentage of Transfers for the Next Day Based on Census

Day	CCU	IMCU
Monday	5%	20%
Tuesday	10%	20%
Wednesday	17%	40%
Thursday	12%	30%
Friday	15%	40%
Saturday	16%	30%
Sunday	14%	30%

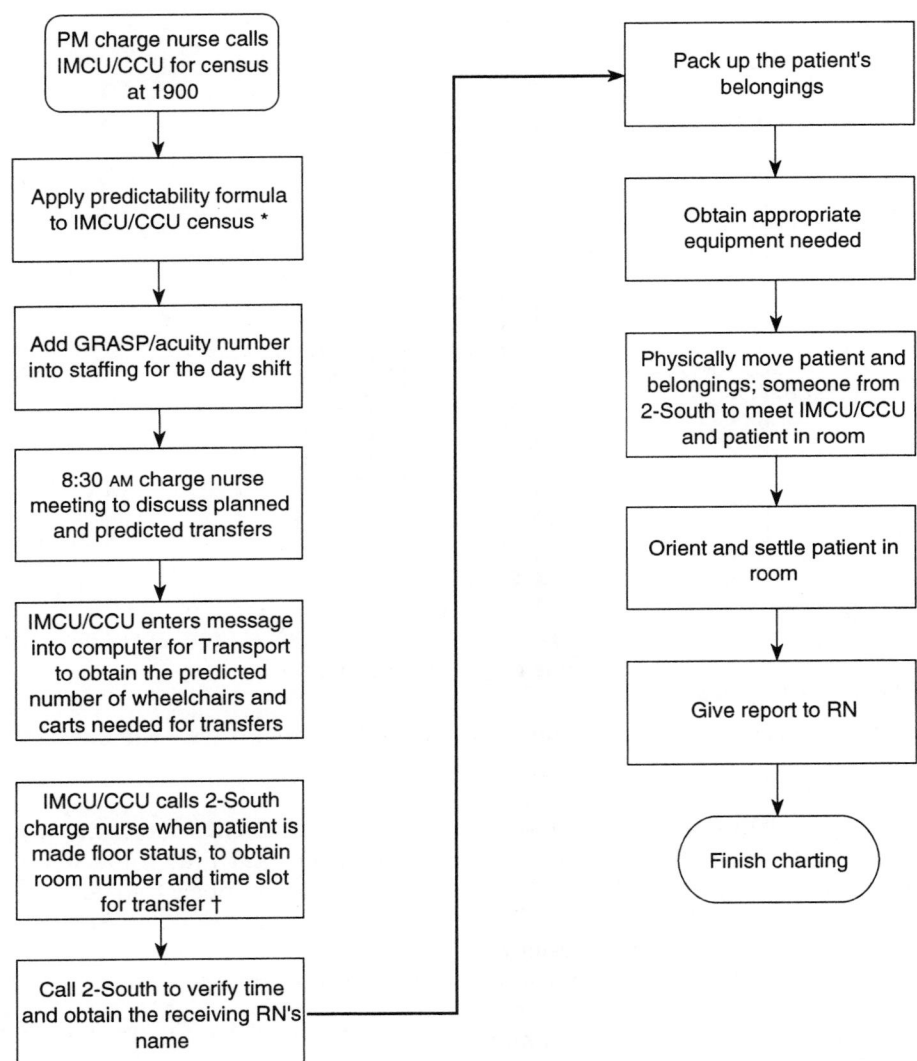

* The predictability formula estimates the total predicted transfers to 2-South for the
next day:
  * Multiply IMCU/CCU census by the respective predictability percentage
    to estimate the total predicted transfers
  * Take 1/2 of the total predicted number of transfers
  * Round up
  * Assign a GRASP/acuity number for each transfer to increase staffing levels

† Ideally at least 1/2 of the predicted transfers will occur in the morning.

Fig. 11-6 New process piloted flowchart.

charge nurses between the units mutually decide whether the patient can wait to transfer until the evening transfer time slot. If CCU or IMCU needs the transfer bed for a new patient or staffing issues arise, the patient can be transferred regardless of the time.

Check: Determine if It Met the Intended Need

After piloting the new process, the team could understand the impact it had made. During the ensuing months, two issues that required attention arose. The first was that valuable nursing time was wasted packing up and transferring the patient between units. The process of packing a patient's belongings and bringing them along with the patient to a new room doesn't require the skill of an RN. The team again called on the Transport Department for assistance. Its people graciously expanded their role by wearing a pager during the designated transfer times; when paged, they would gather the patient's belongings and transfer, settle, and unpack the patient into the new room. The CCU or IMCU RN only needed to give report to the Two South RN, thus increasing the

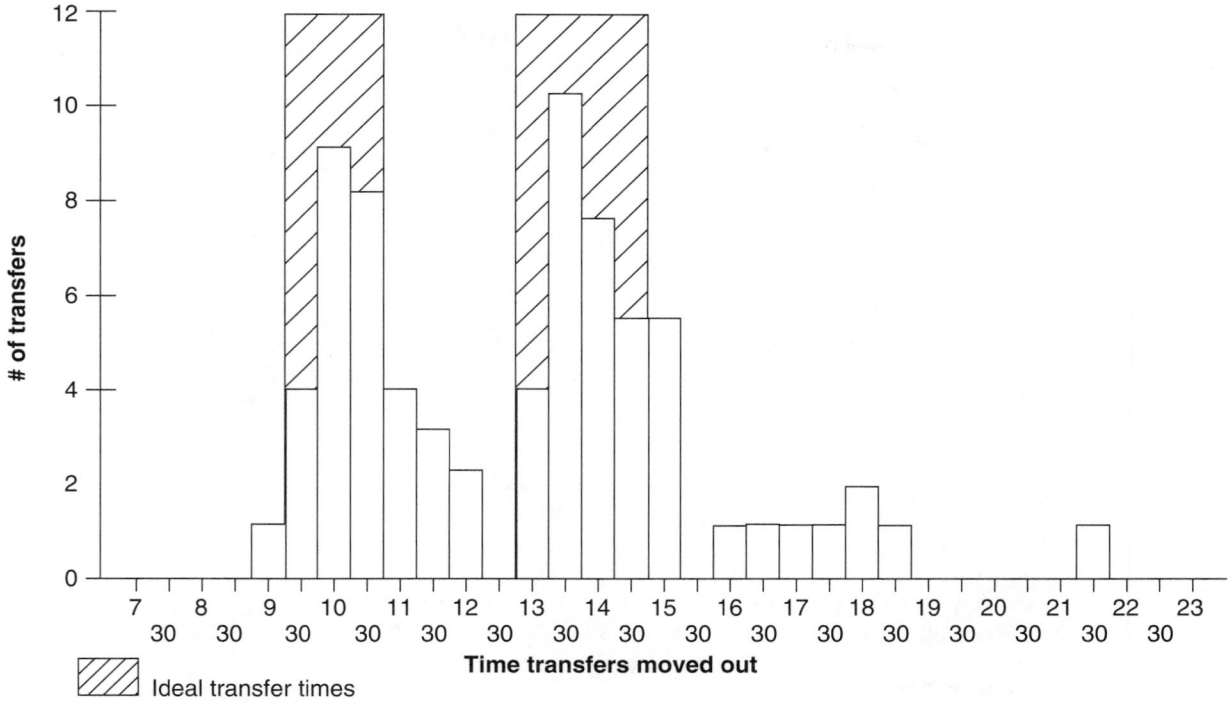

Fig. 11-7 CCU/IMCU transfers to Two South July 9 through July 27, 1990 (19 days, 70 transfers).

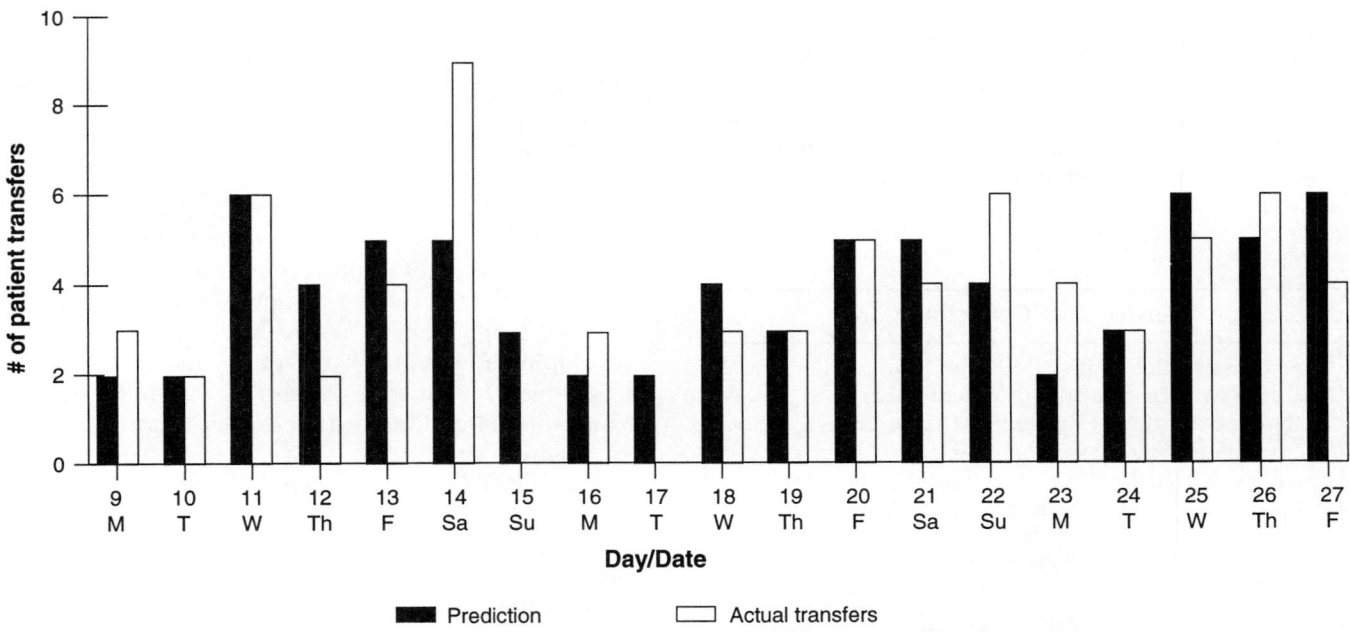

Fig. 11-8 Predicted number of transfers versus actual patient transfers July 9 through July 27, 1990.

efficiency of the new process. The staff of the Transport Department went through a brief transfer orientation in an effort to guarantee a quality patient transfer.

The second and more difficult issue that required attention was a lack of staff understanding. Dealing with this issue was the biggest roadblock thus far encountered. The team spent at least six months educating and reinforcing the process. After verbal re-

inforcements at meetings failed to produce a significant effect, it was seen that more creativity was required. The results of all studies were shared on bulletin boards for staff to see. The transfer time slots were posted on laminated signs in visible locations on all the units. Short items with catchy cartoons about the transfer process were placed in the units' newsletters. The last and perhaps most effective tool de-

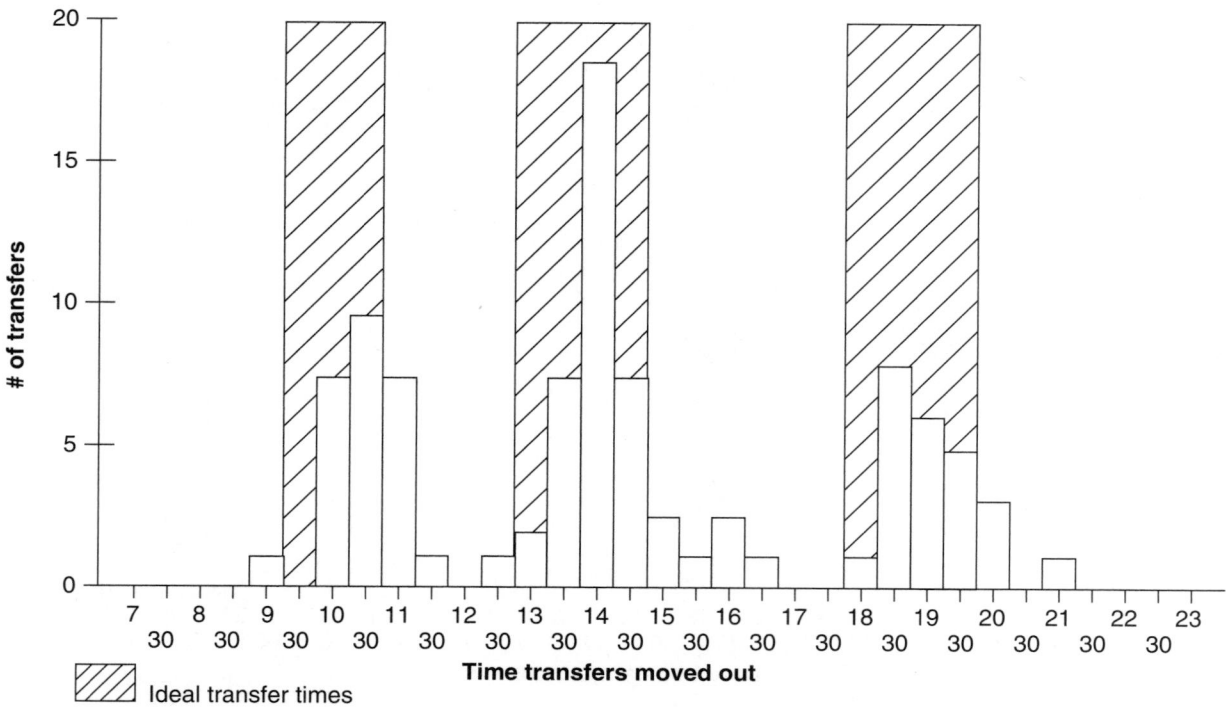

Fig. 11-9 CCU/IMCU transfers to Two South August 13 through September 2, 1990 (22 days, 92 transfers). Third transfer time slot added.

veloped was a transfer card (see the box below) that is attached to the front of a patient's chart when the patient is made floor status. This card has the designated time slots listed and is a constant reminder of this new process. Since development of the card, the

---

Transfer Data Collection Card

Please assist the Transfer Group from CCU/IMCU/2 South in gathering data by completing this short survey at the time of patient transfer to IMCU or 2 South. Leave the completed survey taped on the front of the chart and it will be collected on the receiving floor. Thank you.

TRANSFER TIMES:
0930-1100
1300-1430
AFTER 1800

Time unit or floor received report _____

Time patient was actually transferred _____

If patient report was not given during transfer times, please specify as to the cause of the delay. _____

_____

_____

_____

_____

Patient was transferred from room _____
to room _____

Patient name _____

Date _____

---

process has flowed more smoothly. The journey was slow and trying, but the team seems to have been successful in transforming the attitudes and patterns of the staff in adjusting to this new process.

Act: Hold the Gain; Repeat the Cycle

Although this new process seemed infallible, adjustments and frequent reinforcements were needed and are continually occurring to hold the gain. An initial step the team took to help solidify the change was developing a new policy and procedure for the transfer process. Having the process written in black-and-white eliminated the need for questions as to how the process was to progress. The new policy and procedure could also be used as a reference for new employees unfamiliar with transferring patients.

Maintaining the gains and continued improvement has been the true test of success in beating the transfer tug of war. Vitally important is the continuous review of data to ensure gains achieved are not lost over time. The team's method of data collection is done through survey cards. These cards are placed on the front of each patient's chart when the physician order for transfer is obtained. When the nurse completes the transfer, a check is simply made on the card as to whether or not the patient was transferred and a report to the receiving RN was given within the allotted transfer times. If the answer is no, a brief explanation of the cause or causes for the late transfer is to be indicated. This explanation gives the team

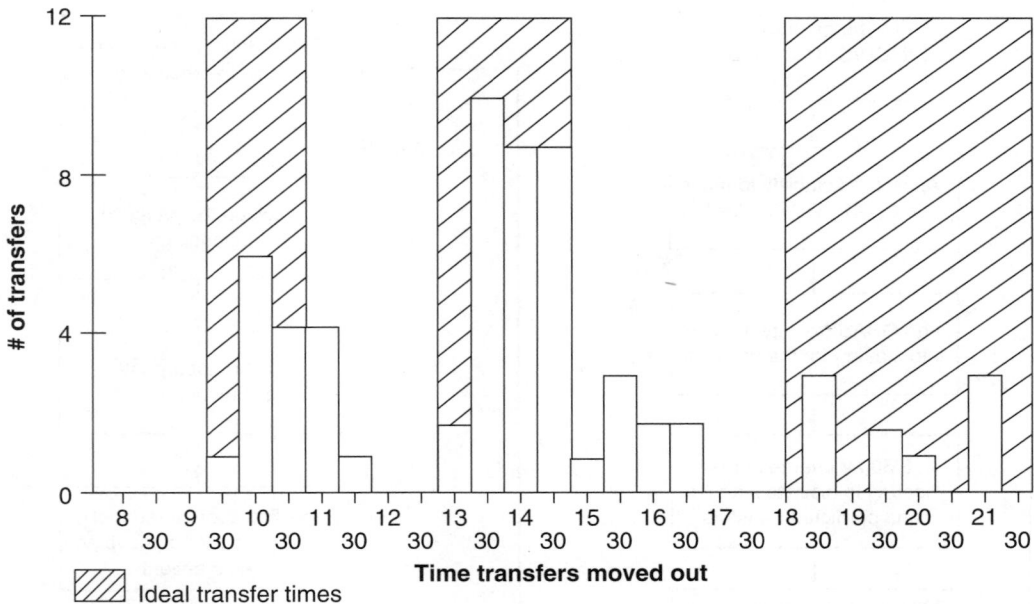

Fig. 11-10 CCU/IMCU transfers to Two South June 10 through July 2, 1991 (23 days, 64 transfers).

identifiable causes for late transfers and allows appropriate intervention. Intervention is taken when more than 20 percent of the transfers fall outside the allotted transfer times. Data is periodically shared with the staff enabling its members to share in gains achieved.

Data collected during June 1991 (Fig. 11-10) uncovered a small but important change that needed to be made in the process. From the graph one might note that several transfers occurred between 10:30 a.m. and 11 a.m. This trend had been seen on previous data collections, with, up until this point, no identifiable cause. The survey cards, having just been developed, were studied, and a cause could now be identified. The timely transfer of, say, a patient with complex needs by an RN having a busy morning by 10:30 a.m. was unrealistic in view of the many tasks the RN had to do in the morning. In an effort to ease the patient transfer in the morning, the transfer time slot was extended to 11 a.m. The team's mission was to be timely and efficient, but not at the expense of Bellin's customers: the patient and the nurse. This was the final adjustment made to the process that is currently in place (Fig. 11-11).

It was also noted from the survey cards that many of the transfers that occurred outside the transfer times were negotiated between the units involved. Negotiated transfers are positive because they ultimately mean the units are communicating in a positive way. The blame rope, so prominent months prior, was fading fast.

Recent data collection shows good and bad news. The good news is that greater than 80 percent of transfers have fallen within the transfer time slots (Fig. 11-12). The bad news is that the reliability of this data was questioned when it was noted that fewer survey cards were being turned in than transfers actually occurring. At one point only 42 percent of transfers were accompanied by a survey card, making the data invalid. Action was taken to educate the staff on the importance of filling out the survey cards. Percentages of cards accompanying transfers have increased, thereby increasing the validity of the data collected.

The formula used to predict next-day transfers is reviewed quarterly. It continues to predict transfers accurately, thus requiring no change or adjustment to the numbers.

+ Recognize and Celebrate

The team's journey through quality improvement at times paused to allow for recognition and celebration. Team recognition was received on a local as well as a national level. Locally, team members presented the project to Bellin Hospital managerial and Board of Directors meetings. Updates could be given at that time and questions answered. Encouraging others to grow in quality improvement, the project was and continues to be used as an example in Bellin Hospital's quality improvement training programs. Most recently the project was featured as part of a breakout session during a daylong conference Bellin hosted for other midwestern hospitals interested in total quality management. Sharing the team's accomplishments with the nation was the biggest thrill. In October 1991 the team was selected as one of three across the nation to present at the National Demonstration Project's annual conference in Atlanta, The National Forum on Quality Improvement in Health Care. All eight project team members were privileged to attend

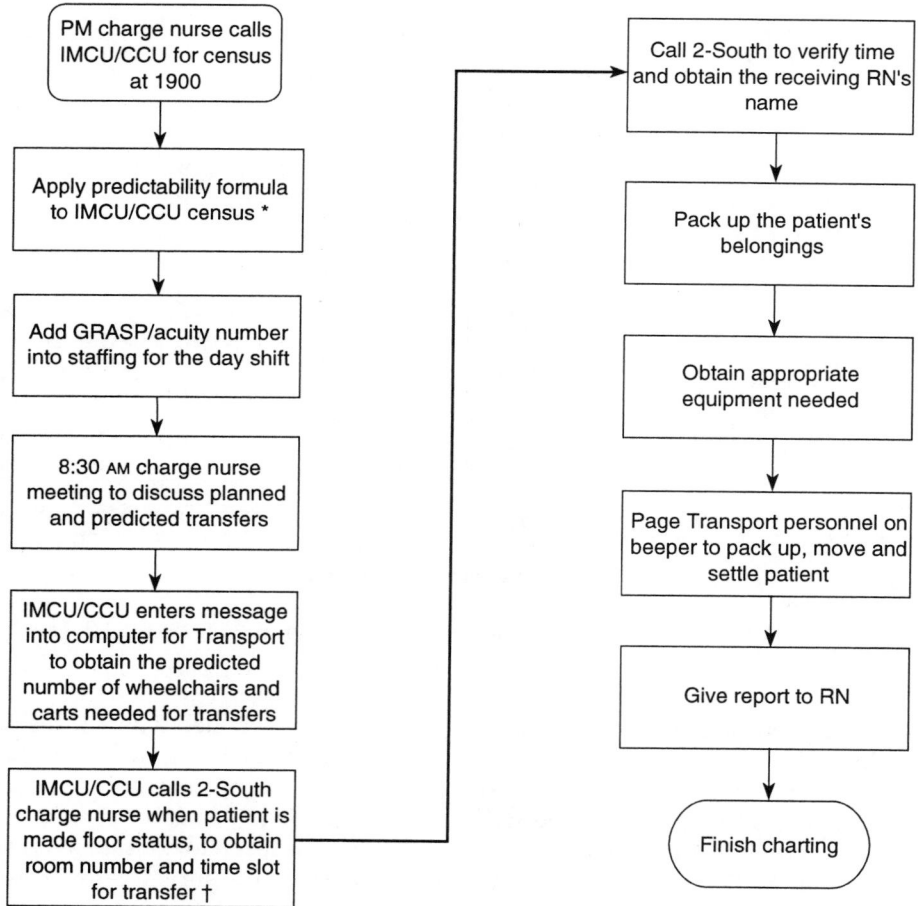

* The predictability formula estimates the total predicted transfers to 2-South for the next day:
    * Multiply IMCU/CCU census by the respective predictability percentage to estimate the total predicted transfers
    * Take 1/2 of the total predicted number of transfers
    * Round up
    * Assign a GRASP/acuity number for each transfer to increase staffing levels

† Ideally at least 1/2 of the predicted transfers will occur in the morning.

Fig. 11-11 Flow diagram of current process.

the conference, with two of the eight presenting. The project was well received, with many questions and positive comments.

Another celebration that took place early on in the project included the team going out to lunch with Bellin's vice president of nursing and senior vice president of hospital operations. This lunch provided an opportunity for the team to share informally with upper management current activities and activities yet to come. A true sense of support was felt by the team, giving its members the will and energy to continue on till journey's end.

The added benefits gained along the way were numerous, but two stand out above all others. First, despite some hardships faced along the way, the project was fun for all involved. A true camaraderie

that is perhaps unobtainable through other means developed between team members. This camaraderie extended through to the units the team members represented. Improved interdepartmental communication is the second added benefit. The three units could now openly discuss common problems instead of immediately resorting to blame. Perhaps this improved communication will pave the way for future QI projects that may develop between the units.

CONCLUSION

This quality improvement journey uncovered hidden truths along the way, some more complex than others. The first lesson the team would learn was that

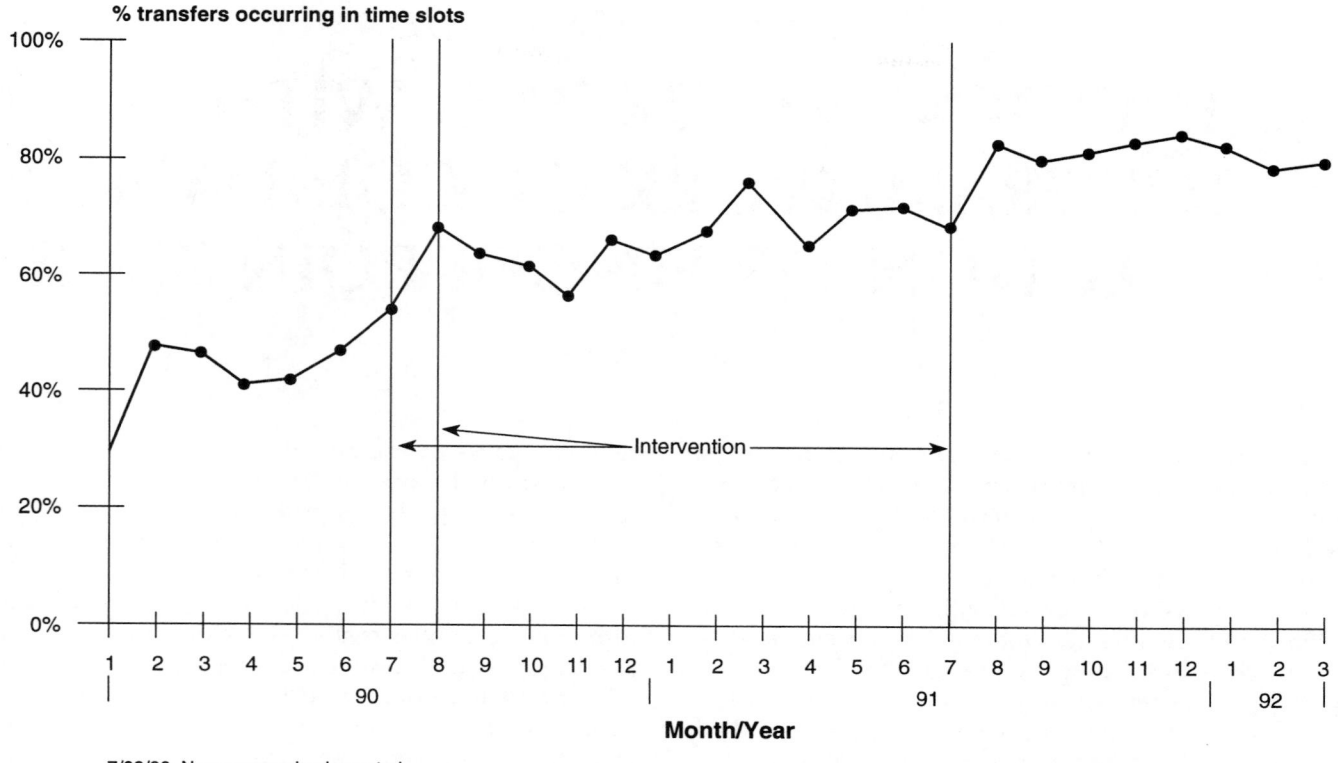

Fig. 11-12 CCU/IMCU transfers to Two South. Monthly record is to show progress and is currently used to determine maintenance of goal.

just because a process has been around a long time does not mean one has to live with it. Change is good. The only way this team could recognize needed change was by creating new paradigms. An early paradigm the team encountered was learning to understand and eventually accept the concept that the problem was with the process, not the people. This idea was a major obstacle for the team to overcome, but was vital to the creation of team spirit and the destruction of the blame rope. After developing the cause and effect diagram, the important concept of people versus process gained acceptance by all.

The most difficult lesson learned was that holding the gains is difficult and may at times seem impossible. Frustration, the common-thread emotion plaguing all team members, was endured for a long six months while the team struggled to hold gains already achieved. The struggle continues, but to a much lesser degree than initially perceived.

Not all lessons learned were so difficult and painstaking. The most unexpected lesson was that problem solving can be fun. Fun times were not only experienced during times of celebration, but could also be experienced at team meetings. The level of festivity grew as the friendships created by team spirit grew.

A final, but very important, lesson was that the unit manager was required to assume a new role. The role has changed from one of active problem solving to one of support. None of the problem-solving activities developed by the team could have been enacted without the support of each unit manager.

There can only be speculation as to whether the blame rope has truly been destroyed. The only sure thing is that the team's mission is complete, instilling a sense of pride in the hearts of all team members for gains achieved.

CHAPTER TWELVE

INCIDENT REPORTING WITHIN THE FRAMEWORK OF CQI: DATA COLLECTION OR FINGER POINTING?

Lenard L. Parisi

"Incident reports" strike a note of terror in the hearts of many practicing nurses. These tools have been traditionally used to capture retrospective information about negative patient events such as accidents, mistakes, and errors. They have been used to statistically track numbers of incidents without any consistent follow-up to create improvement. The nursing staff is often reluctant to complete the form for fear that reporting an incident somehow implies its involvement in the event. Another deterrent to reporting is that initiating an incident report involving another practitioner suggests blame and constitutes "finger pointing," both inconsistent with the concepts of continuous quality improvement. In general, identification of pertinent factors surrounding a patient incident is not viewed as data collection used to identify opportunities to improve care. When the data are reflective of professional practice errors, documentation is often used punitively against practitioners. Some examples of common punitive actions are documented counseling sessions regarding practice, with an entry into the practitioner's personnel file, closer supervision of the staff member's practice, and limitation or suspension of practice privileges.

Deming, in his 14 points, strongly states that fear prevents employees from reporting problems (Walton, 1986). Nurses are usually taught what *not* to write on incident reports and in nurse's notes, for fear of discovery. Reporting medication errors induces fear, as the result is usually some form of disciplinary action against the involved practitioner. Accidents, mistakes, and errors can only be prevented, however, if we have sufficient information to change the process. Staff members must be encouraged to report incidents and participate in processes to create improvement. In his discussion on reducing human error, Juran emphasizes the need to collect data and identify and prevent the most common types of errors (Juran, 1988). If incidents are to be used as opportunities to improve care, the fear of reporting must be eliminated.

According to Juran, there will always be human error. Whenever an individual is expected to perform repetitive tasks over a period of time, the results, at some point, will vary from the expected outcome (Juran, 1988). As health care professionals, however, we must not lose sight of our responsibility for patient safety. Each patient incident must be objectively evaluated to determine appropriate prevention in the future. Some examples of this are an implementation of a falls-prevention protocol in response to patient falls, staff education related to identified knowledge deficits, and staff brainstorming sessions to identify opportunities to improve care and reduce patient risk. When incidents are related to errors in practice, there is a professional responsibility to hold the practitioner accountable and appropriately intervene to prevent similar occurrences in the future.

The existence of a quality program that interprets incident data does not eliminate the need for a comprehensive risk management program. A coordinated systematic approach of these two programs will decrease the number of errors and improve care. The two are interdependent in that quality programs utilize the data to identify opportunities to improve care, and risk management utilizes the data to minimize risk in the future and decrease the liability of the organization (Fiesta, 1991).

Incident reporting, in some fashion, in hospitals will likely never be eliminated. There will always be a need to identify occurrences not consistent with the routine operations and procedures of the institution. What is needed, however, is an incident reporting system whereby data is gathered, communicated, interpreted across departments, and used as an opportunity to improve processes. What follows is an account of the QI processes used to improve the data collection trending and reporting system for negative variances in practice and negative patient outcomes.

THE SETTING

The implementation of QI processes is in the beginning stages at The New York Hospital. The hospital is a 1000-bed tertiary health care facility located in New York City. With more than 38,000 admissions per year, the patient population is varied. The scope of service includes many clinical specialties such as cardiothoracic surgery, burns and trauma care, neonatology, AIDS care, and oncology. The Division of Nursing, accountable to a vice president for nursing, contains six clinical nursing departments encompassing 44 inpatient units. Each unit is directed by a nurse manager who reports to one of the six clinical nursing directors. Each nursing department has a QA coordinator responsible for developing and implementing the quality assurance program. Integration of QA activities throughout the entire Division of Nursing is accomplished through the Nursing QA Coordinating Committee. This committee is chaired by the assistant director of nursing quality assurance, who is responsible for ensuring that there is consistent and relevant monitoring and evaluation across the entire Division of Nursing.

Using the Incident Report

An incident report is completed when an event occurs on hospital premises that is not consistent with the routine operations or care for patients. The report form is most often initiated by the involved patient's primary nurse, on the unit where the incident occurred. The nurse manager or nursing supervisor is notified of the incident. It is the supervisor's responsibility to ensure that the form is completed appropriately and that all pertinent nursing information surrounding the event is included on the form. The nurse manager or nursing supervisor also ensures that any immediate corrective action has been appropriately initiated and documented. The physician responsible for the patient's care is immediately called to examine the patient. The physician then completes the form entering the results of the physical examination findings and indicating any prescribed treatments or diagnostic tests as a result of the incident. After the report is completed it is forwarded to the departmental nursing office, where it is reviewed by the nursing director. The nursing director or designee ensures that all immediate action plans have been implemented and that appropriate intrahospital communication has occurred. The report is then forwarded to the nursing QA coordinator for tracking and trending.

Historically, the QA coordinator in each clinical nursing department was responsible for tracking and trending incident data. When an incident report that contained information relevant to another department was generated, the QA coordinator forwarded a copy of the report to the appropriate department. The departments most often involved were Medicine, Surgery, Pharmacy, Biomedical Engineering, and Respiratory Therapy.

Hospital incidents are most often handled as individual events rather than systems problem. As a result, little information is derived to effect quality improvement or systems changes. Clarification of processes surrounding the incident report have resulted in formal systems of communication to the Risk Management department and Patient Services Administration, the patient advocacy department. Risk Management is notified of all hospital incidents. Patient Services Administration is told of all incidents that result in harm to a patient and of a patient's or significant other's expressions of dissatisfaction and if the type of incident meets reporting requirements of the New York State Public Health Law.

Intrahospital communication of findings related to incident reporting is defined in the Division of Nursing QA plan. Reporting throughout the organization up to and including the Board of Governors is accomplished through written reports and minutes of executive committees that address incident report data. Incident reports are treated as any other QA indicator and listed in QA plans under the important aspects of care: *Medication Administration* and *Patient Safety*.

The Need for Change

The Nursing QA Coordinating Committee was first to identify the need to change the incident report form. Each coordinator was well aware of the deficiencies in collecting data from the incident report. Impediments to data collection included were difficulty in tabulating demographic data because of its disjointed location on the form, lack of documented causal factors related to medication errors and patient falls (important information to create change), and documentation of radiographs or diagnostic tests required as a result of the occurrence. The previous form required filling in the blanks, which often resulted in incomplete information. A brainstorming session was conducted by the QA Coordinating Committee to generate ideas for revising the incident report form. Many of the QA coordinators shared the same frustration when collecting data using the form. It was clear that there was a need for change. One Nursing QA coordinator was chosen to coordinate the project, although the entire committee worked closely together throughout the process.

Initiating a change of this magnitude required support from senior administration. Legal concerns regarding the use of the tool also needed to be addressed. A meeting with the vice-president of risk management and legal affairs was held to elicit support and further insight. Using the points raised during the initial brainstorming session, the need for change was outlined. Some of the reasons were:
- Additional analysis sheets were required to collect information on cause and effect of patient falls and medication errors.
- There was insufficient space to completely describe the incident and include actions planned and actions taken.

- Diagnostic tests or medical and nursing interventions required as a result of the incident were not clearly identified.
- Photostatic copies were required to share information with other departments.
- Terminology on the form was outdated.
- The form was not user-friendly and did not guide the user through the process of including essential information to ensure follow-up and data collection for trending and formation of action plans.

The meeting produced overwhelming support for the project, and a hospital attorney from Risk Management became an ongoing project team member.

The Project Team

The project team was named the Incident Report Task Force. One of the first concerns was to determine the membership on the committee. The form to be developed was to be used hospitalwide, so it was essential that all department users had representation. The first task was to determine who the form users would be.

The Division of Nursing is the predominant user of the incident report. Other departments include Radiology, Food and Nutrition Services, and the Pharmacy. There are several users of the report form that do not necessarily initiate its use; however, they were still included on the task force. These users include Patient Services Administration, the Department of Risk Management and Legal Affairs, the physicians, and Hospital Quality Assurance. Input from these departments was required, to ensure that all required information they obtain by reading the report and evaluating patient incidents was included. All departments had representation on the task force with the exception of the physicians. It was decided that the physician group was too diverse to allow for identification of one representative. Physician input was therefore obtained by soliciting feedback from several different house staff members and attending physicians as the project moved along.

Initial Efforts

The group began by clarifying the role and function of the task force. All members agreed to represent their respective departments and share information in them after each task force meeting. This ensured widespread user input during the design of the new form. The task force decided it would design the form and write the plan for its implementation. At the suggestion of the Department of Risk Management the form was titled "Non-employee Occurrence Report"—replacing "incident" with "occurrence." This change was strongly supported by the task force members. It was apparent that the negative connotation of the "incident report" was somehow lifted just by removing "incident" from its name. The name

change also represented the hospital's philosophical change in its approach toward incident reporting. As the occurrence report was a quality assurance document consistent with the concepts of QI, the Legal Affairs representative advised that a statement be included on the new form that read "for quality assurance purposes only" and that a reference be included to the public health laws protecting quality assurance documents.

Content of Tool

Prior to the revision of the incident report, three years of incident data had been analyzed by the nursing QA coordinators. The coordinators were the "experts" in tracking and trending the data and were most knowledgeable of the types of incidents, the frequency, patient demographics, environmental factors, cause and effect, and action plans developed to prevent future occurrences. Such information is an essential part of tracking, trending, and using the data to create improvement.

Space limited the number of categories that could be listed on the form. To determine the types of incidents that have occurred and to assist in determining which ones should be included on the revised form, a Pareto chart was created. The chart illustrated the number of incidents in discrete categories and helped to identify the types that occurred most frequently. A Pareto chart helps in planning what issue to address first (See Fig. 12-1).

The most common incident types were patient falls, medication errors, variances in blood product administration procedures, variances in treatment interventions, intravenous infiltrations in pediatric patients, burns, elopements, operating room count discrepancies, and equipment malfunctions. Causal factors related to patient falls and medication errors were included as a category of their usefulness in pointing out the reasons patients fall and why medication errors are committed.

Other items included on the revised incident report are general patient demographic data, medical diagnosis, surgical procedure, fall-related factors such as activity orders, a brief assessment of the patient's physical condition, medication administered prior to occurrences, and medication-administration variables such as the type, route, and classification of medication.

Format of Tool. The form is printed in triplicate, eliminating the need to make photocopies for forwarding to other departments. There is a check-off box next to each category on the form to facilitate completion and help capture as much information as possible surrounding the incident. Certain categories were enhanced with a fill-in-the-blank format so that a staff member completing the form would be prompted to

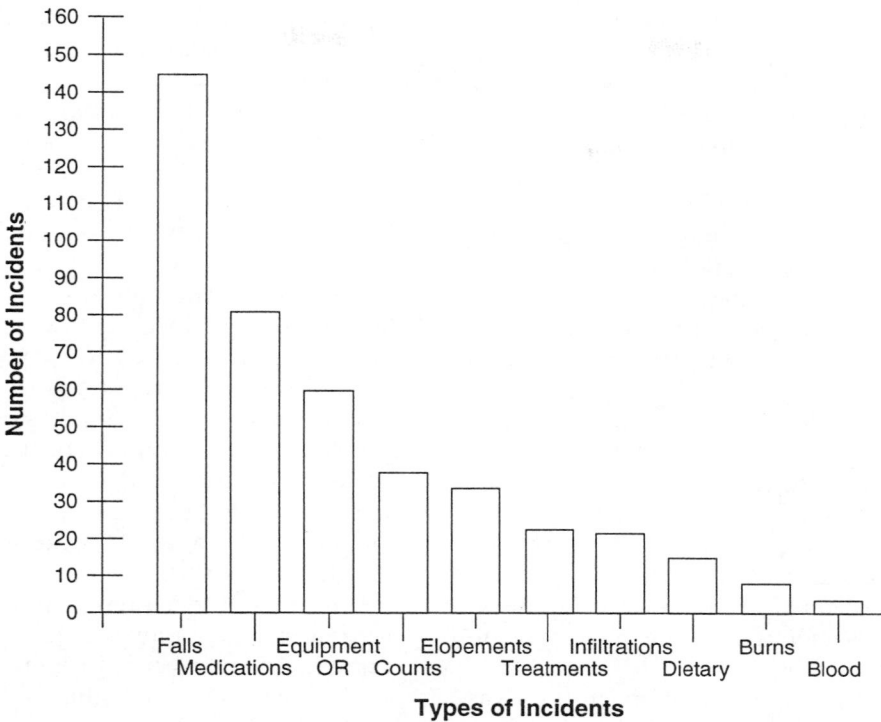

Fig. 12-1 Pareto chart illustrating incident data. (For purpose of illustration only—not reflective of actual data.)

include pertinent information. An example of this is incidents related to equipment where a space for the serial number, something frequently overlooked yet important for tracking, was included. This change has proven useful in conducting follow-up investigations and in meeting reporting regulations for equipment malfunctions of the New York State Department of Health and the federal government.

Use of Tool. The revised occurrence report facilitates tracking of incidents and ensures thorough communication and follow-up. It was decided by the project team that Hospital QA be brought into the communication loop by being provided with a copy of each completed occurrence report. This would provide them with the data to establish a system for tracking hospitalwide occurrences through a data base. The original copy of the report is forwarded to Risk Management, and the second copy retained by the initiating department. A space on the bottom of the form is for the name of any other department that is sent a copy of the report. An additional check-off was included to identify if Patient Services was notified. This department is the liaison between the hospital and Risk Management. It is responsible for coordinating information about incidents reported to the state Department of Health. In the absence of Patient Services' participation, the hospital administrator is responsible for collecting the information.

The Process of Change

The Incident Report Task Force functioned effectively as a quality improvement team. Many of the discussions of what to include on the revised report led to discussions about needed systems changes. Examples of changes that were initiated by this task force included streamlining the reporting process and improving access to information. Hospitals in New York state are under strict regulation to report certain incidents that have potential for or result in harm to a patient. These incidents may be related to treatment or equipment and include patient elopements.

It was important that the momentum of the task force be maintained throughout the form-development process. Regular meetings were scheduled. Departments were consistently represented. Several revisions to the original draft form were made. As the form neared completion, the guidelines and procedure for its use were written. All the decisions and system changes that were made throughout the form-design process were included in the guidelines. A decision was made to print an abridged version of the form completion guidelines on the back of each form.

The final drafts of the Non-employee Occurrence Report, the guidelines, and the policy and procedure were completed, and the material was professionally printed. Although feedback was solicited throughout the project, task force members were asked to formally solicit feedback on the final draft of the incident report from their respective departments. Further suggestions were welcomed; however, departmental representatives were asked to bear in mind the many discussions, at earlier project team meetings, to decide the various types of information that would be included on the occurrence report. Many suggestions were made throughout the design process and the committee spent much time sorting out and prioritizing ideas when making form revisions.

Preliminary testing of the form was conducted by the nursing staff. Using information from previously completed incident reports, staff nurses and nurse managers were asked to complete a sample of the new occurrence report. The response to the new form was overwhelmingly positive. Staff were delighted that the form was simplified, concise, easy to read, and complete. Customer feedback indicated that few changes were necessary. From a cost-containment perspective, the revised occurrence report replaced three other forms, which now were no longer required. As a result of widespread input and support, senior management overwhelmingly accepted the new tool.

The next step in the implementation process was staff education. To accomplish this, a hospital informational bulletin, which advised all employees of the revised incident report complete with ordering information, was distributed. Attached to the bulletin was a copy of the Non-employee Occurrence Report, with the revised policy and guidelines. As the Division of Nursing was the predominant user of the form, it was decided that a more detailed explanation on the use of the form was required. A decision was made to have the nurse managers hold an inservice for the staff on the use of the form, with an emphasis on the narrative description of occurrences. The nursing QA coordinators offered to serve as facilitators in implementing the process as needed.

Evaluating the Process of Change

The implementation of the revised incident report has proven to be successful. Feedback was informally solicited by the project team members from the form users in their departments. At this writing, the form has been in use for six months, and no problems with its implementation have been identified. (See Fig. 12-2.)

The nursing staff, the predominant users of the form, have identified ways in which the revised incident report and process have benefited them. The identified benefits of the revised report were the following:

- The form is more clearly written and easier to complete.
- The form guides the user to collect specific data related to the type of occurrence.
- The data collected at the time of the occurrence provides information to effect immediate improvement.

- The revised form eliminates the need to complete three forms previously used to collect similar data.
- Interdepartmental communication is clearly documented, so that when referred to later the form identifies a clear paper trail.

Nurse managers have been able to discuss and clarify the staff nurse's role in incident reporting during unit inservices on the use of the form. This change process was an excellent opportunity to teach the staff how to document events objectively on the occurrence report and in their progress notes.

The nursing staff reported that the physicians have been satisfied with the changes on the form, as there is a clearer understanding of the circumstances surrounding the reported occurrence, and the physicians are guided through their required documentation process. As a result, usage and completion of the form has improved.

The revised occurrence report has clearly improved documentation of interdepartmental communication. The number of incidents reported to Patient Services has increased; this is supported by documentation on the occurrence report. It is expected that early intervention by the patient representative, when a patient is involved in an incident, will increase patient satisfaction.

Another successful change was to provide the Department of Hospital Quality Assurance with a copy of the report early in the reporting process. This department will track and trend incident data for the entire hospital. This has fostered a hospitalwide approach to QI as it relates to gathering data relative to incident reports and taking a hospitalwide perspective on opportunities to improve care.

CONCLUSION

Implementation of the revised Non-employee Occurrence Report has heightened awareness of the importance of reporting unusual occurrences and variances in practice. Through the processes of education and discussion, staff members became increasingly aware of patient care issues to report. This has resulted in increased reporting. The increase is related to the reporting of systems-related occurrences other than the usual patient falls and medication errors. This has been a benefit in collecting data in the attempt to create improvement in systems and processes.

The most notable improvement resulting from this project has been enhanced interdepartmental communication and the resultant elimination of barriers. During committee discussions of the incident reporting process, each department was able to articulate its need for certain types of data. This has resulted in a hospitalwide approach to collecting data that does not necessarily benefit the department initiating the

THE NEW YORK HOSPITAL
NON-EMPLOYEE OCCURRENCE REPORT

FOR QUALITY ASSURANCE PURPOSES
PROTECTED UNDER EDUCATION LAW § 6527, PUBLIC HEALTH LAW § 2805, j.l.m.

GENERAL INFORMATION

DATE OF OCCURRENCE	TIME OF OCCURRENCE	☐ AM ☐ PM	DATE OF ADMISSION	SEX ☐ M ☐ F	AGE	

(PLATE STAMP OR HISTORY NUMBER, NAME, ADDRESS)

☐ IN-PATIENT ☐ OUTPATIENT ☐ VISITOR ☐ OTHER (SPECIFY)

UNIT	LOCATION (BLDG., FLOOR, RM.)	DEPARTMENT/SERVICE
DIAGNOSIS		SURGERY (DATE)

OCCURRENCE TYPE (CHECK ONE)   FOR FALL* or MEDICATION** complete related section below.

☐ FALL*   ☐ BLOOD PRODUCTS   ☐ TREATMENT   ☐ BURN   ☐ COUNT DISCREPANCY   ☐ EQUIPMENT–SERIAL NO. _____
☐ MEDICATION** ☐ INFILTRATION   ☐ DIETARY   ☐ ELOPEMENT   (O.R. ONLY)   ☐ OTHER (SPECIFY) _____

DESCRIPTION OF OCCURRENCE

WITNESSES (NAME, TITLE, DEPT./ADDRESS)	PHYSICIAN NOTIFIED (NAME)	TIME ☐ AM ☐ PM

PHYSICIAN'S ASSESSMENT AND TREATMENT

SIGNATURE	PRINT NAME	I.D. CODE	WAS TREATMENT REQUIRED? ☐ YES ☐ NO	WERE DIAGNOSTIC TESTS REQUIRED? ☐ YES ☐ NO

*FALLS–RELATED FACTORS (CHECK ALL THAT APPLY)   ☐ OBSERVED   ☐ UNOBSERVED

☐ GOT OOB UNASSISTED   ☐ TRANSFER BED/CHAIR   ☐ UNASSISTED AMBUL.   ☐ RELATED TO TOILETING   ☐ PATIENT ON STRETCHER
☐ CLIMBED OVER SIDE RAIL ☐ OOB IN CHAIR   ☐ ASSISTED AMBUL.   ☐ RELATED TO COMMODE   ☐ PATIENT DID NOT FOLLOW INSTRUCTIONS
☐ WET FLOOR   ☐ OTHER (SPECIFY) _____

MED. ADMIN. WITHIN 24 HRS.	GENERAL ASSESSMENT: (PRIOR TO FALL)	ACTIVITY ORDER: (PRIOR TO FALL)
☐ SEDATIVE/HYPNOTIC ☐ ANTIHYPERTENSIVE	☐ CALL BELL IN REACH ☐ VISUAL DEFICIT	☐ OOB AD LIB ☐ OOB/BRP
☐ ANALGESIC/ANESTHESIA ☐ VASOACTIVE	☐ ALL SIDE RAILS UP ☐ MOTOR DEFICIT	☐ OOB W/ ASST. ☐ BEDREST
☐ PSYCHOACTIVE AGENT ☐ NONE OF THE ABOVE	☐ ALTERED MENTAL STATUS ☐ RESTRAINTS IN USE	☐ OOB TO CHAIR
	☐ HEARING DEFICIT ☐ AT RISK TO FALL	

**MEDICATION–(CHECK ALL THAT APPLY)   TOTAL NUMBER OF OCCURRENCES _____

OCCURRENCE TYPE:
☐ OMISSION ☐ WRONG DOSE ☐ EXTRA DOSE ☐ WRONG TIME ☐ WRONG MEDICATION ☐ WRONG ROUTE ☐ WRONG PATIENT ☐ OTHER (SPECIFY)_____

ROUTE:
☐ P.O.   ☐ I.V.   ☐ I.M.   ☐ S.Q.   ☐ TOPICAL   ☐ P.R.   ☐ S.L.   ☐ OTHER (SPECIFY) _____

CLASSIFICATION:
☐ ANALGESIC   ☐ ANTICONVULSANT   ☐ CARDIAC   ☐ HYPOGLYCEMIC   ☐ NARCOTIC/SEDATIVE   ☐ STEROID
☐ ANTIBIOTIC   ☐ ANTIHYPERTENSIVE ☐ DIURETIC/CATHARTIC ☐ I.V. FLUID   ☐ PSYCHOACTIVE AGENT ☐ PARENTERAL NUTRITION
☐ ANTICOAGULANT ☐ BRONCHODILATOR   ☐ OTHER (SPECIFY) _____

COMPLETED BY	(SIGNATURE)	PRINT NAME	TITLE	DATE
REVIEWED BY	(SIGNATURE)	PRINT NAME	TITLE	DATE
DEPT. HEAD	(SIGNATURE)	PRINT NAME	TITLE	DATE

WAS PATIENT SERVICES ADMINISTRATION NOTIFIED? ☐ NO ☐ YES ☐ A.O.C. COPY SENT TO: _____

41055 REV. (4/92)   LEGAL AFFAIRS - WHITE   ORIGINATING DEPARTMENT - YELLOW   HOSPITAL - WIDE QA - PINK

Fig. 12-2 Non-Employee Occurrence Report. *Copyright 1992, The New York Hospital.*

report, but that does result in an opportunity to improve the care and services provided in other departments.

The implementation of change using the concepts and processes of continuous quality improvement has been effective. A negatively charged issue, incident reporting, was turned into an opportunity to improve patient care. Barriers to interdepartmental communication were broken through the establishment of a common goal and the use of a project team to create improvement.

REFERENCES

Fiesta J (1991): QA and risk management: reducing liability exposure, *Nursing Management* 22 (2).

Juran JM (1988): *Juran on planning quality*, New York, Free Press.

Walton M (1988): *The Deming management method*, New York, Putnam Publishing Group.

CHAPTER THIRTEEN
"IF ONLY THEY WOULD"
Creating Change through a Quality Initiative

Nancy E. Miller

Boston's Beth Israel is a 504-bed teaching hospital of the Harvard Medical School. Its mission is "to deliver patient care of the highest quality, in both scientific and human terms" (Beth Israel Hospital, 1983). Beth Israel first published a Rights of Patients statement in 1972 and has gained international recognition for its philosophy of patient-centered care.

INTEGRATED CLINICAL PRACTICE

At Beth Israel, nursing is recognized as a professional department and, as such, is accountable for advancing practice in keeping with the overall mission of the hospital. The purpose of the Nursing Services is congruent with the mission of the hospital; that is, "to ensure that each patient receives professional nursing care that is patient-centered and goal-directed while supporting nursing and other health care education and research" (Clifford, 1990, pp. 51-52). Since 1974, Primary Nursing has been the vehicle for the delivery of patient-centered care, and the relationships between the patient/family and the primary nurse continue to be the foundation for the development of the Professional Practice Model at Beth Israel (Horvath, 1990). Continuity and accountability for care by a professional nurse are the hallmarks of professional nursing practice.

In October 1990, Beth Israel's model for improving patient care, "Integrated Clinical Practice," was selected for implementation by the Robert Wood Johnson Foundation and the PEW Charitable Trust under its national initiative, "Strengthening Hospital Nursing: A Program To Improve Patient Care." This national program supports hospitalwide restructuring and systems evaluation that will provide better care to patients (SHNP, 1992). Integrated Clinical Practice focuses on how best to care for patients given the complexity of the health care environment and the availability and expertise of health care providers. The goals of Integrated Clinical Practice are to improve continuity of nursing care, restructure hospital nursing practice in order to keep well-prepared nurses in direct-care positions, enhance nurse-physician collaboration, and develop patient-centered support systems (McCausland, 1992).

The goal of developing patient-centered support systems is accomplished through the Work Analysis Structure. An interdisciplinary Work Analysis Advisory Committee provides direction and support for this goal. Three separate work groups are examining the roles, structures, and communication systems that support the delivery of patient care at Beth Israel. The Missing IV Medication Work Team is analyzing the structures and processes that support the nursing-pharmacy system.

Prepare 21

It is important to mention that in 1989, Prepare 21 was established at Beth Israel. This participatory management program challenges the providers of direct patient care as well as those who support patient care to discover better ways to do their work (Rabkin and Avakian, 1992). Using the inherent principles of quality improvement, interdisciplinary and/or interdepartmental project teams are formed to continuously improve a work process. In the spirit of "P21" and Integrated Clinical Practice, The Missing IV Medication Work Team is using the methods and tools of quality improvement to understand and improve the process of ordering, filling, and delivering an IV medication.

HISTORY OF THE PROBLEM

Each day about 800 IV medications are used in the treatment of patients at Beth Israel Hospital. Four satellite pharmacies provide medications for a cluster of patient care units. From 5 p.m. until 7 a.m. on weekdays and throughout the weekend, the main pharmacy supplies medications for the 504-bed inpatient service. It is a complex process regularly carried out by pharmacists, pharmacy technicians, and pharmacy students.

For some time there has been a growing awareness on the part of both hospital pharmacists and nurses that IV medications are missing or unavailable when they are due to be administered to patients. Phone calls or special requests for IV medications from nursing to pharmacy indicate that medications are reported "missing" daily. Members of the Nursing Pharmacy Committee, an interdisciplinary standing committee of the hospital, have tried for many years to "fix" the problem on their own through traditional problem-solving approaches such as informal and formal communication in newsletters and memos. However, the problem never seems to improve. Why is this a persistent problem for pharmacists, nurses, and patients? It is certainly not a trivial concern. IV medications are expensive, preparation is time consuming, nursing time is increasingly scarce, and therapeutic outcomes are compromised when medications are not available on a timely schedule. Each discipline is aware of its job and carries it out according to departmental policy. The first goal was to understand why IV medications are missing.

In the spring of 1991, the Work Analysis Advisory Committee requested the help of the Training and Development Department at Beth Israel. The hospital's internal quality improvement consultant was asked to provide training for the team and to coach the team leader in the use of quality improvement methods and tools.

Education and Team Building

Our team of seven nurses works on a 22-bed medical unit and an 18-bed surgical unit. The pharmacists represent the fifth- and sixth-floor satellite pharmacies, which service the clinical areas involved. These units were selected as the project sites because their people were interested in improving the process, had tried traditional channels for problem solving, and had management support for the project.

In June the quality improvement consultant began to educate the team, its members' managers, and others who would be involved in quality improvement at Beth Israel. She provided a two-day course on the quality improvement process. It was an opportunity for interdepartmental team building and problem solving and an informal way for people to get to know each other over lunch. Most of the participants heard for the first time the principles and processes of quality improvement and learned to use the tools in an actual practicum.

Education and team building were ongoing. By and large, the training was informal and "just in time" so that most learning took place in the meeting as team members interacted and discussed how best to vote on a decision or stratify the data. Team building was a part of every meeting. An ice breaker or climate-setting exercise was a ritual (Scholtes, 1988). These exercises provide a mechanism for team members to separate from the realities of a busy pharmacy or nursing unit, and allow the team to focus on the task of working together to solve an agreed-upon problem. The team gained invaluable insight into the complexity of our systems and the perspective of our customer. The nursing-pharmacy work team spent the better part of our first two meetings working exclusively on team building, establishing ground rules, and sharing our hopes and concerns for the project.

Coaching the Leader

Education of the team leader is also ongoing. At Beth Israel we realized that many early teams fail because there is no ongoing training for the team leader. After the initial training session, a coaching model was designed to support the decision making of the team leader. Specifically, the model was developed to provide an opportunity to team members to learn the principles of quality improvement while engaged in an ongoing project, to ensure the success of this early quality improvement project, and to expand the number of successful team leaders.

In our model, a one-hour coaching session is planned before and after each team meeting. Initially, the focus of each session is educational in that the exchange of information is largely from the coach to the team leader. The quality coach offers invaluable insight into group process, team building, and skills necessary for effective team meetings. She continually emphasizes the effect of both the content and the process of each team meeting on the success of the project. As the work of the project team unfolds, the role of the quality coach becomes consultative as well as educational. The content of each coaching session is driven by the leader's objectives for the next team meeting and by the leader's need for "just in time" training. Ongoing education of the team leader is active and participative as the quality coach and team leader discuss the "what if's" and "how to's" of each phase of the quality improvement journey.

PROBLEM IDENTIFICATION AND ORGANIZATION

Soon after the initial training, we began to think about a single process in the Nursing-Pharmacy system that needed improvement. A customer survey and brainstorming exercise helped to identify and exhaust the list of possible processes. The team agreed that the processes for ordering medications, obtaining narcotics, administering medications, stocking and storing medications, and communicating between nursing and pharmacy would be amenable to the quality improvement process. A project-selection matrix was used to identify the process that would be the focus of this work team (Fig. 13-1).

The team agreed to weight three criteria in the selection of the process. It was important that the pro-

Project Criteria (***weighted)						
Important to external customer						
Important to internal customer ***						
People in process agree it's important						
People in process will cooperate						
Limited scope						
Problem is defined as a process for study, not solution						
Not currently being studied						
Not currently being changed						
Short process cycles, measurable daily						
High visibility ***						
Emotionally appealing ***						
Initial data is easy to obtain						
Potential demonstration value						

Fig. 13-1 Project selection matrix. *Adapted from the National Demonstration Project on Quality Improvement in Healthcare, 1990.*

cess be emotionally appealing for team members, highly visible on a daily basis, and important to the internal customer. Then, as a team member scored each process using the criteria in the matrix, two points were added when a weighted criterion applied to the process, one point was given for any other criterion, and no points if the criteria did not apply to the process. Each member scored the potential processes for improvement. The issue of missing doses emerged as the focus for the team. By a consensus vote, the scope of missing doses was narrowed to missing IV medications because the team agreed they are more expensive to replace, require more preparation, and interrupt work flow and patient therapy when they are not available. In this project, a missing IV medication was defined as any IV medication that was unavailable at the ordered administration time.

Over the period of about two meetings, the team began to develop a Mission Statement. We knew it would be important to clearly state the problem, expectations, and support for this early quality improvement project (see the box on p. 140).

THE DIAGNOSTIC JOURNEY

In order to have a better understanding of the process before flowcharting, the team walked through the actual process of ordering and distributing an IV med-

ication. A "field trip" to see the process and the work place was invaluable. We learned firsthand how the process varies among nurses as well as among pharmacists. The variation and complexity of the process were evident; it was obvious where the process would break down. The benefits of this exercise were far-reaching. The field trip provided an opportunity to better appreciate the needs of the customer as well as to learn the perspective and constraints of the supplier. It was an extremely positive team-building experience, one which set the tone for a truly collaborative attempt to chart the process as it actually occurs.

Initially, a simple overview flowchart was developed (Fig. 13-2). This flowchart provided a seven-step description of the process that would guide the development of more detailed flowcharts. Information from the field trip was discussed in an attempt to understand the process and learn more about the variation in some of the handoffs. The process of "posting an order" (Fig. 13-3) and "filling an order" (Fig. 13-4) needed further definition through detailed flowcharts.

Having gained an understanding of the process as it existed, brainstorming was used to determine breakdowns in the process. With this information from the brainstorming, the fishbone diagram was easy to build with Man, Machines, Methods, and Ma-

---

**Missing IV Medications Work Team
Mission Statement**

Problem

IV medications are often not available when they are due to be administered to patients. This has adverse implications for both patients and employees. It leads to sub-optimal medical therapy and extra cost, interrupts work flow, causes excess paper work, and is frustrating to both nursing and pharmacy.

Team Members

Ed Bezarro, RPh   Joe Fulcher, Pharmacy
                                         Technician
Catherine Armstrong,   Mary Morabito, RN
   RN
Maureen Burns, RN   Lester Chow, RPh
Tina Ledoux, RN   Anne-Marie Gold, RN
Carol Colliton, RN   Peter Hinterreger, RPh
Debbie Tobojka, RN   Margarita Pagan,
                                         Pharmacy Technician
Mary Young, RPH   Nancy Miller, RN Team
                                         Leader
Teresa Chao, RPH   Daryl Juran, Quality
                                         Coach

Expected Outcome

To improve the IV medication order and distribution process

Measures of Success

Decrease in the number of missing IV medications
Decrease in the cost of IV medications
Increase in satisfaction with nursing/pharmacy systems

Constraints

No additional money or resources

Expectations and Support

ICP Work Analysis Advisory Committee
Support the project team
Review the progress regularly
Support the implementation plan

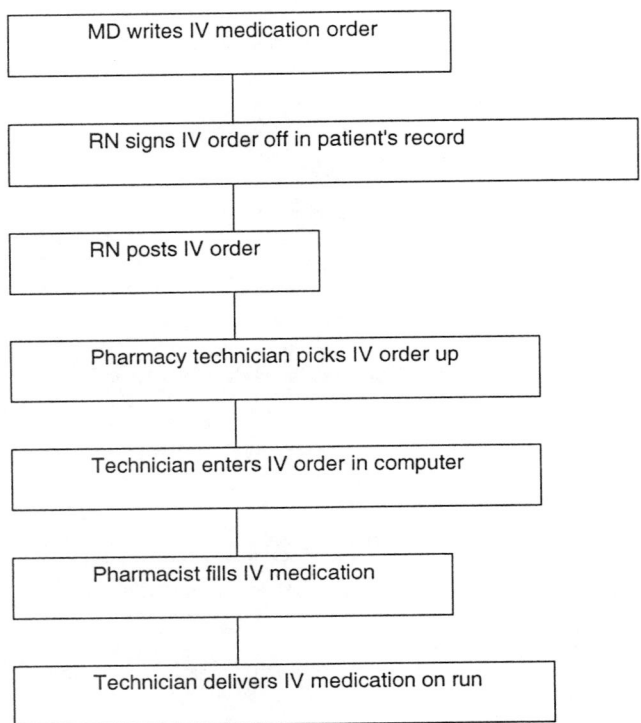

Fig. 13-2 Overview flowchart of the order, fill, and delivery process.

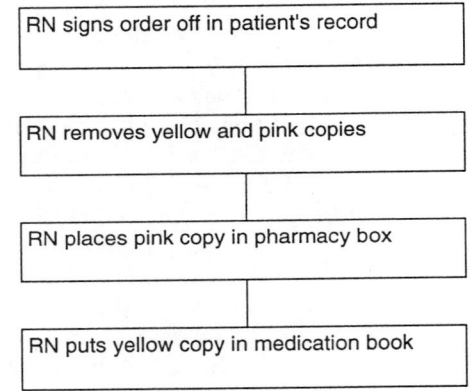

Fig. 13-3 Flowchart of the posting process.

terials as the bony structure. This chart, with any number of possible areas of breakdown, depicted the complexity of the process. The coach recommended a multivote for the most likely root causes of a missing IV medication. Each team member was asked to identify five potential breakdown areas in the process from the fishbone diagram which he or she believed most frequently resulted in a missing IV dose. The following reasons were beginning to emerge as potential root causes of missing IV medications:

- Time to start the medication is missing.
- RNs take medication orders off at routine periods of time each day.
- Large number of meds on run impact the turnaround.
- Special preparation is required for some IVs.
- Order has incorrect information.
- Order missed the run.
- Drug is nonformulary.
- Drug not stocked in the satellite.

- Medication isn't ready.
- Patient is transferred.
- RN can't find the medication in the refrigerator.

These process breaks were arranged on a simple cause and effect diagram and became the leading hypothesis for data collection in this project (Fig. 13-5). Initially, data collection would focus on the time when the nurse transcribes or posts a new IV medication order and also whether or not the nurse assigns a start time for the first dose when she or he posts the order.

Developing the Tool

Our coach recommended that we begin by asking the right questions about the hypotheses. That is, what

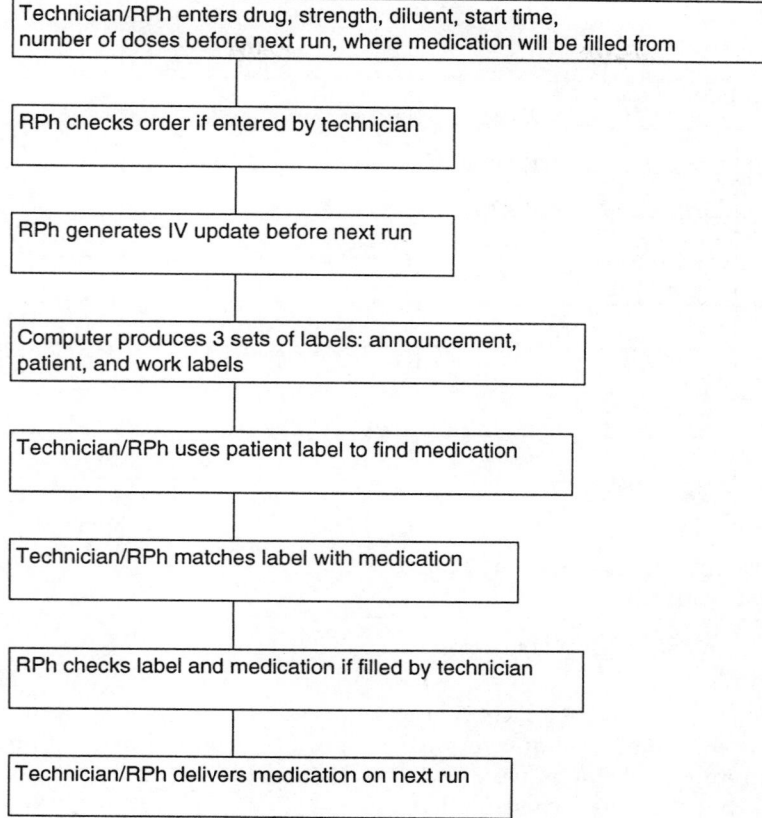

Fig. 13-4 Detailed flowchart of the IV fill process.

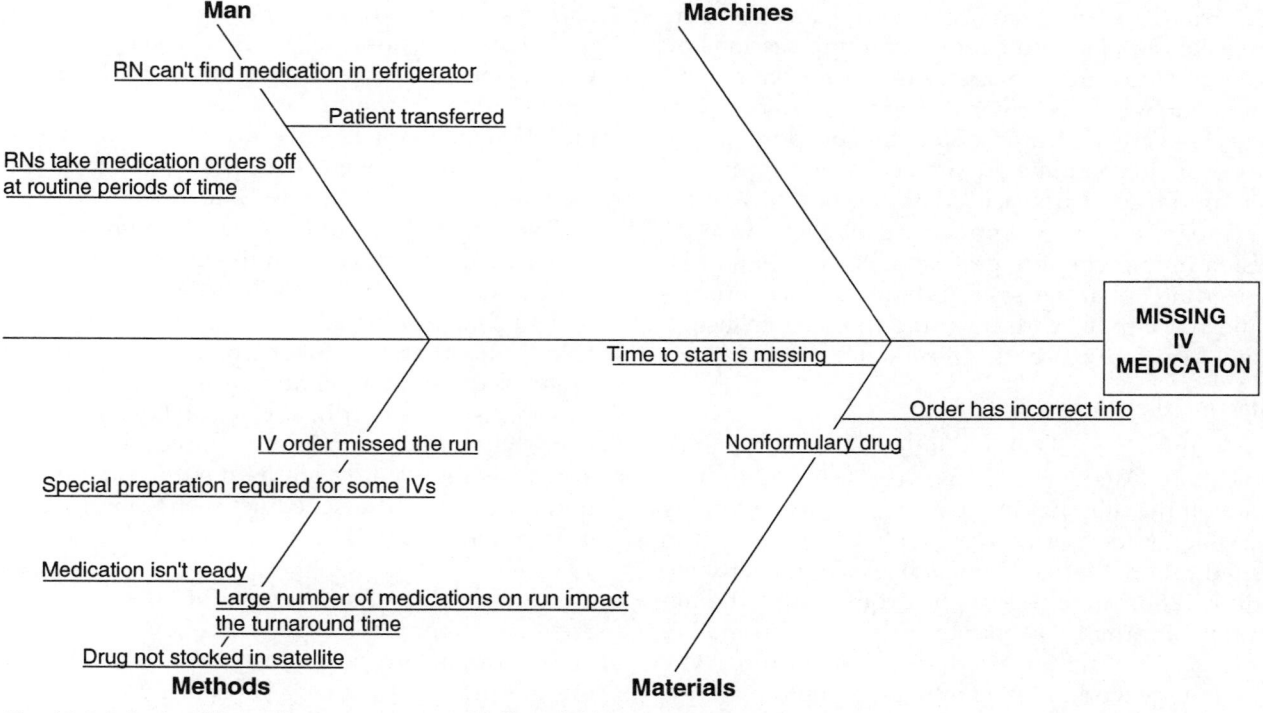

Fig. 13-5 Missing IV medication: cause and effect fishbone diagram.

Date _____ Unit _____												
Time RN Looking For IV Med	Medication	Time Scheduled on MAR	Patient	New Order	Recurring	Dose Chg	Sched Chg	Called	Walked	Sent Req	Borrowed	Other
SAMPLE 11:45 a.m.	ampicillin	noon	John Smith	x			x					
SAMPLE 7:40 p.m.	gentamicin	8 p.m.	Mary Jones		x						x	
CHANGE THE DATA COLLECTION SHEET QD AT 6AM PLACE IN PHARMACY OUT BOX												

Fig. 13-6 Missing IV medication data-collection sheet.

do we want to know? Why do we want to know it? And, where will we find the data? The answers to these questions were extremely helpful as we developed our data-collection tool. Initially, we struggled with the notion of trying to collect as much data as possible about each hypothesis. We continued to learn more about the complexity of the process, and we were hampered by our persistence about making the tool comprehensive. Finally, after many drafts of the tool, we agreed that the tool should be *simple.*

Prior to the start of data collection, team members were asked to plan and conduct training sessions on their units for the pharmacists, technicians, and nurses who would be involved with the project. Data collectors were informed about the purpose of the study, how to complete the data-collection form, and the importance of unbiased data (Plsek and Arturo, 1989). Team members emphasized that we were interested in knowing the process as it exists, and that nurses and pharmacists working in the process should not tamper with it during the data-collection period. We were ready to collect data.

Collecting the Data

During the data-collection period, the Missing IV Medication Data Collection Sheet (Fig. 13-6) was placed on the nursing unit in an agreed-upon, highly accessible location. When a nurse was looking for an IV medication that was unavailable at the ordered administration time, he or she would enter the appropriate information about the missing dose and her actions at the time on the data collection tool. At 6 a.m., a nurse working the night shift would place the data sheet in the pharmacy bin. The data sheets were picked up on the 6:30 a.m. pharmacy run and compiled in the pharmacy until we met to interpret the data.

Interpreting the Data

Data were collected for four weeks from 3/17/92 through 4/19/92. Two hundred and fifty four courses of IV therapy were written for 188 patients during the data collection period. Forty-five IV doses were not available when they were due to be administered to patients. Of the 45 unavailable IV doses, 31 doses were recurring doses (Fig. 13-7). Twenty-four of the unavailable recurring medications did not have a start time written by the nurse when the order was first posted (Fig. 13-8). Twenty-two of the missing recurring medications were ordered to be given on an every-eight-hours schedule (Fig. 13-9).

The initial data confirm our hypothesis that IV doses are unavailable when the intended start time is not posted by the nurse. When the start time on the patient's medication administration record is unavailable to the pharmacist as he or she enters the initial order, a different schedule is often selected by the pharmacist based on his or her ability to fill and deliver the medication. In our sample, the IV medication schedule entered on the medication administration record and the schedule in the pharmacy were different in 34 (76%) of the 45 unavailable doses (Fig. 13-10).

The data show that every-eight-hours medications are most often unavailable. We believe this is the case because an incorrect number of doses is delivered on the morning and evening IV exchange. The number of recurring doses needed in a 12-hour period is de-

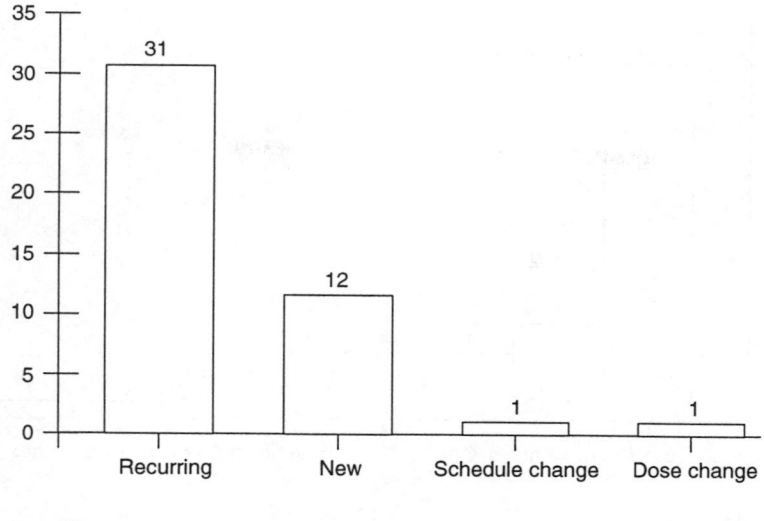

n=45

Fig. 13-7 Missing doses by type of order.

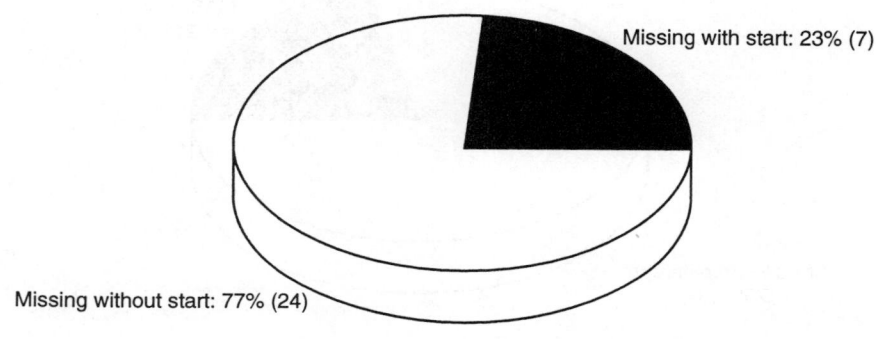

n=31 recurring medications

Fig. 13-8 Missing recurring doses with and without start times.

termined by the pharmacist's computer schedule. In order to receive an accurate number of IV doses, the pharmacist's schedule in the computer and the nurse's schedule on the medication administration record must be the same. This is extremely important in the case of IV doses on a q.8 hour schedule. For example, the nurse is expecting a 12 midnight and 8 a.m. dose on the evening IV fill for an IV medication scheduled at midnight, 8 a.m., and 4 p.m. The pharmacist sends only a 2 a.m. dose because his schedule for this IV medication is 2 a.m., 10 a.m., 6 p.m. The nurse who is administering the IV medication uses the 2 a.m. dose at midnight and finds the 8 a.m. dose is unavailable. Then, the 10 a.m. and 6 p.m. doses are delivered on the morning fill. The nurse needs only a 4 p.m. dose. One dose is wasted or returned to the pharmacy. This process occurs daily.

THE REMEDIAL JOURNEY

Our data support what pharmacists have tried to reinforce to nurses for a long while at Beth Israel: that a start time is crucial to the IV medication order and distribution process. However, as we discussed the idea of finding a way to include a reasonable start time when an IV order is posted, we realized that more information about actual pharmacy run times, delivery patterns, and turn-around time was necessary.

We believe it is still premature to make a recommendation about how to improve until we have a better understanding of the process. An informal survey of nurses revealed large variation in their knowledge of pharmacy run and IV delivery times. The nursing staff responded that it is unable to assign a start time when the order is posted because they cannot predict the time when the medication will be

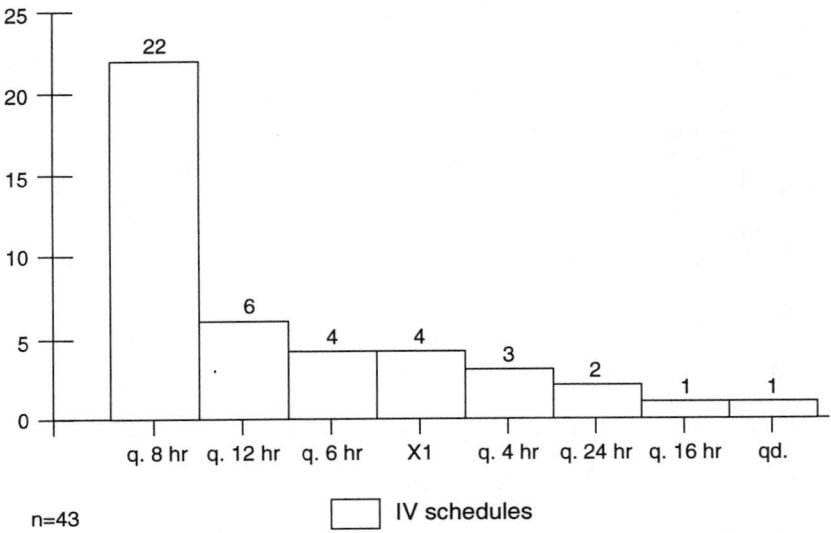

Fig. 13-9 Missing doses by medication schedule.

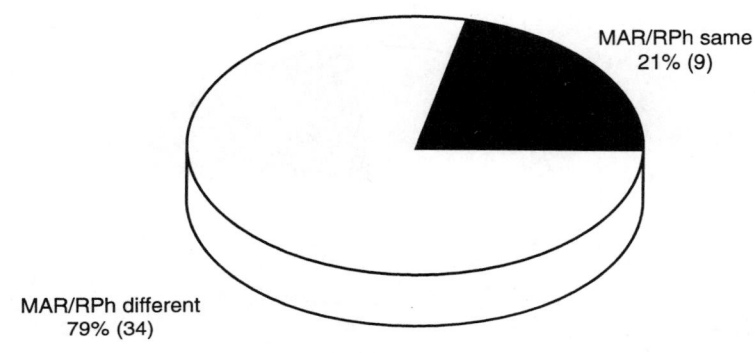

n=43

Fig. 13-10 Variation in RN's medication administration record and pharmacist's schedule.

available. The team is currently collecting data in an effort to explain our process and predict a reasonable timetable for the delivery of IV medications.

CONCLUSION

At the beginning of this project, a number of challenges faced the Missing IV Medication Work Team; many were not new problems. The frequency and length of each meeting seemed unrealistic in a hospital environment. Off-shift and weekend schedules threaten regular attendance. Would it be more advantageous to have a large team with inconsistent attendance or a small team with consistent membership? In our organization, it seemed important to involve as many as possible and plan for good communication. Most often, at least one nurse from each nursing unit and a pharmacist and technician from each satellite pharmacy have been able to attend our weekly meet-

ings. We have been extremely fortunate to have an excellent support staff who perform not only the role of scribe but also develop and circulate meeting minutes each week. This has been very important, as minutes provide up-to-date information on the work of the team.

The ability to work as a team took time and effort to develop. Those of us with experience as project team members knew the value and spirit of a working team. Team-building exercises were extremely helpful in the development of the project team and eventually in allaying our concerns about the organization, communication and commitment of team members to the project. Sometimes, the team-building experiences were seen as silly or irrelevant. However, they were an essential component of our development because they allowed each team member to share his or her knowledge of the process freely, to listen to the perspective of the client objectively, and to work to solve the problem collaboratively. The power of team building cannot be overstated. It is fundamental to the quality improvement process, as it transforms the group into a working team.

Most teams come together to understand and improve a specific, mutually identified process. The Missing IV Medication Work Team was formed to use quality improvement methods and tools in a demonstration project. Although most pharmacists and nurses would agree from the start that many processes in the nursing-pharmacy systems could be improved, the idea of an advisory committee forming a team to solve a problem may have introduced some fear, especially during the early team meetings. Only when the team developed an understanding of the process, and began to trust that a missing dose was not the result of the performance of an individual nurse or the IV room technicians, were members able to commit to improving the process.

Many new skills are needed for all members of a quality improvement project team (Berwick, Enthoven, and Bunker, 1992). The ability to remain silent and listen so that others may offer their knowledge about the process is critical to the success of a team. In this project, we established ground rules at our first team meeting. Not only do they establish boundaries for acceptable behavior in the team meeting, but also they provide an agreed-upon set of expectations for the team leader to refer to as she or he moves the team through the various stages of development. As a new team leader, I was challenged to moderate the comments of a defensive or talkative participant while I persuaded the silent member to share her/his ideas. The coaching model that I described earlier was extremely helpful in these situations.

Lastly, we have learned it is important to celebrate success. At Beth Israel, the Missing IV Medication Team is sharing its work to date through presentations at Beth Israel, at local quality improvement forums, and as part of the Strengthening Hospital Nursing initiative. The excitement about the interdisciplinary and interdepartmental trust, openmindedness, and respect for the work of people in the process are a constant source of energy for the team and enthusiasm for the organization about the power of the quality improvement process.

REFERENCES

Berwick DM, A Enthoven, JP Bunker (1992, January): Quality management in the NHS: the doctor's role—II, *British Medical Journal*, (304): 304-308.

Beth Israel Hospital (1983): Mission statement.

Clifford JC (1990): Professionalizing a nursing service: an integrated approach for the management of patient care, Appendix, Boston's Beth Israel Hospital Division of Nursing Statement of Philosophy and Purpose. In Clifford JC, KJ Horvath, editors, *Advancing professional nursing practice: innovations at Boston's Beth Israel Hospital*, New York, Springer Publishing Company, 51-56.

Horvath KJ (1990): Professional nursing practice model, In Mayer GG, MJ Madden, E Lawrence, *Patient care delivery models*, Rockville, Md, Aspen Publishers.

McCausland MP, editor (1992): If it ain't broke, fix it! *Integrated Clinical Practice News*, Beth Israel Hospital, Winter, 1(1).

Plsek PE, O Arturo (1989): *Quality improvement tools. Data collection*, Wilton, Conn, Juran Institute.

Rabkin MT, L Avakian (1992): Participatory management at Boston's Beth Israel Hospital, *Academic Medicine* 67(5): 289-294.

Scholtes PR (1988): *The team handbook*, Madison, Wis, Joiner and Associates Inc.

SHNP (1992): *Strengthening hospital nursing: a program to improve patient care. Gaining momentum: a progress report*, St. Petersburg, Fla, National Program Office of the Strengthening Hospital Nursing Program.

CHAPTER FOURTEEN

MOVING FROM QA TO QI

Getting Started

Lisa A. Bonadonna

ORGANIZATIONAL CULTURE

An organization must change its culture to adopt QI as a management philosophy. Culture, in this context, can be described as an organization's values, beliefs, ideals, norms, practices, mission, and overall climate toward change. Experts say that the transformation to QI takes three to five years, reasoning that a major paradigm shift and an acceptance of new sets of rules must occur. Change causes distrust, anxiety, and, almost always, opposition. Cultural characteristics and historical trends need to be examined in order to determine potential resistance to the change process. Openness to the principles of QI hinges on organizational readiness to change familiar and habitual ways of managing and doing business.

Identifying cultural attributes that may help or hinder the change process is an important step in determining those that may facilitate or create barriers to change. Previous redesign projects can serve as concrete examples of revolutionary change and an organization's response to it. QI initiatives emphasize education and training as essential, thereby reinforcing the importance of analyzing practices regarding formal education. The value of caring both for patients and for each other, interdepartmental collaboration, and communication patterns are integral pieces of QI policy deployment that require appraisal. Implementing strategies that enhance positive attributes and reduce hindrances can begin the journey of cultural change.

Nursing's Power Base

Readiness for change as a cultural attribute can be assessed by examining historical episodes of redesign that have occurred within an organization. The Medical University of South Carolina (MUSC) Medical Center hired a major health care consulting firm to help redesign the Department of Nursing three years before. This restructuring resulted in the department achieving a position of influence within the organization. All members of the nursing management team were notified that their current positions were abolished, and any member was invited to "apply" for new management positions, which were posted both internally and externally. Despite early protests from existing managers and directors, a dynamic department emerged, built with hand-picked, talented individuals. The Department of Nursing is now led by assertive, educated, visible, and empowered nurses who have decision-making ability at all levels within the organization. This example of redesigning an entire department shows an organization soliciting controversial change, bestowing power to a group that historically had little, and viewing change as a necessary move toward organizational improvement. Having participated in this tumultuous process, the nursing QA coordinator became an initiating force behind the transformation to QI.

Formal Education

Another cultural attribute is that of education. Part of any plan to implement QI includes extensive education and training. For employees to become empowered, innovative, and active participants on project improvement teams, they must have knowledge of change and problem-solving processes, and be well versed in statistical thinking. The mission statement of the organization speaks to the importance of education as a primary goal. The value of formal educational pursuits is clear in the close affiliation that the hospital has with medical, dental, nursing, pharmacy, and health-related professional schools. Students are considered a vital external customer group. When organizations are mandated to trim budgets, often the educational resources are deleted first. However, in this university teaching-hospital setting, formal education is valued and rewarded and resources are aligned in support of it. Informal education of employees about QI requires a significant commitment of time and money. The same importance that formal education has within an organization must be given to informal staff education about QI.

Value of Caring

Just as education and knowledge are essential components of organizational culture, caring is an attribute that must be valued. Every day, health care teams demonstrate expert caring for patients, where technology, planning, and the therapeutic use of self assist in meeting patients' health care needs. Dedication toward patients, our most important external customer, is seen and felt every day within this hospital setting. There are pockets of excellence where employees at all levels and in various departments work in harmony toward meeting and even exceeding expectations of patients, families, and each other. In the movement toward QI, examples of such excellence and caring must be recognized and built into systems, job designs, and key processes so that work can be done right the first time and every time.

Interdepartmental Collaboration

The culture of an organization can also be assessed by looking at ways in which groups work together and employees become involved to solve problems. Interdisciplinary project improvement teams are described as the catalyst that makes QI come alive within organizations. A powerful display of teamwork and interdisciplinary collaboration occurred during the hospital's preparation for and recovery from a natural disaster. After Hurricane Hugo directly hit MUSC Medical Center, turf issues between departments disappeared as executives labored next to housekeepers, physicians helped transport patients, and nurses created a makeshift day-care center for the employees' and the community's children. Response to this disaster revealed that interdisciplinary groups could come together and solve problems, share responsibility, eliminate internal competition, and be innovative. The current transformation that organizations are facing with the adoption of QI needs to become as strong an impetus for initiating change as was preparation for a hurricane!

Communication

Another cultural trait is communication. Recent employee satisfaction survey results showed that the vast majority of employees felt that communication was infrequent, top-down in direction, and often confusing. There are only sporadic open employee meetings where top executives answer questions, and there are no regular newsletters that describe the organization's financial or quality status. It is suggested that poor communication and ill-informed employees can result from an authoritarian management style that stresses control, a lack of team focus, and a bureaucratic design. Building a new culture of continuous improvement requires an atmosphere that facilitates employee involvement and decision making on the front lines. This new work paradigm must foster a liberal, two-way communication flow, one that keeps employees aware of the organization's progress and direction (Marszalek-Gaucher and Coffey, 1991, p. 152-153).

Quality Redesign Task Force Members
Nursing QA coordinator (chairperson)
Assistant director of pharmacy
Director of quality management
Hospital administrator residents (2)
Department of Medicine QA coordinator
Special projects assistant to the executive medical director

QUALITY REDESIGN TASK FORCE (QRTF)

This chapter describes early work of an interdisciplinary Quality Redesign Task Force (QRTF) at MUSC, a 610-bed teaching facility. This group was formed to begin analyzing quality management practices. Selection of QRTF members was easy because of an already established network of QA professionals within the organization. Many members had worked together on QA projects, participated in groups such as risk management and safety committees, and served as resources to each other in managing their own department QA programs (see the box above). Since each QRTF member had experienced some dissatisfaction and frustration with the current status of the housewide QA program, interest in exploring the issues that plagued QA efforts was high. The collective knowledge of the group members was immediately evident. Most had done extensive reading, attended conferences on QI and knew about the sweeping QI transformation that was occurring in hospitals across the nation. Those who were less informed were soon brought up to date. Books, films, and periodicals from both the industrial and the health care setting were distributed and discussed.

Many group members had successful track records associated with implementation of QA in their own departments. The Nursing QA Coordinator had established a unit-based QA program that successfully passed a JCAHO survey and had widespread nursing management support. The assistant director of pharmacy had been both a designated facilitator and leader in the QI transformation that occurred at another university teaching hospital. The director of quality management was well versed regarding the medical staff's efforts in QA and regulatory standards related to quality. The acquired knowledge of the QRTF and the cumulative experience and demonstrated success of individual group members were a positive force in the emergence of a mature, productive, and goal-directed work group.

QRTF Activity

The purpose of the QRTF was to conduct an organizational assessment of existing QA practices and to

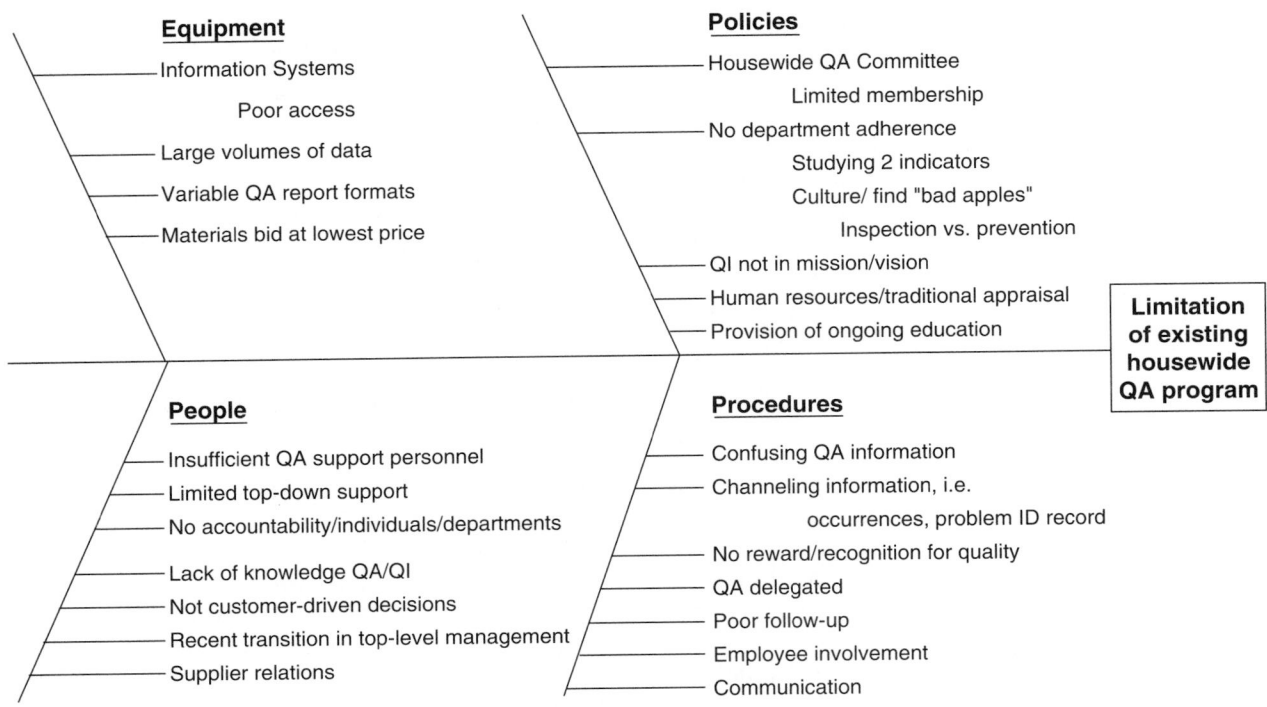

Fig. 14-1 Limitations of existing housewide QA program: cause and effect fishbone diagram.

make recommendations on moving toward QI. Because of the complexity of the project and desired pace that QRTF members established, meetings were scheduled every one to two weeks, over a period of six months. The Nursing QA coordinator, as chairperson of the group, set the agenda and assigned minute taking to different group members. Support from the members' own department heads provided freedom to negotiate time away from their already existing duties. Meetings were lively and often heated. Numerous group conflicts arose from differences of opinion as to whether quality problems were due to knowledge deficits, poor system design, or individual practitioner performance. QI problem analysis tools, such as the cause and effect diagram (Fig. 14-1), and flowcharts were helpful in categorizing causative factors contributing to the undesired outcome of ineffective QA practices. The chairperson welcomed overt disagreement, guided discussions toward quality problems and poor system design, and discouraged blaming of specific people and departments.

Group decisions were made based on consensus. Honest sharing of ideas, a passion for the subject, and frequent collaborative confrontations resulted in a highly cohesive, motivated work group. Although QRTF members came from a variety of disciplines and had varied self-interests, a common goal was reached. The QRTF agreed to explore causative factors that contributed to poor quality, and to make recommendations toward redesigning quality management practices.

The QRTF became internal consultants for QI. As the QRTF proceeded, it was realized the scope of the redesign project was immense. The mere size of the university teaching hospital seemed overwhelming: 610 beds, 19 medical departments, 50 nursing units, a growing ambulatory service, and innumerable support departments.

Despite the diversified scope of service, it was apparent that hindrances in achieving QA success occurring in one department were often repeated in several. So, identifying global trends, such as no assignment of QA responsibility, had greater value in the overall organizational assessment than specific department issues. In order to analyze multiple disciplines' efforts in QA, it became clear that the interdisciplinary nature of the QRTF was an asset, if not a necessity.

Data for organizational QA assessment was derived from brainstorming sessions within the QRTF, examination of QA meeting minutes, feedback from staff, physicians and management, JCAHO survey recommendations, and comparing and contrasting the current QA program with models in other teaching hospitals that had begun incorporating principles of QI. Analysis of committee and organizational structure helped in the formation of the recom-

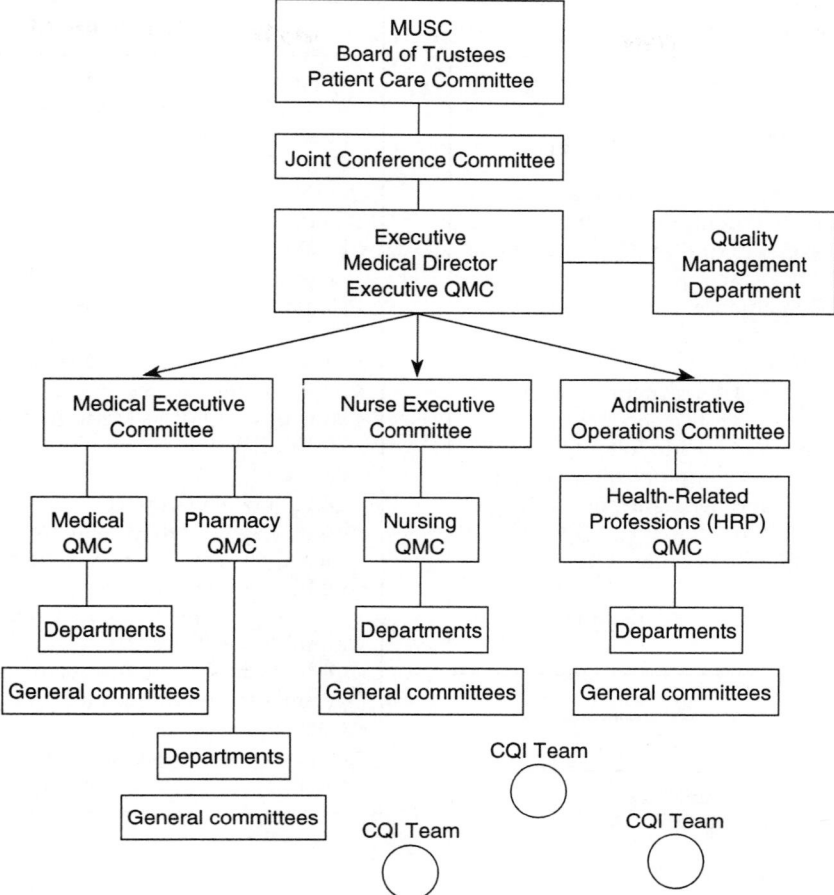

Fig. 14-2 MUSC Medical Center Quality Management Program Information Channeling Chart.

mended Quality Management Information Channeling Chart (Fig. 14-2).

QRTF Support

Initial support from top-level executives was an important factor in the QRTF success. Because of QA recommendations made from a JCAHO survey, the executive group began to demonstrate an increasing realization of the problems linked with current QA practices and an increasing curiosity about QI. Both the executive director of nursing and the newly appointed executive medical director were particularly vocal allies about the need for organization transformation toward continuous improvement. Peter Scholtes describes "the demography of change" as an important strategy for making change. He says that to lead change it is imperative to identify powerful individuals within the organization so that they can champion the transition to QI (Ernst & Young, 1990 p. 56). The executives were beginning to show evidence of becoming quality champions. They began to

meet regularly to discuss the QI transformation, their vision, and their role in it. Individuals were selected to serve on a formalized QI steering committee, which included most of the members of the QRTF. The QRTF began educating the executive group by circulating articles about QI, as well as periodic executive summaries of the QRTF activities. QRTF members began getting invitations to select executive meetings both to share their progress and to further gather data on attitudes and practices related to quality. Management commitment is an imperative as a means of leading cultural change toward QI.

QRTF RECOMMENDED ACTIONS

Implementation of CQI Plan

The results of the organizational assessment led the QRTF to design a quality plan that takes into account the existing weaknesses of the housewide QA program, as well as begins to incorporate principles of CQI. (See the boxes on p. 150.)

Purpose of CQI Plan

- Reaffirms commitment of top-level management and the Board of Trustees to pursue an active course toward CQI and hold departments accountable for continuous improvement of patient care and services
- Defines framework of Ten Step Model and other problem-solving tools that departments will use to monitor and evaluate quality and appropriateness of care
- Provides ongoing documentation, and review of improvements in patient care and systems that impact patient care
- Establishes interdisciplinary CQI structure for leaders to oversee CQI activities
- Centralizes CQI activities to provide follow-up of improvement efforts, enhanced communication, recognition of accomplishments, and avoidance of duplicated effort
- Coordinates and integrates existing QA activities within CQI structure
- Complies with standards of the JCAHO and other regulatory bodies

Objectives of CQI Plan

- Continual improvement of patient care
- Identification and review of opportunities to improve patient care
- Initiation of actions that resolve problems
- Identification of customers, their expectations, and efforts made in exceeding those expectations
- Detection of trends in patterns of performance, knowledge deficits, or interdisciplinary system problems
- Development of CQI educational program
- Documentation and communication of improvements

Scope of CQI Plan

- Encompasses all hospital departments and designated committees
- Focuses on the structure, process, and outcomes of patient care
- Includes system improvements and availability of resources

Authority

The chief quality officer (formally the executive medical director) at the request of the Board of Trustees, and as chairperson of the Executive Quality Management Council (E-QMC), has authority for overseeing the CQI plan. The line executive committees delegate the monitoring and evaluation activities to specific departments and are responsible for acting on the reports and recommendations from the Quality Management Councils.

Quality Management Councils (QMCs)

- The E-QMC membership includes the chief quality officer, executive director of nursing, chief executive officer, and director of pharmacy services.
- Chief financial officer, director of quality improvement, and chairpersons of the four QMCs are ad hoc members.
- E-QMC provides strategic short- and long-range planning and direction through the Quality Improvement Department, addresses issues unresolved at the QMC level, designs CQI budget, solicits outside CQI consultants as needed, and assigns and approves Project Improvement Teams.
- Four other QMCs (Medical, Nursing, Pharmacy, and Health Related Professions) are responsible for coordination of all department CQI activities.
- QMC membership consists of representatives from each hospital department, with the chairperson from each QMC serving as ex-officio members.
- QMC members review department minutes/reports, and prepare a synopsis for scheduled presentation at monthly meetings.
- QMC members provide feedback and education to departments they represent.
- QMC minutes are reviewed by QMC members, QMC chairpersons, designated executive committees, and the Executive QMC as needed.

Unit-based/Departmental CQI Plans

- The manager/department head is responsible for implementing and evaluating a unit-based CQI plan within his or her department.
- Unit-based CQI committees forward quarterly reports using an approved standardized format, on two important aspects of care through their line management channel, designated QMC, and Quality Improvement Department.
- Interdisciplinary Project Improvement teams are unit/department-based or are initiated centrally with approval of the Executive QMC.

General Committees (such as Infection Control, Pharmacy and Therapeutics, Standards of Care, and Blood Usage)

Designated general committees are accountable to their respective line executive committees and submit a semi-annual report of their activities and accomplishments to a designated QMC.

Quality Improvement Department

- The director of Quality Improvement reports directly to the chief quality officer and coordinates, ensures follow-up, and evaluates all CQI and QA activities within the hospital.
- Quality Improvement support staff serve as consultants and facilitators to the QMCs and individual departments.
- Coordinates CQI education.

Vision Statement: Ambulatory Quality Improvement Team

Values	Challenges
Respect	Space
Quality care	Faulty systems
Patient and employee satisfaction	Communication
Accuracy	No cooperation
Timeliness of service	Poor staffing/resources
Strategies	**Guiding Principles**
Training/education	Efficiency and effectiveness
Motivation/commitment	Customer-driven decisions
CQI measurement	

The Ambulatory Quality Improvement Team values and is committed to customer satisfaction (both internal and external), which is determined through measurement and improvement of key processes that impact patient care.

Comparison of CQI Plan to Existing QA Practices

Management Support. Acceptance of the CQI plan by top-level executives showed that there was a readiness to move in the direction of quality improvement. The plan was scrutinized and modified several times until there was consensus among the executives that the structure and functions described were workable. There was early realization that successful implementation would require a time commitment, long-range planning, major shifts in the organizational mission and structure, changes in management attitudes, and resource allocation. The executive medical director presented portions of the plan to the president of the Medical University and the dean of the Medical School. Formal assignment of responsibility for CQI was assigned to the executive medical director as well as a title change to chief quality officer. Encouragement was received from the president to pursue this direction and to establish a budget.

The CQI plan would require top management to become educated and lead the way. The managers' own education began by having the QRTF hold focused discussions describing the CQI plan, and review of the guiding principles of QI. The chief quality officer attended an extensive advanced business seminar at Harvard Business School that focused on the practices of QI. Members of the QRTF gave a half-day seminar to department heads and middle and top managers on the topic. The Executive QMC and members of the QRTF then visited the University of Michigan to learn about Michigan's experiences in planning for CQI. Early evidence of top management commitment was apparent.

Accountability and Follow-up. The CQI plan offered a structure for the leaders to oversee QI activities. Feedback from the chairpersons of the QMCs would allow the Quality Improvement Department to track improvements and make recommendations to the Executive QMC. Aspects of the plan that needed further development were the issues of rewards, recognition, incentives, communication channels, information systems, performance standards, and management expectations. The QRTF recommended the assignment of task forces to further explore these issues.

Change in Scope. Traditional QA practices focus primarily on clinical outcomes. The move towards QI expands the scope to include interdisciplinary improvement in systems and key processes as well. Instead of having one housewide QA committee, four QMCs coordinate and review the CQI activities within designated departments. All chairpersons of the QMCs served on each QMC to provide continuity across services (see the Quality Management Councils box on p. 150).

Quality Improvement Department. The reporting relationship for the director of Quality Improvement was changed. Previously, this position reported to the director of the Medical Records Department. In order to enhance visibility and alignment with top-level executives, the director of Quality Improvement, as manager of the Quality Improvement Department, now reports to the chief quality officer.

Creation of the Quality Improvement Department included the integration of existing quality-related functions. Risk management, utilization review and PRO activities, patient satisfaction and complaints, and existing QA support staff now come under the Quality Improvement Department. The addition of support staff positions to facilitate the QMCs and department CQI activities was approved.

Pilot Project Improvement Team

Despite being in the early phases of CQI planning, it was recognized that there were numerous opportunities for improvement that could begin to be addressed. A pilot interdisciplinary Ambulatory Quality Improvement Team (AQIT) was formed and co-

Identification of Customers

Internal	External
Attending physicians	Patients
Medical Records	Referring physicians
Secretaries	Third-party payers
Lab	Patients' families
Radiology	Area hospitals
Pharmacy	Community
Central Supply	Vendors and suppliers
Nursing	

Defining Customer (Patient) Requirements

Employee knowledge of systems
Clinical competence
Timeliness of service
Treatment with dignity and respect
Convenience

Brainstorming List of Ambulatory Problems

Lab results in a timely manner
Medical record access
Environment
Lab request process
Referral of patients
Scheduling
Delay in service
Patients arriving without appointment
Lack of patient-focused care

chaired by the Nursing QA coordinator. It was realized that the AQIT needed to receive CQI education, define its mission and areas to be improved, collect data, institute actions, evaluate those actions, and ascertain if the improvement was successful.

The Nursing QA coordinator held a formal inservice on the principles of QI. Ground rules were shared and agreed to by the team such as attendance, conduct during brainstorming, recording minutes, and commitment to the problem-solving process. A vision framework was devised by brainstorming what values, challenges, strategies and guiding principles that the group had in determining its vision of continuous improvement (see the box on p. 151).

After education and defining a group mission statement, ideas were solicited from the group as to the definition of their internal and external customers, defining customer requirements, and what was needed to exceed those requirements. Brainstorming then revealed a list of problems that the team in the ambulatory area encounters (see the three boxes on this page).

Through multivoting technique, team members then selected two problems that they viewed as high-volume, high-risk and problem-prone. The highest-priority problem that the group identified was the ordering of lab studies in the ambulatory area. A cause and effect fishbone diagram (Fig. 14-3) was used to elicit causative factors that contribute to patients having wrong studies done, omitting studies that were ordered, and studies not being on the patient's chart upon their arrival at the clinic. A flowchart helped the group to determine where in the process breakdowns in communication or flow of information occurred (Fig. 14-4). After group analysis

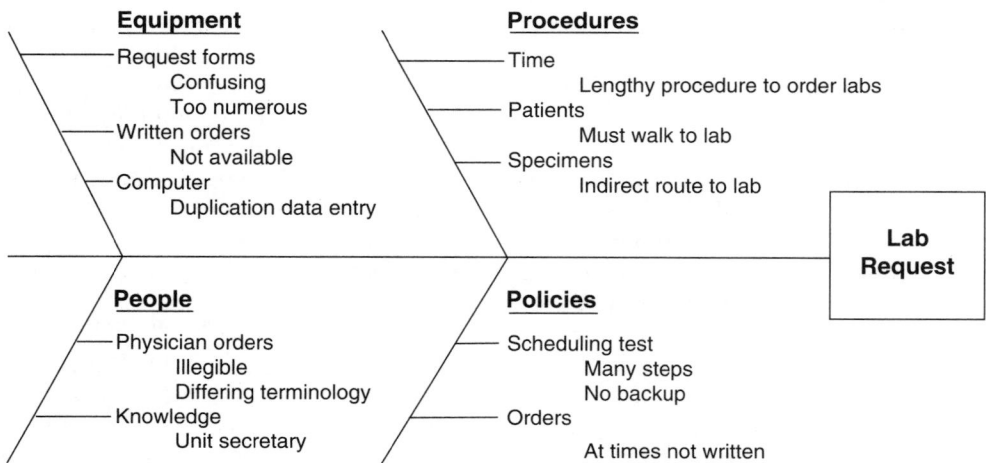

Fig. 14-3 Lab request: cause and effect fishbone diagram.

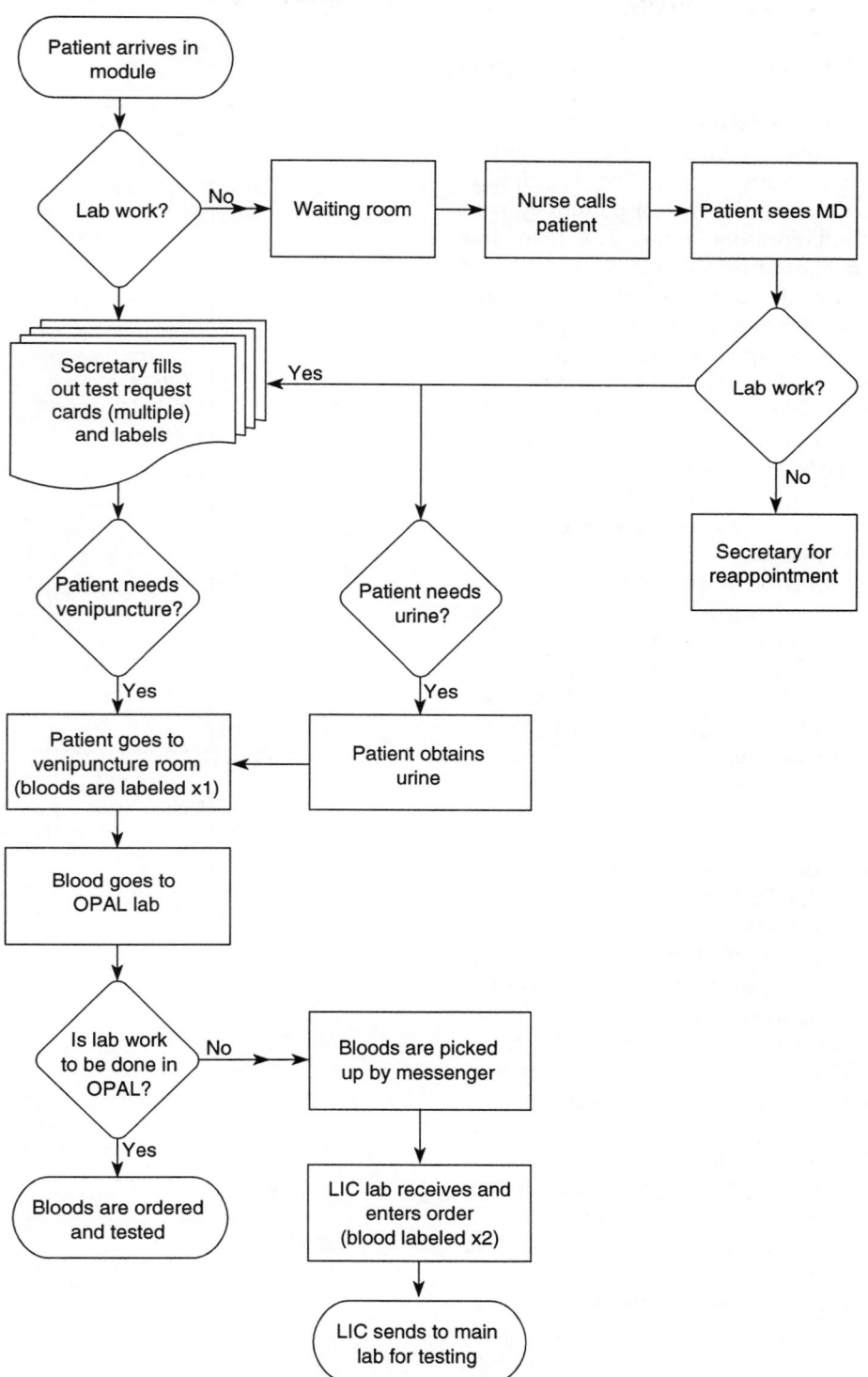

Fig. 14-4 Flowchart: current procedure.

the process was again flowcharted with recommended changes (Fig.14-5). A data-collection tool was then designed to ascertain the frequency of lab request cards being completed inaccurately, or sent to the wrong laboratory, and if patient location was listed (Fig. 14-6).

Through use of CQI tools and techniques, conclusions, recommendations, actions, and evaluation of those actions are now being determined. Originally, 16 lab request cards were being completed by unit secretaries to order laboratory work. The team has now designed and piloted one lab request card that lists clusters of lab profiles to be ordered. It was discovered that some patients were being charged twice for their visit because of duplication of lab-order entry into the computer, a problem that also has been remedied. Additional office space was allocated for order entry. Another venipuncturist was hired, and venipuncturists now carry beepers—which eliminates patients having to travel to the lab from the clinic office. Further analysis is under way to determine the efficacy of these interventions.

Use of QI tools and techniques demonstrated to the Ambulatory Project Improvement Team and the executive group that improvements can be accomplished with a planned approach to change, the empowerment of staff, willingness to collaborate, and placing customer expectations first. This example can be used internally to help educate others about the benefits of QI.

Strategies for Success

In addition to the commitment and knowledge of group members, the QRTF success can be attributed to several variables. A thorough organizational analysis allowed the QRTF to effectively devise the CQI plan. The group spent approximately 80 percent of the time on diagnosing system problems and 20 percent of the time on devising action plans. Examination of all existing QA components was done, including methods used to handle occurrence reports, information systems available, and adherence to JCAHO standards. This attention to detail proved extremely helpful in presenting recommended actions to the executive group. When probing questions were raised regarding our rationale for adding additional support staff to the QM Department, our responses were well thought out and supported with factual, persuasive data. This degree of preparedness facilitated acceptance of the CQI plan. Another strategy that helped with acceptance of the CQI plan was the manner in which the plan was presented. The QRTF selected several small groups of key executives representing areas of medicine, nursing, administration, medical records, and pharmacy services. Several meetings were scheduled with time devoted to edu-

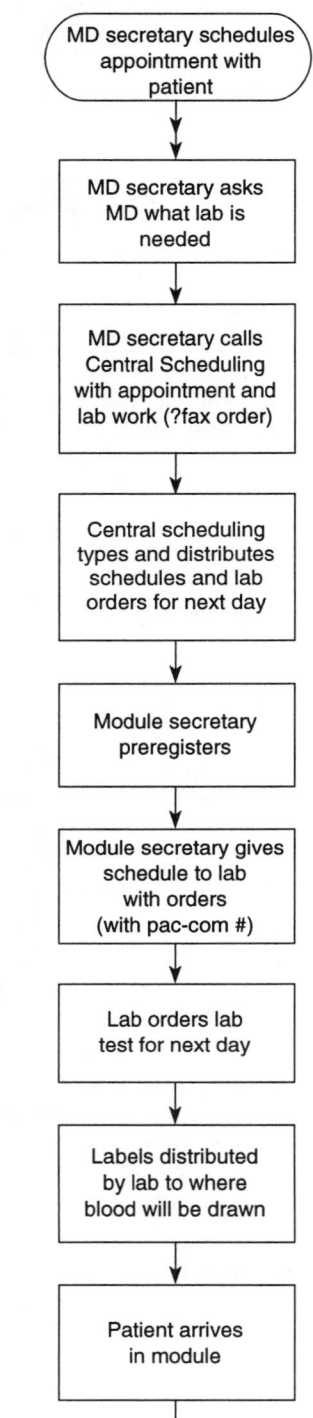

February 24, 1992
Recommended Revision Procedure for Lab Testing for Ambulatory Private Patients

Continued.

Fig. 14-5 Flowchart: recommended revised procedure.

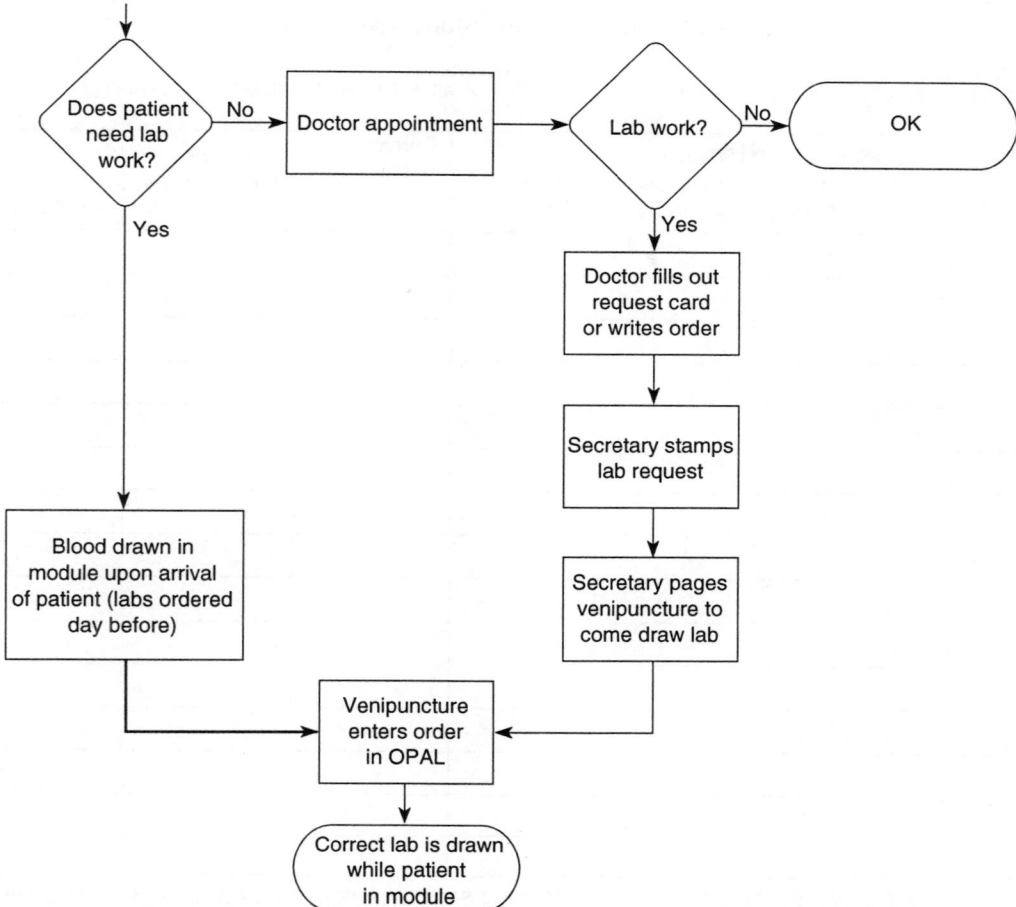

Fig. 14-5, cont'd. Flowchart: recommended revised procedure.

cation, presentation of the CQI plan, and discussion. When it was detected that certain executives were confused, uncertain, or showing resistance, a separate meeting with a few QRTF members was arranged for them.

Presentations of the CQI plan were succinct, polished, and always supplemented with audiovisual support in the form of slides. Hard copies of the plan were placed in binders with tabs, and distributed to the executives prior to the meetings. Accompanying the plan was a cover letter summarizing the content and asking that the executives read the material and come prepared with questions. One section of the distributed material housed articles on QI from industrial, medical, and administrative perspectives. Points and questions that participants raised were recorded, and follow-up was done by the QRTF. Suc-

cessful presentations entail knowing the audience, educating its members, and soliciting participation and feedback.

CONCLUSION

Adopting CQI as a management philosophy will require organizations to thoroughly examine their current methods of managing quality and to begin taking significant steps towards change. Quality experts within the organization can begin to analyze existing QA practices and initiate organization redesign toward QI. The QRTF at MUSC Medical Center was a catalyst in beginning to transform the organization from one that practices traditional QA to that of QI. Plans are under way to devise short- and long-range goals and the required resources needed for this transformation.

QI Blood Requisition Study – Ambulatory

System Outcome: Lab requests are completed accurately.
Special Instructions: Data collected by LIC or OPAL on all delinquent lab slips during 2 week period
_____.

Date	Time	Location (Module or Preregistration)	Patient Classified Correctly	Ordering MD Listed	Correct Test Request Card (If No, List Test & Card)	Nurse VP Labels Card & Tube Correctly	% Cum.	

CONFIDENTIAL: THIS REPORT IS INTENDED SOLELY FOR QUALITY ASSURANCE AND WILL BE USED ONLY BY AUTHORIZED INDIVIDUALS.

Fig. 14-6 QI blood requisition study—ambulatory.

REFERENCES

Crosby PB (1984): *Quality without tears—the art of hassle-free management*, New York, New American Library.

Ernst and Young Consulting Group (1990): *Total quality, an executive's guide for the 1990s*, Homewood, Ill, Dow Jones-Irwin.

Goal/QPC (1988): *The memory jogger plus +*, Goal/QPC, Methuen, Mass.

Marszalek-Gaucher E, RJ Coffey (1991): *Transforming healthcare organizations, how to achieve & sustain organizational excellence*, San Francisco, Jossey-Bass Publishers.

Meisenheimer CG (1992): *Improving quality, a guide to effective programs*, Gaithersburg, Md, Aspen Publishers.

Pinkerton SE, P Schroeder, *Commitment to excellence, developing a professional nursing staff*, Gaithersburg, Md, Aspen Publishers.

CREATING A CORPORATE QUALITY CULTURE THROUGH 100 PERCENT EMPLOYEE INVOLVEMENT

Catherine J. Buck
G. John Pandl
Jean A. Walters

INITIAL EFFORTS IN QUALITY MEASUREMENT

Froedtert Memorial Lutheran Hospital, a 300-bed tertiary care facility affiliated with the Medical College of Wisconsin in Milwaukee, began its journey toward continuous quality improvement in 1988. The hospital's strategic plan that year included a goal to "Establish a management/medical staff task force to devise a method for measuring the quality of Froedtert Hospital's clinical programs." Responsibility for completion of this goal was assigned to the vice president, patient care services.

The task force formed consisted of four members of the upper management team and four members of the hospital's medical staff. The management representatives included the vice president, patient care services, the assistant vice president, quality assurance, the assistant vice president, ancillary services, and the director of pulmonary cardiology. The physician representatives included the senior vice president, professional and academic affairs, the chairman of the hospital's utilization review committee, the physician responsible for quality assurance for the Medical College of Wisconsin, and a general surgeon. The task force began by formulating a working definition of quality and examining all quality efforts currently in existence on the Medical Center Campus. In pursuit of a model for quality measurement, standards from the Joint Commission on Accreditation of Healthcare Organizations, the Wisconsin Administrative Code for Hospitals, the Wisconsin Peer Review Organization, and other regulating bodies were studied. Computerized severity-of-illness systems including Medisgroups, Apache, Cost Quality Management System, Systemetrics, and others were carefully examined.

Late in 1988, an associate professor of biostatistics from the Medical College of Wisconsin was invited to join the task force. It was at his suggestion that the task force examined a computerized quality review process, under development by the Health Care Financing Administration (HCFA). Known as the Uniform Clinical Data Set (UCDS), this project was intended to expand and improve the ability of an agency to assure the quality of care delivered to Medicare beneficiaries using peer review organizations (PROs) as the principal mechanism. The task force examined this system to determine if it could be modified for use in hospitals to improve both the quality of care and the utilization of resources.

Uniform Clinical Data Set

In 1989, the Quality Measurement Task Force decided to enter into an agreement with HCFA to investigate whether the Uniform Clinical Data Set could be customized for use in hospitals. Two components of the UCDS of particular interest to Froedtert Hospital were (1) an extensive, detailed clinical data base and (2) a comprehensive set of computerized algorithms, a sequence of contingent or branching criteria that utilize this data base to determine whether there are opportunities for improvement in patient management. Three full-time nurse abstractors were hired to begin abstracting patient records and entering information into the UCDS. To start, three years' worth of medical records containing select diagnoses were reviewed. All patient records having a diagnosis of pneumonia, stroke, GI bleeding, or closed cranial trauma were entered into the system. The data base for each diagnosis was then analyzed with the assistance of the hospital's medical staff as well as faculty from the Department of Biostatistics at the Medical College of Wisconsin. This process constituted initial attempts in the area of quality improvement with the hospital's medical staff.

Productivity, Resource Utilization, Customer Satisfaction

The following year, the hospital continued its efforts in the area of quality measurement. The 1989 corporate strategies included direction to revise the hospital's productivity system in an effort to provide more meaningful data and useful management tools. The topic of appropriate utilization of resources was becoming one focus of the Quality Measurement Task Force. The annual strategies also called for the performance of market research to address the perception of the consumer regarding quality and the levels of consumer satisfaction, the results of which were used by the Management/Medical Staff Task Force on Quality Management.

It became increasingly apparent toward the end of 1989 that these three separate and distinct initiatives of productivity, customer satisfaction, and quality measurement were looking to one another for information, consultation, and overlapping representation. Discussions took place as to how the efforts could be effectively integrated. The solution was not clear until the hospital's president heard a speaker from Rush Presbyterian St. Luke's Medical Center in Chicago tell of its experience with total quality management. That organization had entered into a relationship with the 3M Company to learn from the experience of industry the principles and practice of total quality management. The president directed the administrative team to investigate this concept as a potential integration solution for the productivity, customer satisfaction, and quality measurement strategies. Site visits were made to two hospital institutions credited with pioneering the concept in healthcare.

Introduction to Total Quality Management

In 1990 quality remained Froedtert Hospital's number one corporate strategy. More specifically, the hospital's corporate plan called for an implementation plan to initiate the total quality management process through unification of the quality management, service management, and productivity programs. Additionally, the plan called for enhanced efficiency in the delivery of health care at Froedtert Hospital by eliminating the overuse of resources through the integration of cost/quality management concepts. More specifically, the administrative team was to develop a cooperative medical staff and management plan to identify specific target areas, communicate to clinicians, monitor applications, and document results.

Implementation Plan

A total quality management steering committee, with representation from the productivity, customer satisfaction, and quality measurement groups, was formulated. An implementation plan for this new concept was developed (see the boxes above).

Unsure of exactly how to proceed, the committee, named the Continuous Quality Improvement (CQI) Steering Committee, prepared a request for proposal

---

TQM/CQI* Implementation Plan: 1990	
1/90	Send requests for proposals (RFPs) to training/ consulting firms
2/90	Develop employee reward program
3/90	TQM/CQI management introduction meeting
4/90	Evaluation of RFP responses
6/90	Select training approach
8/90	Upper management training
10/90	Middle management training
12/90	Employee orientation to TQM/CQI

*The hospital moved away from the phrase *total quality management* and adopted *continuous quality improvement* in its place.

CQI Implementation Action Plan: 1991	
1/91	Employee orientation to TQM/CQI
3/91	Team leader training
3/91	Kickoff
6/91	Develop model for MD role in CQI
6/91	Educational needs assessment
6/91	CQI director in place
9/91	Evaluation of recognition program
10/91	Six-month financial performance report
11/91	CQI Team of the Year Award dinner
11/91	Board/management/physicians CQI retreat

---

to obtain assistance in the establishment of such an effort at Froedtert Hospital. Eight requests for proposals were sent to various companies, including 3M, the Juran Institute, and Avatar International, known for their commitment to 100 percent employee involvement.

Much consideration was given to choosing the quality improvement approach and model most consistent with the organization's culture. Deming's philosophy that revolutionized Japan was of intense interest to the steering committee. His 14 points seemed a well-defined road map for the changes that needed to take place at Froedtert Hospital. How exactly to apply and use Dr. Deming's methods, however, became the source of significant conflict among the committee's membership. With the allocated resources, the steering committee was faced with the question of which and how many employees to involve. Provide intensive training to a select group such as the management team or involve other layers of the organization? The advantages and disadvantages of each approach were considered.

The management kickoff/introduction to continuous quality improvement occurred in March 1990. Patrick Townsend, author of *Commit to Quality* (1986), led a Froedtert Hospital retreat sharing his

---

Vision Statement for the Continuous Quality Improvement Process

Quest
Froedtert Memorial Lutheran Hospital

Froedtert Memorial Lutheran Hospital is committed to the pursuit of continuous quality improvement to build upon our reputation as an outstanding academic health center. *All* individuals associated with Froedtert Hospital are involved in our foremost objective, which is to meet the needs and expectations of those we serve. We strive to provide an exceptional work environment where:

Quality Underscores Every Single Task

---

experience in quality improvement and commitment to 100 percent employee involvement. He professed that rather than asking the question "who can we get to volunteer for this stuff?" one should ask, "who can we afford to leave out?" He stressed the need to examine if the organization was "doing the right things" as well as whether the organization was "doing things right." His amusing, anecdotal stories drove the point home that conformance to customer expectations 100 percent of the time was a reasonable goal.

Through 1990, the steering committee met two to three times monthly as it worked on the implementation plan. Patrick Townsend was employed to train the upper management team in the principles of quality improvement. Avatar International provided three days of training to the middle management group in preparation for initiation of the quality improvement process.

Continuous Quality Improvement: The Vision

The continuous quality improvement vision statement was shared with the employees and displayed in each department. The process was titled QUEST, an acronym for Quality Underscores Every Single Task. The vision statement for the continuous quality improvement process is shown in the box above.

FMLH Model

The Froedtert Hospital model was patterned after Patrick Townsend's model as described in *Commit to Quality.* All hospital employees were to be members of a quality improvement team. The components of the QUEST process were (1) quality improvement teams, (2) 100 percent employee involvement, (3) ongoing training, (4) customer surveys, (5) communication, (6) cross-functional analysis, (7) integration of quality assurance and quality improvement, and (8) recognition.

Physician involvement in the process occurred when the physician was part of the problem or part of

the solution. Additionally, the medical staff was forming departmental teams to examine opportunities for improvement as revealed by the Uniform Clinical Data Set. In essence, two efforts were running side by side, the QUEST process and the UCDS initiative. To date, integration is slow but occurring.

Organizational Chart

The QUEST process began with 100 percent employee involvement. It was decided by the steering committee that all Froedtert Hospital employees would participate in and contribute to the CQI process through membership on a quality improvement team.

The staff constitutes the quality improvement teams, which are each made up of 8 to 12 members. Each department, depending on its size, has one to six teams. Because management has made a strong commitment to this effort, team members consider their participation a priority responsibility, not an intrusion on their real jobs.

The team members are responsible for contributing to and acting on opportunities to improve. This is accomplished through sharing knowledge and expertise, participating in meetings and discussions, carrying out assignments between meetings, interviewing customers, observing processes, gathering data, writing reports, and so on.

Each team has an appointed team leader. This individual facilitates the team process, arranges logistical details, and prepares documentation. The leader is the contact point for communication between the team and the rest of the organization, including the quality improvement director.

The QI director serves in an advisory role to the teams. This individual focuses on team process rather than product, and is concerned with how decisions are made and what decisions are reached. The director assists teams in structuring or breaking down a task into individual assignments. The QI director also serves as an expert in continuous quality improvement philosophy as well as in data collection and analysis techniques.

The Quality Improvement Steering Committee was initially responsible for defining the procedures that frame the structure of the quality process. The committee now assists in guiding the QUEST process as it evolves and serves in an advisory capacity to the QI director as well as to the quality improvement teams. The steering committee members are key CQI resource people within Froedtert Hospital.

Fig. 15-1 illustrates the initial organizational model employed by the hospital.

Training

The first important part of implementing CQI was training. The steering committee hoped that if all hos-

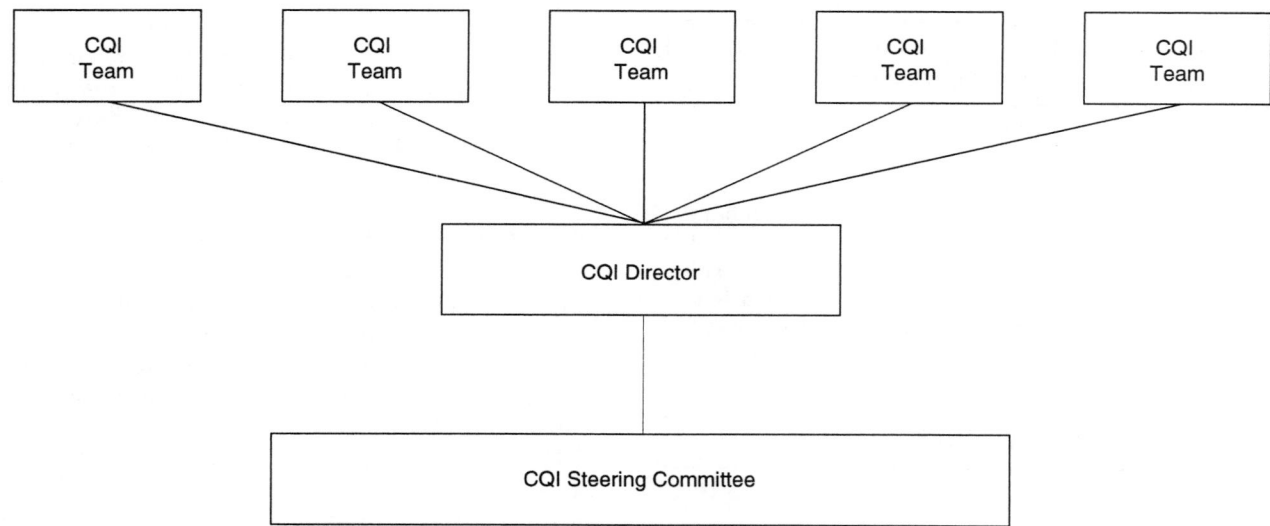

Fig. 15-1 Organizational model for the continuous quality improvement process at Froedtert Hospital.

pital employees received a firm foundation in the principles of QI, they would better understand how to implement and utilize the process effectively. Much confusion and concern existed about the program. Employees were questioning whether they would really have the power to make changes. They questioned whether management would relinquish their authority.

Orientation began for all employees in December 1990. After much discussion by the steering committee, it was decided that all employees would be given a 90-minute orientation to the process and that additional training could be given at intervals after implementation as necessary. Members of the steering committee volunteered to conduct the training sessions. This initial training described the history, purpose, and techniques of quality improvement, the benefits of such a process, team structure and proposed meeting schedules, how to select opportunities or problems to work on, and the rewards built into the process. Many employees questioned whether the administration would allow them to have this important role in solving problems in the hospital; this was a frequently asked question during training. Another area of concern dealt with how to fit 30 minutes of meeting time each week into an already busy work schedule. Upper management assured the employee teams that time for this process was to be built into their work day.

During the initial orientation, the role of the team leader was discussed. Managers were given the authority to choose team leaders for their area, identifying one Leader for every 10 or 12 employees. Based on the number of employees in the department, the steering committee had tentatively identified how many teams each department would have, but this

was also subject to change at a manager's request. After the initial training, some staff members indicated that they would be interested in being a team leader; they were encouraged to contact their manager concerning this request. Team leaders were given a three-day training program.

The team leader training was comprehensive. Leaders were trained in the actual "how to's" of carrying out the QUEST process. They were taught how to lead a group and what different characteristics team members may play: for example, how to draw out a quiet member, how to work with a complaining member, how to work with the member who takes over the group. In addition, team leaders were introduced to a number of techniques for brainstorming, identifying and refining problems, investigating and studying problems, implementing suggested solutions, and evaluating the results. For instance, team leaders were taught how to conduct surveys, how to use a fishbone diagram to more clearly determine cause and effects, and how to work with a force field analysis to study opposing influences and determine which approach would help to reach the desired situation.

Team leaders were given an opportunity to work in groups to identify problems and carry out each of the steps during the training. At the end of three days, the team leaders had identified actual problems in the hospital and investigated possible solutions for them. A number of solutions were subsequently implemented after team leading training.

The current functions of the Team Leader are to facilitate the team process, arrange logistical details and coordinate documentation for the QI director. It is the responsibility of the Team Leader to communicate regularly with his or her manager and the QI

Director regarding the team's activities and progress. The Team Leader also utilizes the manager and/or CQI Director to clarify whether a proposed change is within the realm of the team's authority.

Survey

A survey of all employees was done in February 1991 to identify opportunities for improvement. Eight hundred forty-five employees responded to the survey, which consisted of 118 questions that could be answered on a five-point scale. The answers were categorized into 14 different categories and then were analyzed by department. Each department's scores were compared to its division and the hospital at large. Areas of strength included community standing, interpersonal relations, working conditions, and overall job satisfaction—which accounted for about 30 percent of the total items. Areas where need for improvement was indicated were administrative style, physician relations, and rewards. The Administrative Team took these results and made changes to increase the visibility of these issues. It also implemented several solutions that improved communication with the Cost Center Manager group. Plans are in place to resurvey all employees 18 to 24 months after the first survey.

75 percent of the employees completed the survey. The survey results were compiled by outside consultants and distributed to hospital administration and to all departments.

Kickoff

The kickoff began in March 1991 after much planning by the steering committee. The steering committee felt that having a well-planned, creative kickoff would be a telling statement to all hospital employees. Managers were available to assist with kickoff activities throughout the entire day. The steering committee organized the activities and assigned managers on all three shifts to various tasks.

The theme was set from the moment the employees entered the hospital. A huge sign told all who entered that they were entering "Q Country" (Quality Country). QUEST balloons were tied throughout the corridors and in the cafeteria. Managers were stationed at the end of the parking lot corridor to give coffee and donuts to all employees and visitors who entered in the morning. Team leaders wore T-shirts with the QUEST logo. Although T-shirts were not part of the dress code, team leaders were allowed to wear their shirts at work on this day in recognition of their new status. Team leaders also had "Team Leader" inscribed on their name tags as a sign of recognition.

Throughout the kickoff day, managers delivered cookies to day and evening shift employees. On the night shift, several managers distributed pizzas.

One highlight of the kickoff were QUEST-O-Grams. A QUEST-O-Gram was a gold piece of paper with "QUEST-O-Gram" at the top, the QUEST logo on the side, and the message, "Thank you for _____ ." They gave employees the opportunity to write a message of thank you, praise, or recognition to any employee or volunteer, highlighting something special which that employee had done. On the day of the kickoff, QUEST-O-Grams were delivered in person by managers to employees at their work places. It took only a little time for the employees to begin utilizing QUEST-O-Grams. Once employees started receiving QUEST-O-Grams and other employees saw the positive benefit, they quickly began to write their own QUEST-O-Grams. More than 2,000 were written and delivered on the day of the kickoff. The QUEST-O-Grams were received so positively that they became a permanent part of the QUEST process.

SOLVE Process

A multistep problem-solving model became the basis of the CQI process. This model, created by Avatar International, involves five primary steps: *S*olvable problems and opportunities, *O*bservable causes, *L*ogical solutions, *V*alidation by peers or management, and *E*mpirical results. At each step, the team identifies many alternatives and narrows them down to one or more specific items based on the data available. This model is displayed in Fig. 15-2.

Fig. 15-3 illustrates the team process from the initial idea to its implementation. Not all steps pictured need to be accomplished with every process, yet each step is considered.

Validation by management is required only if the solution requires money, information, or coordination beyond the team's control. It is advisable for the team leader to inform his or her manager regularly so he or she can be a resource to the team. The team leader may need to gain support from co-workers prior to implementation. Evaluation of the solution is the final step.

Recognition Process

Industry has demonstrated that there are advantages and disadvantages to employee recognition programs. Froedtert Hospital's recognition program was designed to recognize the CQI teams and employees who make the contributions that add to the quality of service. The program was created to be understandable, easy to administer, and flexible enough to be adjusted as the situation dictates. The CQI Steering Committee realized that each person values different types of recognition, the greatest of which comes from the internal knowledge of a job well done.

Team recognition awards are given to the members of the teams who reach the stated levels of ideas or

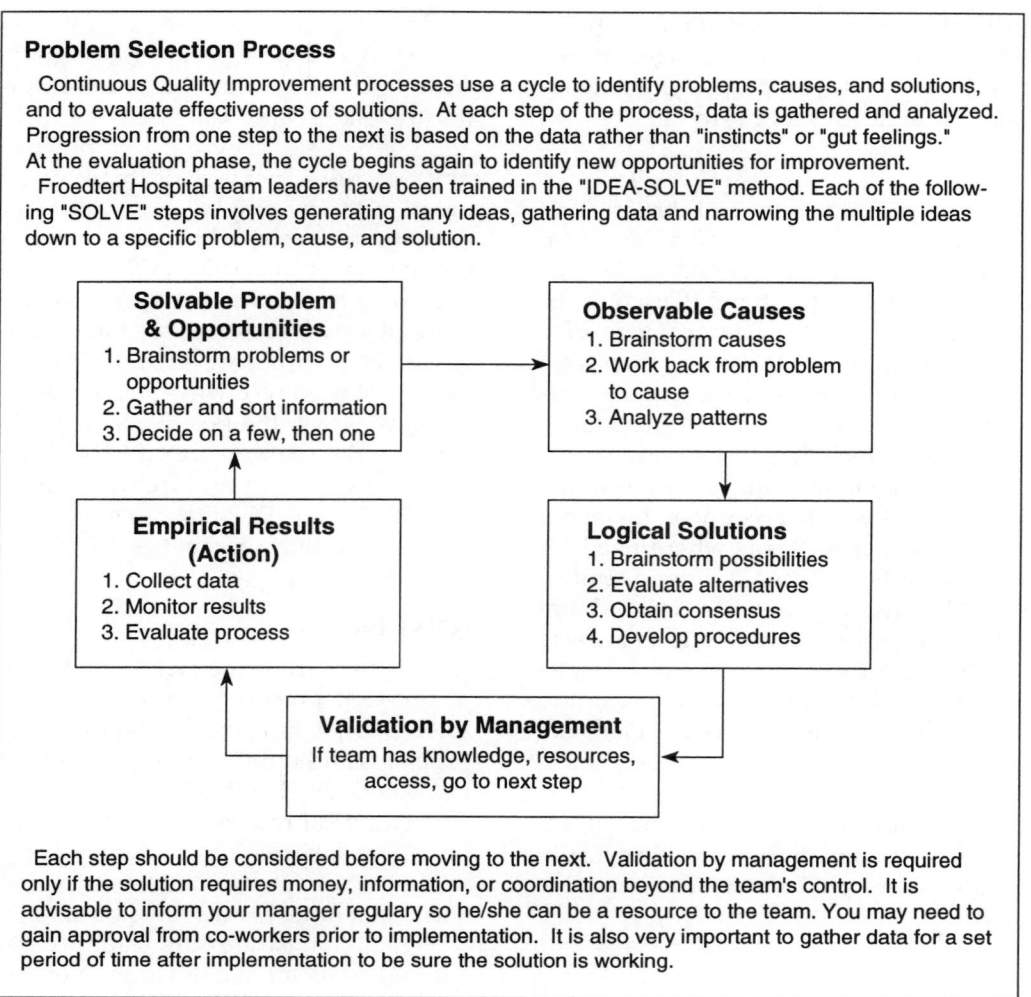

Problem Selection Process

Continuous Quality Improvement processes use a cycle to identify problems, causes, and solutions, and to evaluate effectiveness of solutions. At each step of the process, data is gathered and analyzed. Progression from one step to the next is based on the data rather than "instincts" or "gut feelings." At the evaluation phase, the cycle begins again to identify new opportunities for improvement.

Froedtert Hospital team leaders have been trained in the "IDEA-SOLVE" method. Each of the following "SOLVE" steps involves generating many ideas, gathering data and narrowing the multiple ideas down to a specific problem, cause, and solution.

Solvable Problem & Opportunities
1. Brainstorm problems or opportunities
2. Gather and sort information
3. Decide on a few, then one

Observable Causes
1. Brainstorm causes
2. Work back from problem to cause
3. Analyze patterns

Empirical Results (Action)
1. Collect data
2. Monitor results
3. Evaluate process

Logical Solutions
1. Brainstorm possibilities
2. Evaluate alternatives
3. Obtain consensus
4. Develop procedures

Validation by Management
If team has knowledge, resources, access, go to next step

Each step should be considered before moving to the next. Validation by management is required only if the solution requires money, information, or coordination beyond the team's control. It is advisable to inform your manager regulary so he/she can be a resource to the team. You may need to gain approval from co-workers prior to implementation. It is also very important to gather data for a set period of time after implementation to be sure the solution is working.

Fig. 15-2 SOLVE Process. *Created by Avatar International.*

documented cost savings. Ideas need not necessarily save money for the hospital. However, for those ideas that do save money, cost savings must be documented and measurable in order to receive credit. Projected cost savings are annualized. It is the annualized amount that is used when determining specific awards (see the box on p. 164).

A "Team of the Year" is selected by a committee made up of team leaders. Selection is based on the accomplishments of the team during the previous year.

Individual employee awards are designed to recognize those "moments of truth" when an employee puts forth extra dedication and effort that are recognized by a customer. These honors are called Customer Service Awards and, as such, reflect the times when an employee goes out of his or her way to serve.

The individual Customer Service Awards take the shape of "Quality Coins." The intent is for each manager or designee to distribute these coins in recognition for customer service efforts. Staff may recom-

mend that awards be given to individuals outside of their area. These recommendations are made to the appropriate manager. The coins can be redeemed through the cashier, cafeteria or the gift shop. Each is worth $10 in cash, gifts, or meal passes. Many individuals have also made creative key chains and other items to show off their coins.

The second means of individual employee recognition is through the use of the QUEST-O-Grams, which any employee can send through interoffice mail.

EXAMPLES OF TEAM PROJECTS

Wheelchair Availability in Lobby

One problem addressed was a lack of wheelchairs in the lobby of the hospital for incoming patients. This was a chronic problem, one which became more acute with the opening of the new Ambulatory Care Building, which significantly increased traffic through the lobby to the new outpatient clinics (as well as existing

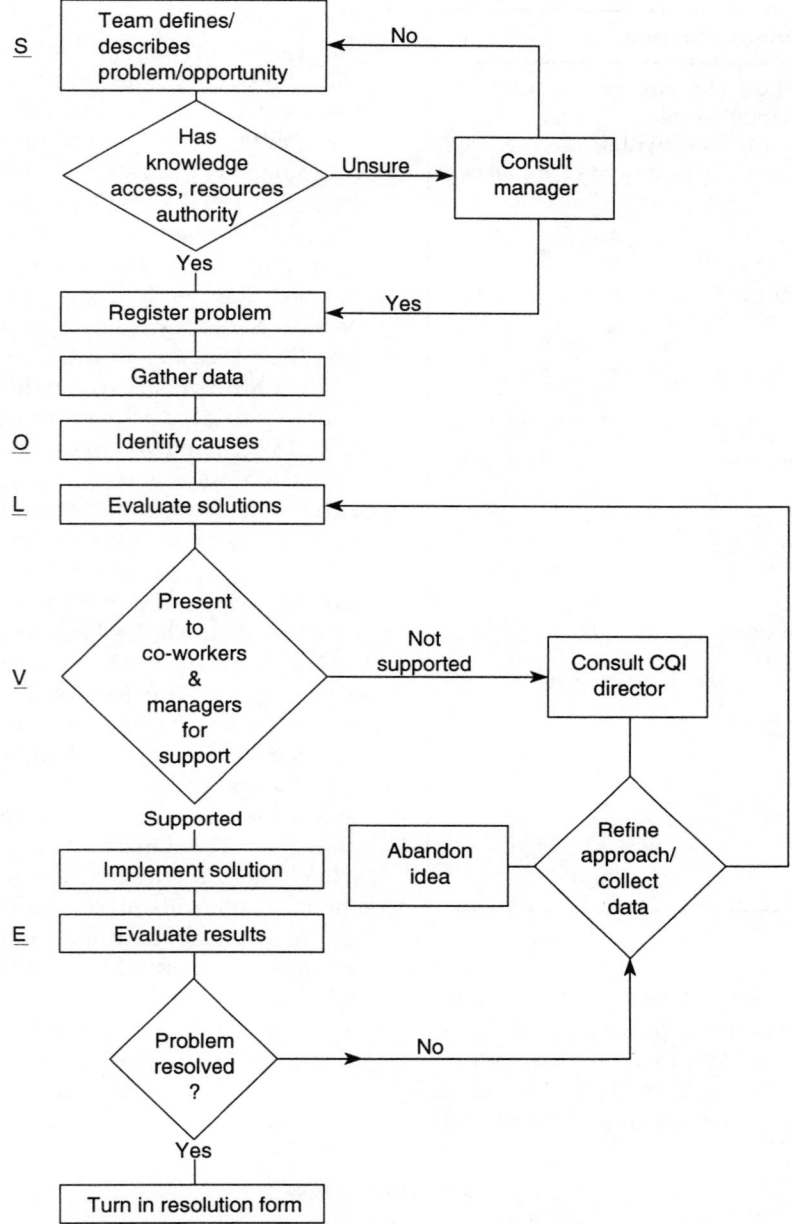

Fig. 15-3 Flowchart of quality improvement team process.

clinics). Past solutions of gathering wheelchairs to the lobby were short-lived, as the wheelchairs soon disappeared. Another solution of purchasing new wheelchairs on an annual basis seemed to alleviate the problem only for a few months, after which time the new wheelchairs were widely circulated and began to disappear like the older ones. The problem was first identified by a multidisciplinary group of managers who were trying to identify problems and opportunities to improve meeting customer needs. This team decided to approach a team of transporters, as they were the users of wheelchairs. The team was also joined by a representative from the Information Desk (Telecommunications Department) and a security guard.

The transporters said the solution appeared to be to purchase additional wheelchairs. However, as the teams met, it became apparent that the answer to several key questions were unknown. What is the traffic flow through the lobby at various times during the day? What is the average number of wheelchairs available at various times? How many wheelchairs are needed to adequately accommodate patients? Where are the wheelchairs going when they disappear? Is there a way to get wheelchairs back to the lobby when taken for patients? The transporters were willing to gather data to answer these questions, and the managers assisted with data analysis.

Recognition Program

The quality improvement director has the authority and responsibility to award credit for ideas or cost savings. The specific awards are listed below and are modeled after the Paul Revere Experience as described in *Commit to Quality.*

Quality Ideas	Award
Bronze	
10 Resolutions or minimum of $10,000 in savings	Bronze Pin
Silver	
25 Resolutions or minimum of $25,000 in savings	Silver Pin & $25
Gold	
50 Resolutions or minimum of $50,000 in savings	Gold Pin & $50
Platinum	
75 Resolutions or minimum of $75,000 in savings	$75
Diamond	
100 Resolutions or more than $100,000 savings	$100
Double Bronze	
125 Resolutions	$25
Double Silver	
150 Resolutions	$50
Double Gold	
175 Resolutions	$75
Double Diamond	
200 Resolutions	$100

Data was gathered on the number of wheelchairs available in the lobby each hour from 8 a.m. to 8 p.m. Monday through Friday during three separate weeks in September through November 1991. The range was wide, from as many as eight to as few as zero.

The combined averages of all three weeks indicated that two to three wheelchairs were usually available (Fig. 15-4). Next, the volumes of clinic visits per hour were calculated. It was determined that 8 a.m., 2 p.m., and 10 p.m. had the highest volumes, and the combined volumes of 8 a.m. and 10 p.m. were enough to occasionally deplete the stock of wheelchairs. The team decided from this data that for the most part, there were enough wheelchairs available to meet the needs if they could be kept circulating back to the lobby. They also decided that six to eight was the necessary number, with six the minimum.

Next a flowchart was made to indicate what happens when a patient is transported in a wheelchair (Fig. 15-5). The team discovered that there were three crucial points where wheelchairs were likely to disappear. These are designated with an asterisk. The team realized a solution had to involve retrieving wheelchairs from Milwaukee County Hospital, an adjoining facility, and getting wheelchairs that were left by patients in clinics back to the lobby.

The team decided to brainstorm other causes for disappearing wheelchairs, and these were organized into a cause and effect diagram (Fig. 15 - 6). The team decided to highlight with an asterisk each cause it felt it had some control over changing, an important criterion for a successful solution. Causes included no place to park wheelchairs in lobby, no set number of wheelchairs for lobby, no formal way to get wheelchairs from Milwaukee County Hospital, patients taking wheelchairs home, and wrong equipment on wheelchairs. Now the team was ready to begin considering solutions.

The team decided on several solutions to address the multiple causes of wheelchairs disappearing from the lobby. First, there were several wheelchairs in circulation that could be easily collapsed, put in a car,

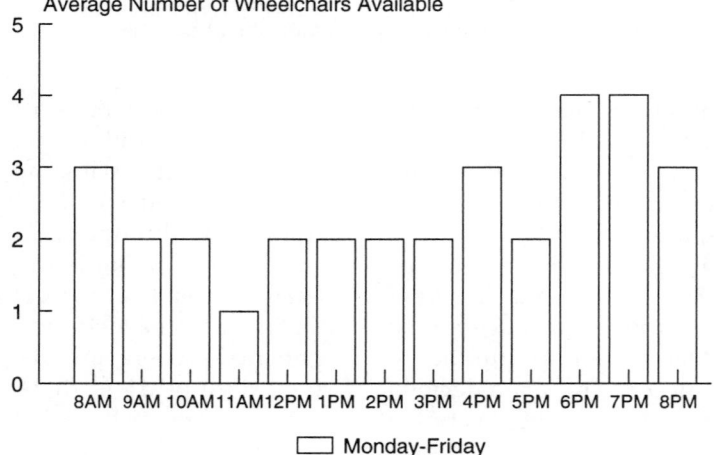

Fig. 15-4 Average number of wheelchairs available each hour from 8 a.m. to 8 p.m.

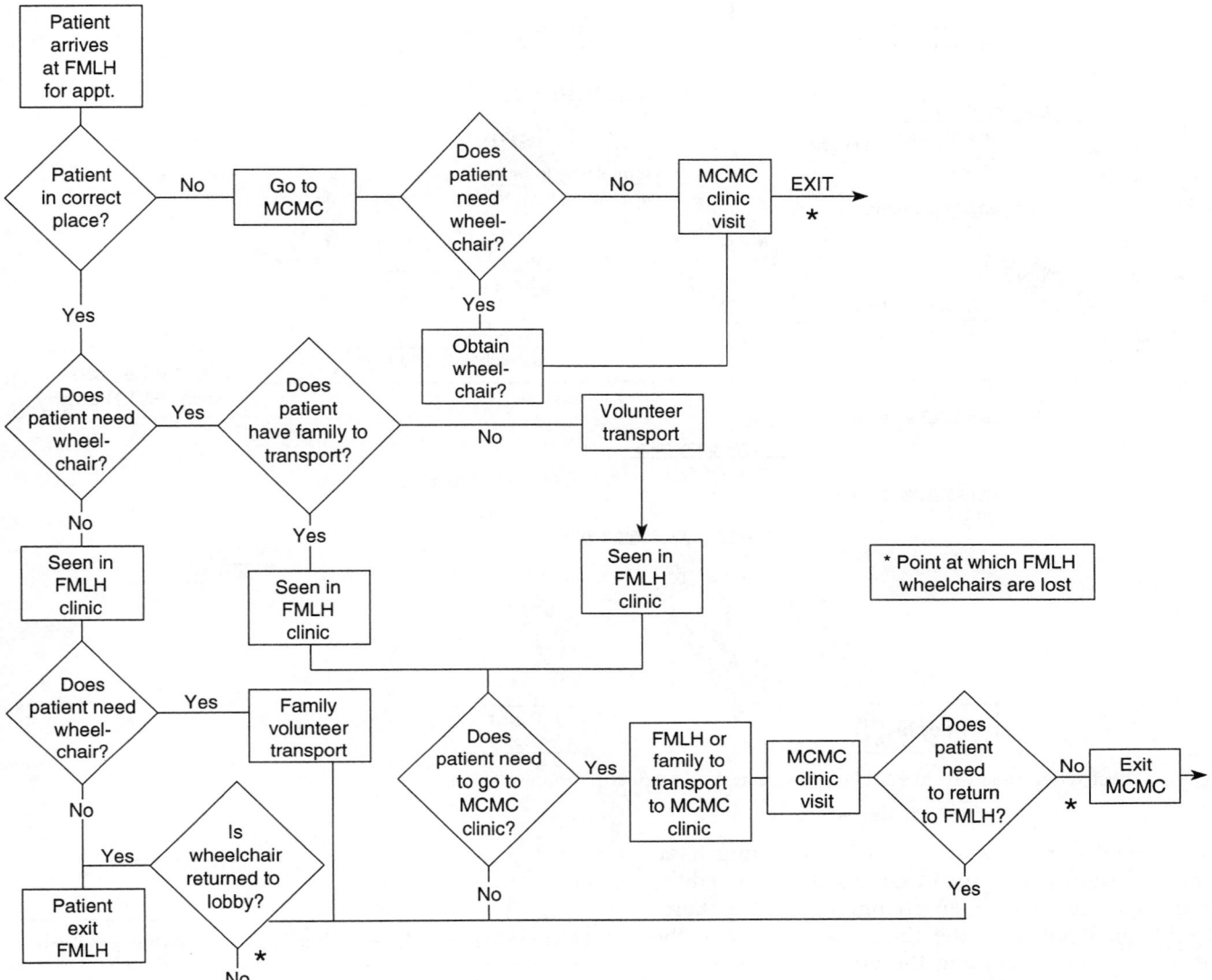

Fig. 15-5 Flowchart: Patients in need of wheelchairs to Froedtert Hospital outpatient clinics. An asterisk denotes a critical point.

and taken. A metal bar was installed in those chairs, preventing them from being collapsed. A space was made available in the corner of the lobby for storage of wheelchairs waiting to go into use. The transporters decided that the transporters assigned to the therapy area would have time to make a run to Milwaukee County Medical Complex in the morning before taking patients to scheduled therapy appointments. A memo was sent to all clinic receptionists and administrators requesting they call the Information Desk if a wheelchair was left in the clinic by a patient or family so someone could come to get the wheelchair. Security and parking attendants were invited to a meeting to address wheelchairs left by the exit to the parking structure—which created a fire hazard. They agreed to return wheelchairs to circulation in the lobby. Finally, it was decided that if the lobby wheelchairs were marked as such, they would be eas-

ily identified and returned to the lobby area. Because many were in need of repair, new backs of seats were ordered in gray, which matched the lobby color scheme and was noticeably different from the blue of the other wheelchairs. On the backs, FMLH LOBBY and a number were painted for additional identification. These changes resulted in wheelchairs being available when needed at all times since March 1, 1992.

Linen-Change Policy

Approximately two months after kickoff, two of the QUEST teams from the Department of Nursing simultaneously identified a problem with the hospital's linen-change policy. The two teams joined forces to tackle the issue. The problem was recorded as, "Too much time, energy and money is spent on unnecessary linen changes." This combined team along with

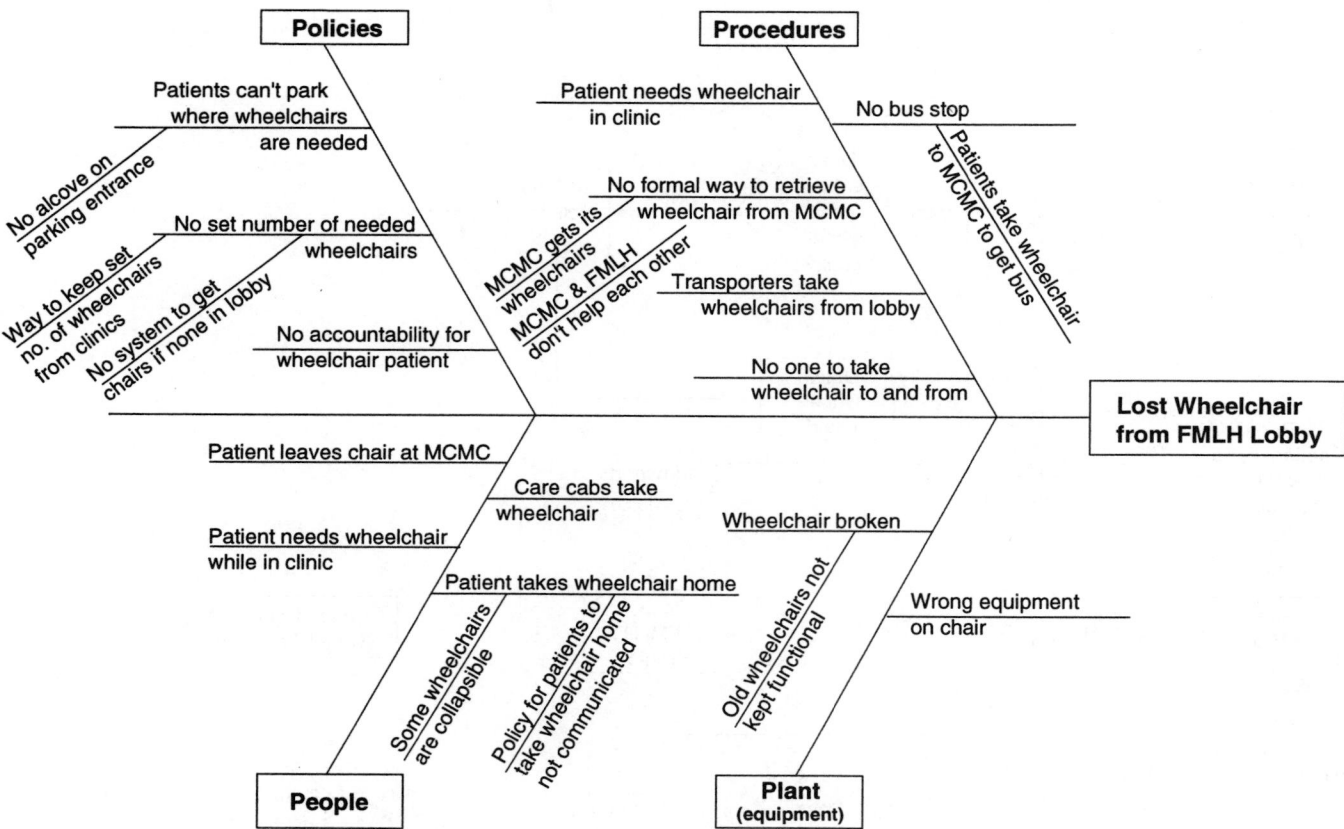

Fig. 15-6 Lost wheelchairs from FMLH lobby: cause and effect fishbone diagram.

the hospital nursing staff began by collecting data. For a four-week period the nursing staff evaluated the need for a complete linen change on each patient. The hospital policy at the time was to change the entire bed daily, including the bedspread. Data collection revealed that 59 percent of patients needed a complete linen change and 41 percent did not. This QUEST team determined that at least 75 patients per day were receiving unnecessary linen changes. A new bed linen-change policy was drafted and approved. A cost benefit analysis was performed (Table 15-1). A nursing staff education program was designed by the QUEST team to help in implementation of the change. The entire process took five months. The anticipated annual cost savings for laundering of linen was anticipated to be $91,572.

This QUEST team received a Gold award for its efforts.

Arranging Clinic Appointments Prior to Discharge

An example of clearly defining a complex problem and breaking it down into specific components can be drawn from the effort to address the excessive amount of time taken by Clinical Systems communicators (unit clerks) to make clinic appointments for patients being discharged. The practice of having the communicator make the clinic appointment for the

TABLE 15-1 Bed Linen Change Cost Savings Analysis

Item	Cost
Linen	
Average linen per patient per day is 8 lb. at $0.21/lb.	$1.68 per day
7 × weekly linen change cost	$11.76 per week
3 × weekly linen change cost	$5.04 per week
Difference per week/per patient	$6.72
Savings per week at approximate daily census (ADC) of 185	$12.43
Annualized savings in linen costs	$64,636
Labor	
Nursing time of 5 min. per complete vs 2 min. per partial bed is a 3 min. per bed savings	
Present situation	1,295 beds/week
Changed to	555 beds/week
37 hours/week saved at $14/hour	$518 per week
Annualized savings in labor cost	$26,936
Total Cost Savings	**$91,572**

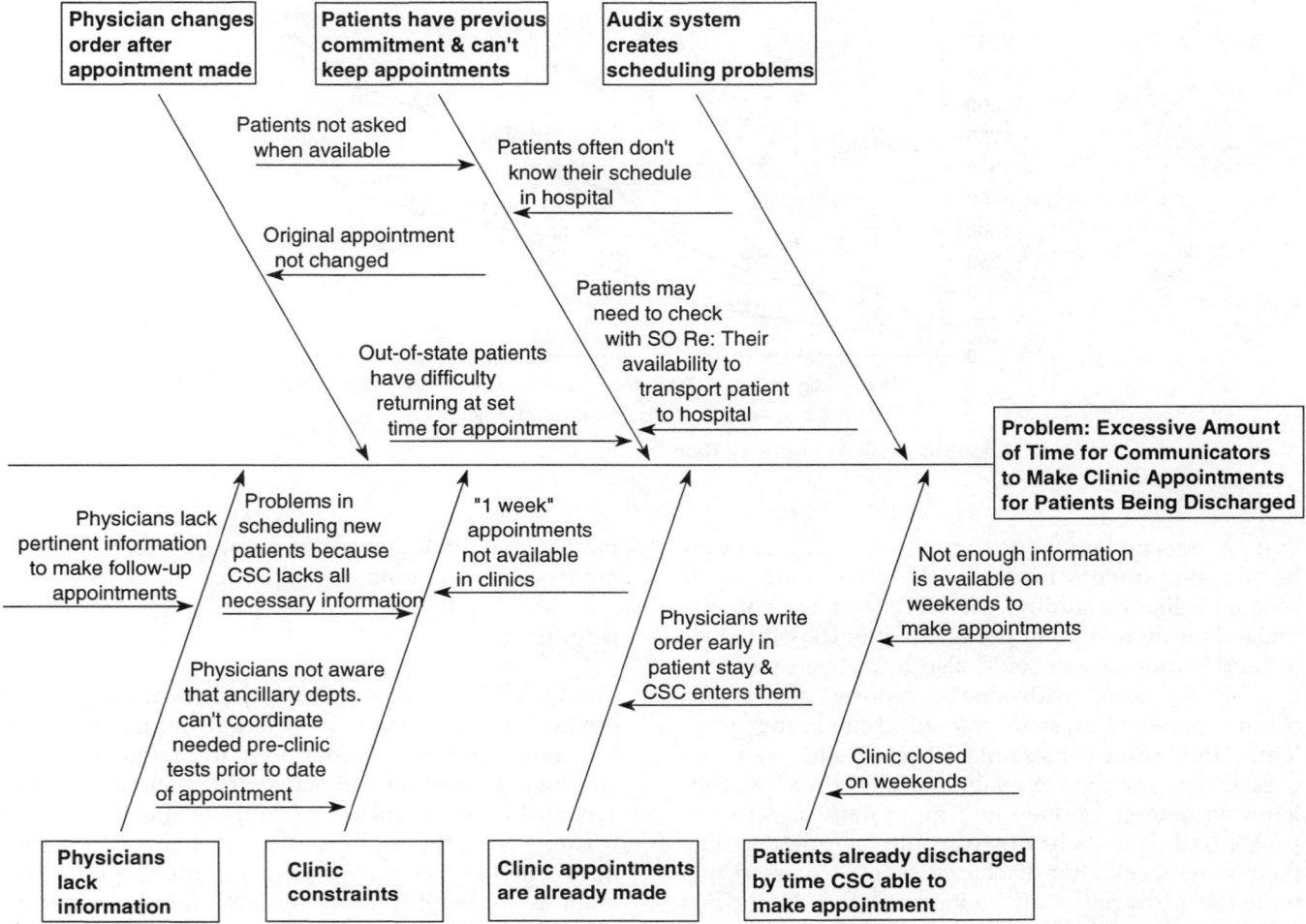

Fig. 15-7 Excessive amount of time for appointment scheduling at discharge: cause and effect fishbone diagram.

patient prior to the patient's discharge had been practiced since the hospital's opening. Numerous problems existed with this system. The communicators frequently had difficulty contacting the clinic to obtain an appointment. The appointment time was not always convenient for the patient, and the no-show rate was very high. The communicators felt that an opportunity to improve existed in this complex issue.

One communicator QUEST team used the brainstorming technique to reduce this broad issue into different, more specific problems. Numerous techniques were used to assess the severity of the problems including a fishbone cause and effect diagram, Pareto charts to determine the amount of time taken to make the appointments, and statistics on average numbers of no-show rates for clinic patients.

The cause and effect diagram helped to examine the multiple causes of this complex problem, such as the excessive amount of time it was taking communicators to make clinic appointments for patients being discharged (Fig. 15-7). The diagram systematically clarified both major and minor causes of the problem and helped define less apparent contributors to the problem.

When evaluating causes identified by the fishbone diagram, the communicators documented the frequency, duration, amount, rate, and percentage for each of the causes. Using a Pareto frequency diagram, they further identified the average amount of time it took to make appointments and determined it to be 15, with 7 appointments made per unit, per day. The range of time spent to make appointments was from 3 minutes to 10 hours (average, 15 minutes). The communicators contacted other hospitals to determine whether unit clerks made appointments for patients at these hospitals. Of the six hospitals contacted, all hospitals had patients or significant others make their own appointments.

No-show rates were also analyzed by contacting the clinics involved. The no-show rates range from 10 to 50 percent, depending on the clinic involved.

In determining solutions, the communicators identified all possible solutions, evaluated them and planned to act on the possible solutions. The communicators analyzed the causes identified on the fishbone diagram in evaluating solutions. The major cause with the greatest number of minor causes was

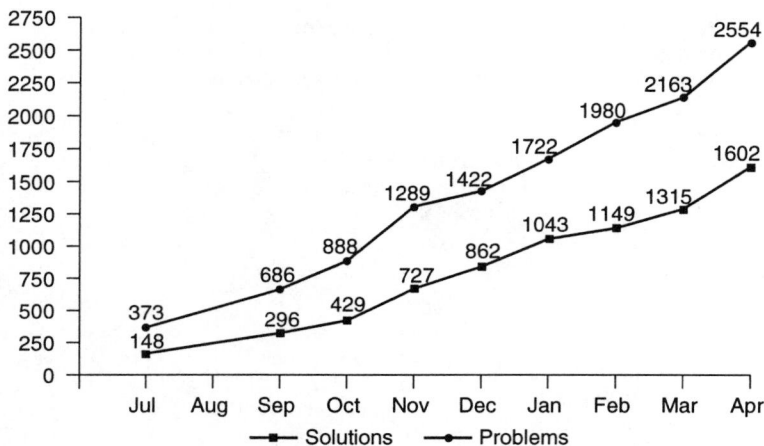

Fig. 15-8 QUEST results to date.

that patients had previous commitments and couldn't keep appointments made by the communicator. It seemed a likely solution, therefore, to have patients make their own appointments. Most of the other major and minor causes could also have been resolved by this solution, with one exception: the Audix (phone message) system created "scheduling problems" and "clinic constraints." These issues were discussed with the clinic managers to alert them to problems with their phone-message system and to the problem of patients having difficulty getting appointments one week after discharge. They discussed this with the physician staff and rearranged their clinic appointment schedules to resolve this problem. The team came to a consensus that the one most effective solution to many of the problem causes was to have patients make their own appointments.

Since this decision was not under the accountability and control of the communicators, the team met with the vice president of medical affairs to share its data and recommendations. He took this recommendation to the Medical Executive Committee. The Medical Executive Committee had reservations concerning making this change without a pilot study. The Neurology Department agreed to be a pilot service for the project. The pilot has been initiated, and now data is being gathered concerning the effectiveness of patients making their own appointments. When the pilot has been completed, the results will be taken back to the Medical Executive Committee for final decision.

While this issue has not yet been resolved, it is an excellent example of a continuous quality improvement team tackling a complex problem, breaking it down into workable components, investigating each of the opportunities, systematically evaluating solutions, and taking the data and recommendations to the next-highest decision-making body. The commu-

nicators have felt a sense of empowerment in working toward resolution of this issue.

RESULTS

The QUEST process has had a significant impact on the hospital after one year. A large volume of activity has come from every department in the hospital. The employees have come to realize that each of them has a contribution to make to improve quality, reduce waste, save time, and increase efficiency. No matter how small or seemingly insignificant the improvement might be, it is important and the team is recognized for its efforts. At Froedtert, we have succeeded in institutionalizing the concept that "Quality is everyone's business" (Townsend, 1986).

The volume of activity has been outstanding. As of March 11, 1992, after almost 12 months of activity, 2,163 problems or opportunities for improvement had been identified and 1,315 solutions had been implemented. These solutions represented a total of $340,217 in annualized savings, which did *not* include time savings. Thousands of hours of employee time have been saved. Time savings have not been tracked initially, but will be included in 1992. Opportunities for improvement are being identified at a rate of about 225 per month, and solutions are being implemented at the rate of 145 per month (Fig. 15-8). About 13 percent of the number of solutions implemented have a clear-cut cost savings.

As the quality improvement teams reach specified intervals of solutions implemented, they become eligible for team awards. From June of 1991 through March 1992, 78 team awards were given, involving 42 of the 135 teams throughout the hospital and a total of about 400 employees. Thirty-three of these awards were at levels where each team member received a cash bonus of $25 or more for his or her efforts. The awards were and continue to be given in the department of the team or at the hospital cafeteria, with attendance by the president, vice president, department manager, CQI director, and the team. In addition, the team's efforts are described in the QUEST newsletter.

Froedtert Hospital participated in a quality of service evaluation in August of 1991, conducted by an independent local marketing research firm. Four hundred recently discharged patients were sent four-page questionnaires with 35 questions dealing with physical facilities, dependability and reliability of performance, communication skills, competency, and overall impressions. Each question could be answered on a five-point scale, and the scores were compared with nine other local hospitals. Froedtert scores were the highest of the ten hospitals in overall impressions, facilities and reliability. Communication and physicians were the second highest and the hospital was above industry standards in 26 of the 31 categories. Since the study was first done in 1988, improvements were seen in 30 of the 31 question areas, with 13 being statistically significant improvements. Froedtert Hospital embarked on continuous quality improvement from a position of strength in quality, but it was felt that Froedtert could build upon this and bring quality to an even higher level.

Success Strategies

In evaluating Froedtert Hospital's approach to CQI, there were several elements that were identified as successful. First, giving the teams the ability to identify the problems they wanted to work on helped to get commitment from a larger number of employees. The teams initially picked problems most significant to them and after solving them gradually began to look at the needs of patients and other internal customer groups. Second, the teams have had considerable latitude to work out configurations or various times to have meetings. The teams have been meeting the weekly requirement of devoting a half-hour to quality improvement activities, but teams might meet weekly, biweekly, or monthly. Third, the teams have learned that making several small improvements can have as significant an effect as solving one major problem. There also is significant satisfaction in solving several problems, which gives the team incentive to continue with more.

PITFALLS AND LESSONS

A few problems also occurred that possibly could have been prevented. Originally, all the managers were placed on teams, and it soon became apparent that most employees were inhibited by their presence. Therefore, at the unanimous request of the team leaders, the managers exited the department teams, and four teams of managers were formed, with patient care directors and ancillary department managers on each team.

The individual awards in the form of Quality Gold Coins created controversy initially, especially among professional employees. This subsided as departments worked out mechanisms to distribute coins.

The QUEST process was modeled after the Quality Has Value program at the Paul Revere Insurance Company as described in *Commit to Quality* (Townsend, 1986). While we have made it work at Froedtert, we have also come to realize how much different and more complex a tertiary care medical center is in comparison to an insurance company. Several strategic directions for 1992 were identified, and they included interdepartmental team work and cross-functional problem solving, integrating QI techniques and processes into committee functions, physician involvement, participation by Medical College of Wisconsin employees, integration of purchasing with vendors who have QI programs in place, and successful integration of QI and quality assurance. A corporate goal has been established: for 90 percent of the teams to reach the Bronze award level (10 solutions implemented), and that 10 cross-functional teams will be formed, with at least five implementing their solution by the end of the year. A three-year long-range plan has also been developed which includes moving toward statistical process control and benchmarking by years three and four.

CONCLUSION

Froedtert Memorial Lutheran Hospital began its quality improvement efforts in 1988. Three years of planning and one year's experience with 100 percent employee involvement have proven to be an enlightening experience for all involved. One hundred forty employee teams have begun the transformation—the transformation of an organizational culture looking for a better way to provide patient service. It is recognized that the journey ahead is a long one. There is no turning back. Froedtert Hospital looks forward to the benefits a sincere continuous quality improvement process offers.

REFERENCE

Townsend PL (1986): *Commit to quality*, New York, John Wiley & Sons.

TOTAL QUALITY MANAGEMENT IN AN ACADEMIC TEACHING HOSPITAL

Early Experiences

Jo Marie Walrath

INSTITUTIONAL OVERVIEW

The Johns Hopkins Hospital is a 1000-bed major academic teaching hospital located in the metropolitan area of Baltimore, Maryland. Approximately 5,600 employees constitute the Hopkins Hospital staff. As part of a tertiary care hospital, the staff provides both inpatient and outpatient services across a wide variety of medical specialties. Table 16-1 depicts the volume of services provided.

A total quality management (TQM) process, based on the key concepts of Crosby, Deming, and Juran, began at the Johns Hopkins Hospital in 1989. The impetus for this initiative came from the hospital president with the expectation that all levels of hospital personnel would be actively involved in the hospital's total quality process.

Quality Management Organizational Structure

The decentralized organizational structure of the Johns Hopkins Hospital makes implementation of the TQM process a challenge. The hospital is organized into ten major clinical functional units and five ancillary functional units as shown in Fig. 16-1. Each clinical functional unit is managed by a triad: a physician, with the title functional unit director, a nursing director, and an administrator. The functional unit director reports directly to the hospital president. The nursing director and administrator report directly to the functional unit director and are in a dotted-line reporting relationship to their respective vice presidents.

An allegiance to the functional units persists. This allegiance is nurtured through strong vertical reporting mechanisms with weaker horizontal integration. Rarely can a functional unit unilaterally improve a "service process." Processes are complex, and quality improvement initiatives require interdepartmental cooperation. Therefore, an organizational structure is required to support a hospitalwide TQM initiative

TABLE 16-1 Key Indicators of Hospital Services

Unit of Measure	FY '91 Volumes*
Patient days	292,900
OR minutes	3,606,000
OR cases	23,900
OPD visits	198,600
ED visits	83,900
Radiology RVU	2,836,000
Laboratory tests	2,305,000

*Rounded to the nearest hundred. *From Johns Hopkins Hospital, Monthly Report of Operations,* 1991.

with representation from both clinical and ancillary units.

A Quality Management Steering Committee was established to direct and coordinate the hospital's TQM program. This committee includes vice presidents, directors, and administrators from each major functional area. The committee serves as the integration point that enhances problem solving and quality improvement. The committee directly reports to the president and executive committee of the hospital.

The steering committee has limited its scope of responsibility to include only issues that are interdepartmental and that require groups across functional units to cooperate in the problem-solving process. The committee identifies, through a variety of mechanisms, specific improvement opportunities within the institution. Although the committee's focus is interdepartmental, all functional unit personnel are expected to identify and implement intradepartmental quality improvement initiatives. Fig. 16-2 illustrates how the TQM process is integrated at the executive level of the hospital.

Hopkins has modified the 10-step JCAHO process into a 10-step quality improvement process (Table 16-2). The steering committee identifies a quality improvement project team, which uses this process in the planning, action, and monitoring phases of a quality improvement initiative. The initiative assigned by the TQM steering committee and pre-

Jerry Reardon, Cochair of the TQM Committee, Karl Bankert, of Management Engineering, and the TQM project team members are acknowledged for their contribution to this chapter.

I. Corporate Management Structure

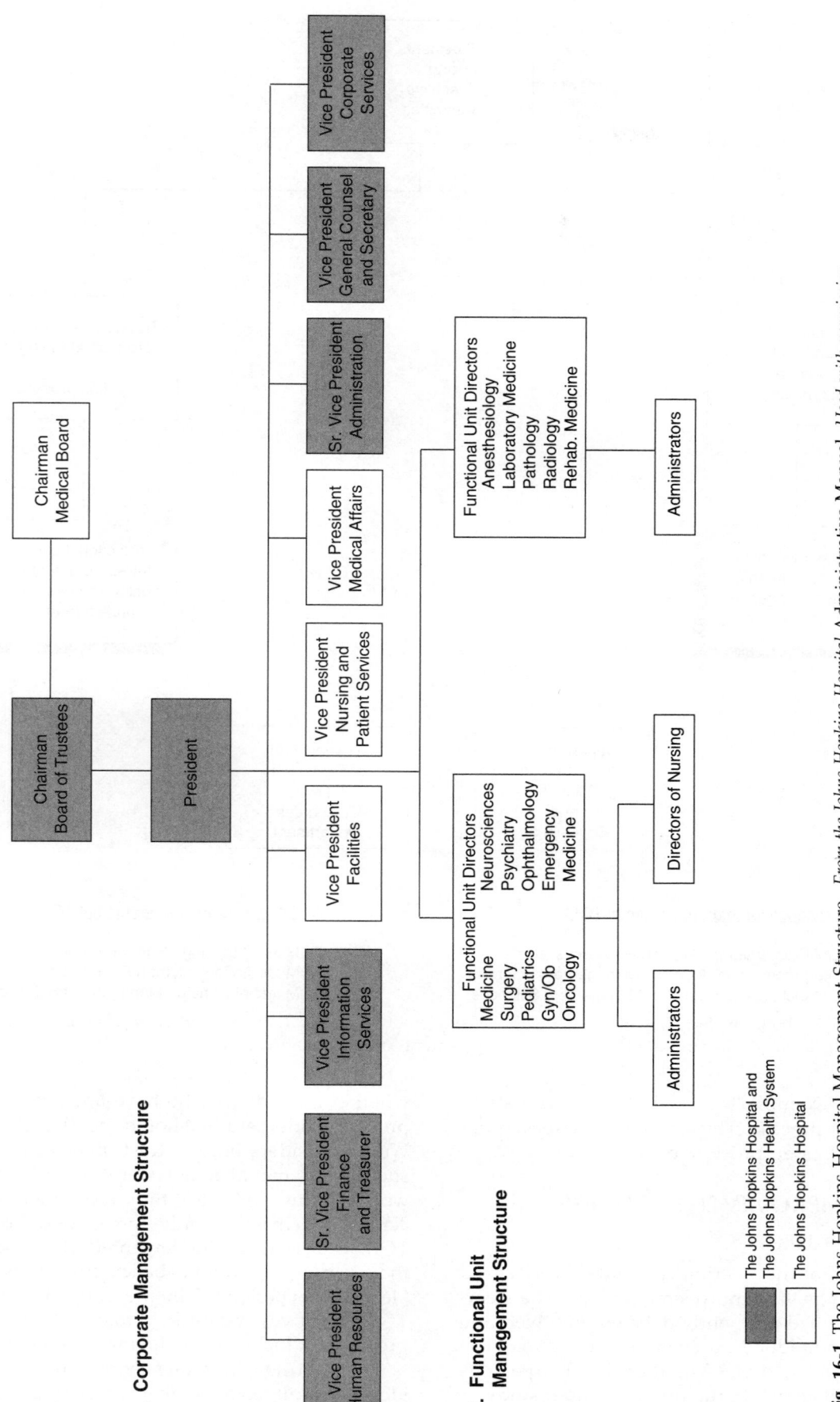

II. Functional Unit
Management Structure

Fig. 16-1 The Johns Hopkins Hospital Management Structure. *From the Johns Hopkins Hospital Administrative Manual. Used with permission.*

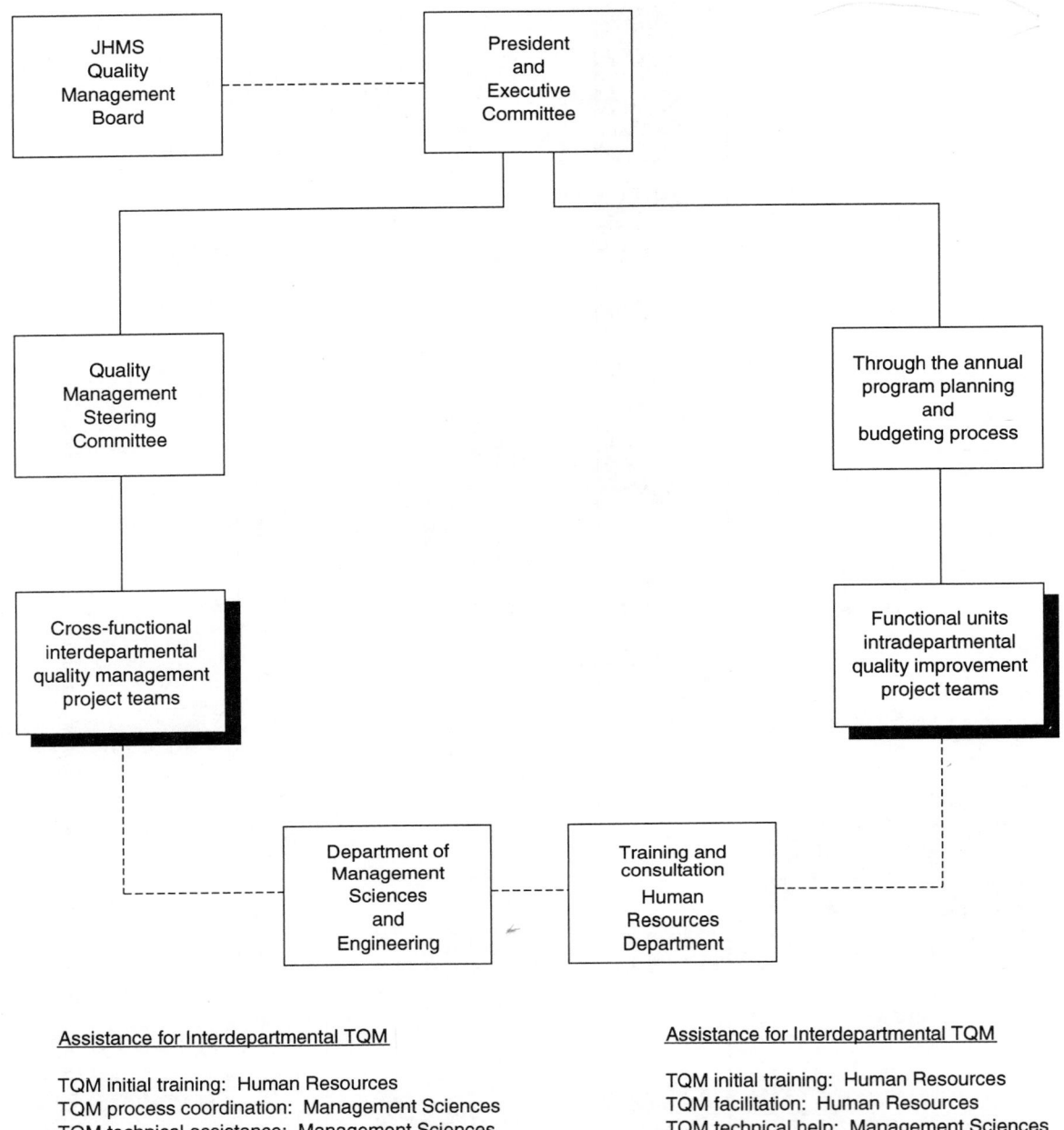

Fig. 16-2 The Johns Hopkins Hospital Quality Management Process. *Courtesy of the Johns Hopkins Hospital Human Resources Department:* Total Quality Management Training Manual.

sented as an example was to improve the patient transportation process. This chapter describes application of the 10-step process to this initiative.

QUALITY IMPROVEMENT PROCESS

Assign Accountability

Two members of the steering committee were asked to cochair the quality improvement team. The steering committee had frequently debated who were the appropriate individuals to chair project teams. The central issue debated was whether the chairpersons should be "outsiders" to the problem under study or whether individuals who have line authority for the process under study should be the chairpersons. Would outsiders bring a fresh perspective to the issue? If line management were not the chairs, how would "buy in" to the recommendations be achieved? This was only the second hospitalwide TQM project to be implemented. The cochairs and the steering committee believed the task to be a "learning experience" in the early development of TQM initiatives and decided to try the "outsider" approach, but included the line managers on the team.

The steering committee charged the cochairs with identifying all team members and completing the im-

TABLE 16-2 Johns Hopkins Hospital Quality Improvement 10-Step Process

Step	Process Steps	Key Outcomes
1	Assign accountability	Determine who is responsible and has authority to accomplish goals
2	Determine customer/supplier relationships	Identify who receives and supplies the service/product
3	Develop customer requirements	Identify customer's expectations
4	Conduct process improvement analysis	Evaluate and analyze the process in order to identify opportunities for improving care/service/problems
5	Prepare quality goals	Identify how customer requirements will be met
6	Establish quality targets	Establish desired results of the work process
7	Complete action plans	Identify major steps required to accomplish the goal
8	Implement change	Initiate solutions to the issue
9	Monitor and take corrective action	Measure effectiveness of solutions implemented
10	Maintain improvements	Identify methods to assure continued achievement of change

Courtesy of The Johns Hopkins Hospital Human Resource Department: Total Quality Management Training Manual.

provement process. The expectations of the steering committee were that the team would provide progress reports at scheduled intervals and would utilize the committee for problem solving. The team was asked to complete its charge in three months.

Environmental Scan

The cochairpersons had learned a very valuable lesson from the first hospitalwide team. *Success depended upon a clearly defined problem.*

The sheer geography of the 45-acre hospital complex creates a transportation challenge. The cochairpersons realized a team charged with "patient transportation" was doomed to fail if the team did not have a narrowly focused charge. The cochairs engaged themselves in an environmental scan of the existing transport system to obtain background information for the team and to limit the project's scope. The cochairs interviewed the major clinical and support departments, including the central transport service, in order to gain a provider and user perspective on this issue. The interviews uncovered a perceived level of dissatisfaction with the service level provided by the central transport service of the hospital. Probably one of the most significant findings from the interviews was the existence of two very defined levels of hospital transport: internal department systems and the central system. Many of the departmental systems evolved to optimize patient care and were an attempt to improve the patient transport system. These interviews led the cochairpersons to the following conclusion: The project of "patient transportation" was indeed too global. The movement of patients throughout the institution was a very complex process. Many variables influenced the transportation process. These included the patient's medical stability, facility design, availability and condition of transport equipment and accessories, workforce productivity, and a mostly unscheduled demand for transport services. All of the major clinical depart-

ments, with the exception of the Oncology Department, identified a need for improvements in both their internal transport systems and the central system. Transportation of patients also involved a variety of individuals. It not only included the defined "escort service" but also nurses, physicians, nursing support staff, security guards, secretaries, and family members.

The chairpersons narrowed the scope of the project team based on their findings in the transport system assessment. The following premises would guide the team's work:

1. Internal transport systems would continue to transport medically unstable patients.
2. No internal transport system would be disrupted until an alternative system was identified.
3. Based on anecdotal evidence, the efficiency and effectiveness of the central transport system could be improved.
4. Inpatient, rather than outpatient, transport would be the priority for improvement.

The focus of the transport issue was narrowed to transportation for the purpose of radiology or inpatient transport needs.

Committee Selection

With the scope of the team's work more narrowly defined, the cochairpersons selected team members who were either customers or suppliers in the radiology/inpatient transport process. Team membership included managers responsible for inpatient nursing units, radiology, and transport services. Membership also included one customer dissatisfied with the current process, a staff member from the Pulmonary/EKG Station. The team also included staff from the Management Sciences department and the department of oncology. Oncology was the only major clinical unit that operated its own escort system. Oncology did not rely on central transport services and

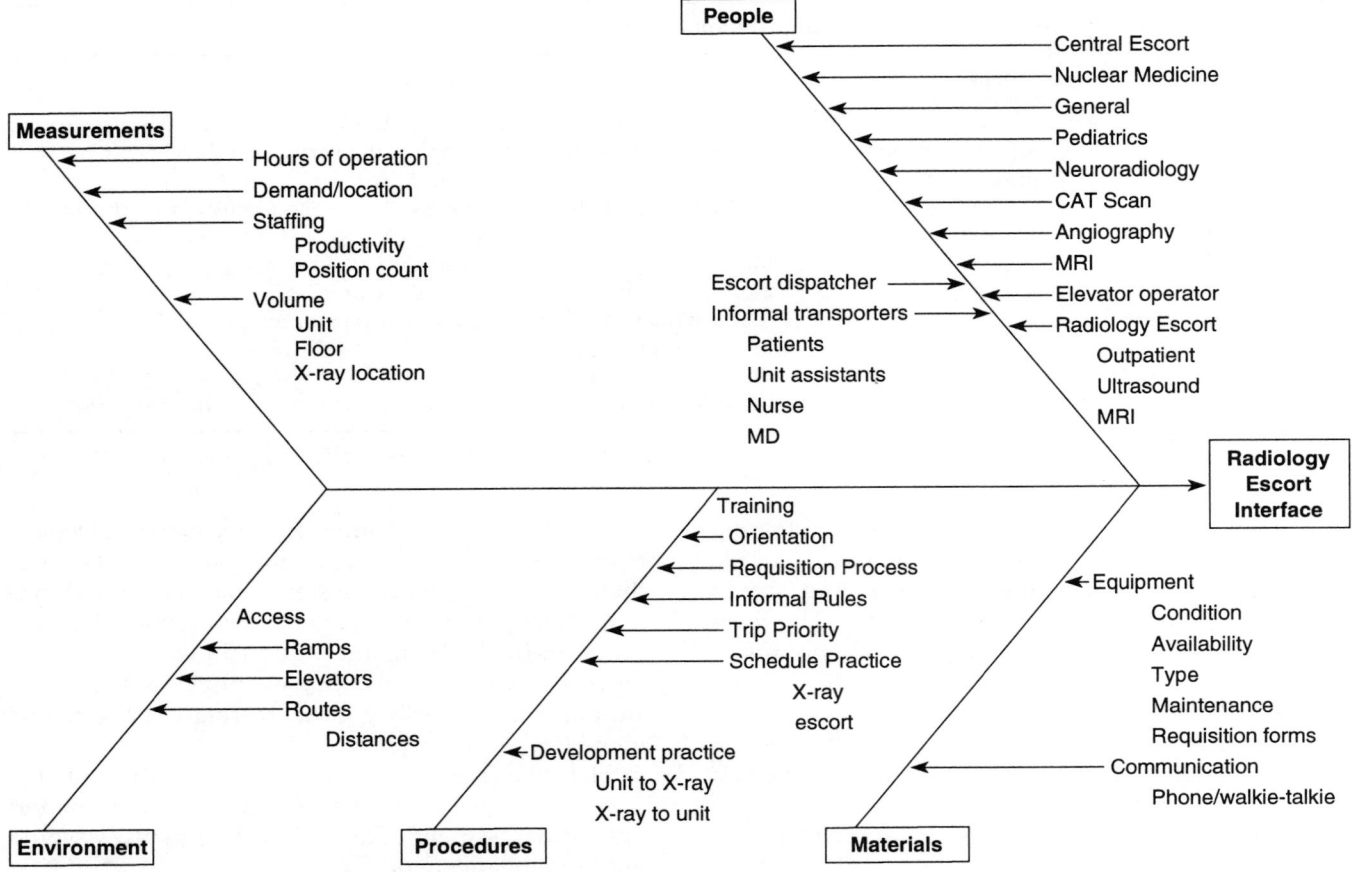

Fig. 16-3 Transport process: cause and effect fishbone diagram.

indicated a high level of satisfaction with the internal system. It was anticipated that these additional members could add varying perspectives to the issues. The chairpersons and team also decided to hold focus groups when appropriate. These groups could provide valuable insight into issues without expanding the committee size to a point where problem solving would be cumbersome.

The team met over a three-month period for two hours per week. The initial meeting was four hours. In this meeting all team members were trained in TQM principles and analytical tools, were given the charge of the steering committee, and began the essential team-building process, which solidified over subsequent meetings. Meeting schedules were coordinated and deadlines established.

The project team was guided by the "operating principles" set out by the steering committee. These are:

- Anticipate and respond to the customer's expectations
- Establish operating standards and productivity measurements
- Assure consistency and accountability to standards

- Support organizational goals as resources are committed

Initial Meeting Focus

In addition to the team learning the content and analytical tools of TQM, early meetings focused on review of existing data. This included the transport system assessment and previously collected data regarding radiology and transport services' utilization.

The first task of the committee was to complete a cause and effect (fishbone) diagram in order to gain insight into the existing interfaces for the transportation process specific to radiology and the inpatient nursing units.

Fig. 16-3 illustrates the variables that affect the existing transport process between the departments. The diagram focused the team in five key areas:

1. *Measurement.* What additional information does the team need to better understand the process?
2. *People.* Who is currently involved in this process and how will changes affect them and be communicated to them?
3. *Environment.* Are there environmental factors that enhance or detract from the transport process?

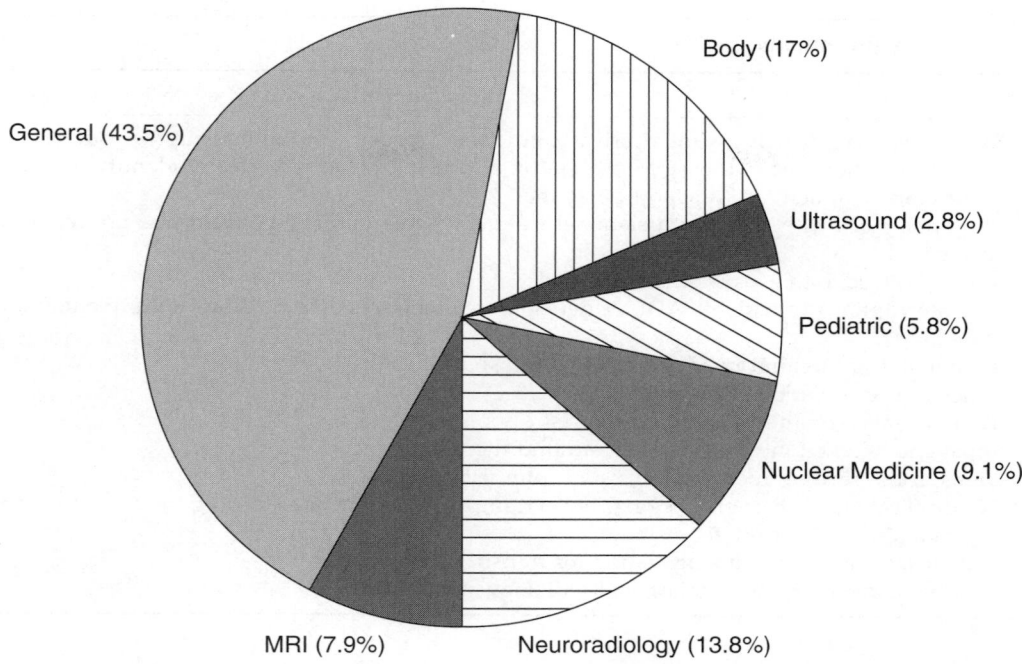

Fig. 16-4 Radiology escort service average trips per week (7/89-2/90).

TABLE 16-3 Supplier/Customer Relationships

Service/Product	Supplier	Customer
Radiology procedure	Radiology	Patient, nurse, physician
Patient transportation	Central escort	Radiology, patient, nursing unit
Radiology requisition	Physician, nursing unit	Radiology, central escort
Transport of requisition	Nursing unit, central escort	Radiology
Radiology schedule	Radiology	Nursing unit, physician, central escort

4. *Procedure.* What policies and procedures, formal or informal, affect the process?

5. *Materials.* What equipment is used during this process?

Constructing a cause and effect diagram serves to raise a variety of issues. Information gleaned from this process kept the project team focused throughout future meetings.

Another preliminary data review of the transport system was undertaken. The findings illustrated in Fig. 16-4 further narrowed the project team's focus. The majority (60.7%) of transports occurred between the nursing units and "general" radiology or Body Scan. The team decided to concentrate its improvements in these areas.

Additional tools of analysis used by the project team are described in the section titled Process Improvement Analysis.

Identify Customer/Supplier Relationships

The transportation of patients between a radiology department and a nursing unit clearly demonstrates the fluidity in the customer/supplier relationship. The customer is defined as the receiver of the service and the supplier as the provider of the service. Table 16-3 identifies that the supplier/customer relationships shift depending upon which part of the radiology/transport process is being discussed.

Team members benefitted from the discussion of customer/supplier relationships. It was evident that most members viewed themselves as "the customer" to the exclusion of others involved, and that none of the group clearly knew what the others expected or wanted.

Establish Customer Requirements

Among the hallmarks of TQM are that customers have a right to have their requirements met and, in order for this to occur, the customer is obligated to communicate his or her requirements to the supplier. Each of the four key groups involved, nursing, radiology, physician, and transport, needed to clarify its requirements. These requirements would become the basis for standard development. Table 16-4 identifies the major customers and their requirements.

TABLE 16-4 Customer Requirements

Customer	Requirements
Patient	We *assumed* that patients wanted privacy, efficiency, respect, and uninterrupted routines. The team violated a major part of the TQM process by not asking patients to clearly identify their expectations.
Nurse	Courteous treatment by transport personnel
	Prompt service with transport personnel waiting on the unit if the patient was not ready when they arrived
	Prior knowledge that x-ray was scheduled
	No interruptions to patients ADL or personal treatments to accommodate an unplanned call from radiology
	Equipment on the unit in advance of the transport
Radiology	Efficient use of radiology suites
	Patient sent to the department on request
	Inpatients worked into the schedule around the outpatients
Physician	Films in the reading room by the 5 p.m. physician rounds
	No duplication of chart entries (e.g. not writing x-ray orders and needing to repeat the same information on the x-ray requisition)
Central Escort	Patient waiting at the nursing station for transport personnel
	Courteous treatment by nursing and radiology staff

There was agreement among team members that the end user of the service, in this case the patient, would be the principal customer.

The team decided to collect more data before standards were identified. The data would help all team members to better understand the actual transport process.

Prepare Quality Goals

Team goals were broadly defined and subject to change as data were collected and analyzed.

- The patient would be the primary customer and would receive prompt, courteous, and efficient service.
- The patient would not be off the nursing unit for routine radiology exams (e.g., chest, limb, and abdominal films) for more than one hour.
- Nursing would be informed in advance that x-rays were being scheduled in order to plan care more appropriately.
- Escort service and nursing would work closely together to ensure that equipment was available.
- Escort service would maintain equipment in safe, good working order.
- Physicians would have films available on rounds.
- Physician documentation of x-ray orders would not require duplication of entries in the medical record.
- Patients would be available for escort.

Establish Quality Targets

The team would consider it had improved the radiology/transport process if the following targets were achieved:

- 100 percent of patients would go to the Radiology Tower (General X-Ray) within their scheduled block of time.
- Turnaround time (i.e., time patient leaves nursing unit until he or she returns from radiology) would not exceed one hour.
- 100 percent of radiology requisitions would be logged onto a unit "planning sheet" by the nursing unit staff.
- 50 percent more requisitions would be picked up the evening prior to the radiology exam.
- Baseline data would be determined for the number of escorts required for transports and distribution of wheelchair versus stretcher transports.
- Perceptions of nursing staff would be improved regarding satisfaction with the transport process between radiology and central transport.
- Radiology procedures would not increase in number from the baseline data.

PROCESS IMPROVEMENT ANALYSIS

The team identified the goals of data collection. Table 16-5 outlines the specific data requirements and tools of analysis. One month of representative data was the basis of analysis.

Complete Action Plan

Team members reviewed and analyzed the collected data. Table 16-6 identifies the key findings and what strategies the team identified to improve the radiology/transport process.

Several action plan items merit further discussion.

A new radiology requisition form was developed. The new form had several improvements. First, a

TABLE 16-5 Process Improvement Goals and Requirements

Goal	Required Data	Tools of Analysis
To gain an understanding of the transport process	Transport system assessment Identify variables affecting process	Report Fishbone diagram
To review current physician practice	Rounds schedule Ordering schedule	Physician interviews

To develop an efficient system that matches radiology and nursing transport resources to volumes	Volume of inpatient/outpatient procedures by:
	  Nursing unit
	  Functional unit
	  Building location
		Bar graph

To determine the type and number of tests that are being done	Types of procedures:
	  Chest x-rays
	  All other x-rays
		Pareto chart

To determine radiology suite utilization	Suite utilization by:
	  Hour
	  Inpatient/outpatient
		Frequency graph

To determine how current form is being utilized	Radiology requisitions	Team review
To determine how existing unit planning sheet is used	Review unit planning sheets	Reports from all functional units
Review flow of requisitions	Requisition process	On-site share-a-day with transporters Flow diagram

Determine how transport resources are currently used	Volume of transport by:
	  Day of week
	  Location
	  Hour
		Bar graph
		Pareto graph
		Frequency distribution

copy would always be retained on the nursing unit so the nursing staff would know their patient required an x-ray. Secondly, it would be logged onto the planning sheet so that proper equipment could be acquired in advance of the test. Finally, physicians wanted the form to replace the need for them to re-write an order.

Concurrent to the team's work, the supervisor of transport services had completed an inventory of equipment, reorganized resources, allocated one individual to do preventive maintenance, and changed the pickup system for collecting equipment throughout the institution. All unit par levels for wheelchairs were reviewed, restocked, and reallocated as needed.

In addition to reviewing volume and resource utilization data, two other customers, nurses and physicians, had requirements to be met. Two major concerns expressed by the nursing staff were unplanned x-rays and inadequate equipment. The team developed a planning sheet to be used on the units by nursing personnel to track scheduled x-rays, equipment needs, and turnaround time—that is, time away from nursing unit. This sheet was intended to improve planning and was also to be used in the pilot evaluation.

The flow of radiology requisitions was reviewed. The current system for moving requisitions between the nursing units and radiology was variable and proved very inefficient. Transport messengers "picked up" radiology requests daily at 7 a.m.; physicians "dropped off" requisitions in radiology randomly throughout the day; and nursing unit clerks called transport throughout the day to pick up x-ray requisitions any time a physician wrote an order. Two team members accompanied escort transporters on their morning requisition "pick-up" rounds. After completing these rounds, only seven requisitions were collected from the nursing units. No sooner had the transporters delivered the requisitions to the radiology dispatch office than the phones began to ring for them to return to the nursing units for additional requisitions.

In addition to reviewing the flow of requisitions, team members reviewed existing physician rounds schedules to ascertain when the majority of requisitions were written. It was found that surgical areas generated requisitions by 7 a.m. and again in the evening by 8 p.m. Medical units, however, were not finished with rounds until 11 a.m., and then there were also requests throughout the day.

Irrespective of the erratic system, all physicians expected routine films to be available for their last daily working rounds.

It became very clear why the requisition escort pick-up system wasn't successful, and it became clear that a new process was needed.

TABLE 16-6 Project Team Findings and Action Plan

Key Findings	Action Plan
1. Patients transported by 3 functional units to the main Radiology and CAT Scan facilities represented the largest number of central transports.	Implement a pilot study to include the departments of Medicine, Surgery, and Neurosurgery. Limit pilot study to patients going to the hospital's main radiology location (i.e., Tower) and to CAT scan (body, head and neck).
2. Outpatient studies superseded inpatient studies. Inpatients were done at times when there were limited transport and nursing resources on the nursing units.	Block-schedule inpatients around peak unit staffing periods.
3. There was no planned communication between inpatient units and radiology.	Deliver radiology schedules for CAT scans the evening before the exam. Develop new requisition with multiple copies. This would eliminate the need for duplicating orders and to alert nursing staff of x-ray orders. Establish block schedules for routine x-rays. Develop a planning sheet to be used in nursing unit to capture x-ray and equipment needs.
4. Inadequate time to plan and mobilize equipment and human resources for the efficient movement of patients to radiology.	Use new "transport" log on each pilot unit to improve planning from unit perspective. Complete time study of transporter's work.
5. Lack of standards to facilitate transportation staffing patterns.	Analyze data from radiology log to determine turnaround time. Establish a standard based on data.
6. Lack of standards for determining equipment (i.e., "fleet" size), composition, deployment, and maintenance.	Implement preventive maintenance schedule. Complete inventory of current equipment. Reallocate equipment based on unit par level.
7. No coordination between physician and transport rounds for pickup and delivery of radiology requisitions.	Request MD write requisitions evening before exam to facilitate radiology's room and resource allocation. Reevaluate "pick-up" schedule for radiology requisitions.

Implement and Monitor Activities

A pilot study was implemented for a three-month period. A variety of data was collected to determine if the changes implemented resulted in reaching the quality targets.

The use of block times was intended to improve use of radiology suites as well as to aid the nursing staff in planning activities around patients' radiology studies. Only 35 percent of all patients were transported during their scheduled block times. On the surface, this strategy appeared to be a failure. However, radiology's and nursing's perception was that the process improved. Transporters were scheduled to specific units and specific suites. The process actually seemed to improve flow: 38 percent of patients went to radiology prior to their scheduled block time. The team concluded that block-scheduling routine exams and assigning transporters to specific units improved the overall process.

The team did not measure turnaround time prior to the pilot. This was viewed in retrospect as a strategic error. It was the perception of the nurses and physicians that the turnaround time was greater than one hour. Pilot findings were that 70 percent of all patients had a turnaround time of less than one hour.

The committee recommended that the standard be established at one hour and that the managers of both radiology and transport services improve on the new standard as the pilot ended and changes became routine practice.

A major concern of the nursing staff was that no patient care planning could occur on the unit because nurses rarely had prior knowledge of scheduled radiology studies. The planning sheet was to aid nursing in planning both for equipment needs and patient care. In only 28 percent of the transports did the staff complete all the data elements on the planning sheet. Nurses reported that having a copy of the requisition remain in the medical record was sufficient. The staff reverted to "par levels" for equipment needs on the units. The team recommended that each unit could determine if it wanted to use the planning sheet after the pilot ended.

Requisition pickup times were rescheduled to occur after physician rounds. An evening pick-up was scheduled because physicians were requested to write orders the evening prior to the test day to facilitate radiology's planning for the next day's work. Physicians' ordering patterns did not change; therefore, the evening pick-up was an inefficient use of resources. However, an unplanned change occurred. The prepilot system required the escort to be called to pick up the requisition and at some later time called to pick up the patient. In the pilot, nursing personnel waited for radiology to call for patients and sent the requisition with the patient. This practice occurred in 58 percent of the transports and did not seem to create any difficulties. The team recommended that one call to the units for both patient and requisition was adequate, thereby improving escort productivity. The team also maintained its recommendation that physicians write orders the evening before the exams; however, compliance to this request remained poor.

The pilot did invalidate transport services' perception that the majority of hospital transports required two transporters. In fact, data collected indicated that only 13 percent of patients required this. It also demonstrated that the majority of these transports came from the neurosurgical units and required stretchers rather than wheelchairs. This study helped central services reexamine its equipment needs and alter par allocations to the nursing units based on these findings.

Physicians were concerned that increasing the ease of requesting radiology exams might result in more studies being ordered. However, the data indicated a decrease in studies during the pilot period. The committee members attributed this decrease in x-ray utilization to another initiative in progress rather than to this initiative.

The implementation of the newly designed radiology requisition did not totally eliminate the need for redundancy of physician documentation. Both the medical records and legal departments required that a brief order be written in the chart; the requisition could not replace the order. All three groups, radiology, nursing, and physicians, found the new requisition format and the fact that a copy remained in the record as an improvement.

Focus groups were held with radiology, nursing, and central transport. Although a major effort was undertaken to include everyone in the planning and ongoing communication regarding the pilot, some staff stated they knew nothing about the effort. Personnel directly involved with the initiative stated a major outcome of the study was their gaining a new appreciation of the work involved in the radiology/transport process. Those involved in focus groups with nursing and escort were more aware of how they personally impeded or assisted in the movement of patients between departments.

Maintain Improvements

At the completion of the pilot project, the supervisors of radiology and central transport services were delegated responsibility and authority for expanding the pilot, monitoring performance against the one-hour standard, and continuing to improve upon the standard. Status reports to the steering committee are scheduled quarterly.

LESSONS LEARNED

There were key lessons learned from this TQM project.
- Fishbone diagrams turn into "Moby Dicks"; that is, the problems are so numerous and complex they can cause group paralysis.
  Key: Keep the committee charge well focused.
- You can never overcommunicate. Every hospital communication forum and all written media were used to present the pilot study and proposed changes. All nurse managers met to discuss the pilot project and their role in its success. Even after much communication, individuals on units stated they were "unaware" of the project.
  Key: Strategize communication plan and include in the action plan. Take time to carefully identify communication strategy when change is complex. Accept the fact that not everyone will know or care about your project.
- Authority and responsibility for designing and maintaining change must be vested in middle managers. The chairpersons of teams become "resident experts" on the issue under study and it becomes difficult to divest from the issue.
  Key: Keeping key department managers involved throughout the process is critical for "buy-in" and continued refinement to the changes. Chairpersons can facilitate the process but responsibility and authority for implementing and maintaining change should be the responsibilities of the manager whose area is under study.
- The process of any "hospital service" is complex, multifaceted; however, it can be improved upon.
  Key: Complex systems cannot be completely changed with one pilot study. Revisit data and continue refining solutions to the problems.
- Team building within a project team is essential.
  Key: Care must be taken to identify chairpersons who are skilled at conducting effective meetings and fostering open communication.
- The TQM process requires interdepartmental cooperation because committee members engage in negotiating, turf-watching and conflict resolution.
  Key: Consider a group facilitator as a committee member to work with the chair.
- The initial problem is often viewed as a "people problem."
  Key: People are rarely the problem. Complex systems evolve to improve processes. How and why they evolve is rarely understood. Clearly defining what the group is aiming to improve will maintain group productivity.

- The TQM project team can take on "a life of its own."
  Key: Chairpersons must keep to the plan. All team members have other responsibilities.
  Disband the team after the plan is developed. Vest implementation and evaluation plan in the managers of the affected area. Reconvene the team as needed. Always keep the team committee informed of important milestones and outcomes.

CONCLUSION

Since the "early experience" described in this text, numerous teams, both intra- and interdepartmental, have completed projects or are in progress with new initiatives. TQM remains an evolutionary process in this major academic center, and it has the potential to create revolutionary changes in the organization. The early experiences of this project team helped both the steering committee and new teams relook at how TQM is implemented, how it can be modified, and how each team's success and disappointments can guide future quality improvement initiatives.

CHAPTER SEVENTEEN

PLANNING AND IMPLEMENTING TOTAL QUALITY MANAGEMENT

Pamela A. Triolo

TQM in health care organizations combines the theory, tools, systems, and organizational models developed over the past four decades in the United States and Japan by Deming, Juran, Crosby, and others. Hospitals and industries that have pursued TQM have distinguished track records characterized by high involvement and empowerment of all staff, not just managers. In view of health care's increasing complexity, team learning is encouraged, data-driven decision making is fostered, and strong, consistent educational efforts support maintenance and improvement of not only the services offered, but the work environment itself.

Implementation of Total Quality Management does not occur overnight. Though it builds on an organization's strengths and existing systems and programs, the customization of TQM to the health care delivery system requires substantial planning. Careful, thoughtful, and patient planning is the key to successful implementation and integration of TQM. This chapter describes the intrinsic role of middle managers in the design and implementation of total quality management in a tertiary health care center. Though senior leadership must support and drive the process, the core strength is the multidisciplinary, cross-functional involvement of middle managers.

PRELIMINARY PLANNING

The University of Iowa Hospitals and Clinics (UIHC) is the largest university-owned teaching hospital in the United States. The staff of 7400 provides a variety of specialty and subspecialty health care services to an annual ambulatory complement of nearly one half million patients and more than 900 inpatient beds.

Two years before the appointment of a TQM Steering Committee, the design team, senior level leadership studied and planned a retreat to determine the state of organizational readiness for Total Quality Management. It was determined that because of the large size of the organization, and the intent to develop a critical mass of change agents at the middle management level, planning for TQM would be preceded by an organizational development program. The purpose of this program was to foster teamwork and networking, as well as to enhance management skills among selected middle managers, including medical staff with management responsibilities.

In 1989, the administrator appointed the Advanced Management Institute Steering Committee. This committee was composed of senior and middle managers from throughout the medical center. The Steering Committee was charged with identifying a target audience for this leadership development program, conducting a comprehensive educational needs assessment, and developing recommendations for the design and format of a weeklong, intensive annual educational program. Working in cooperation with the Graduate Program in Health and Hospital Administration and the College of Business, a curriculum was crafted that flowed from the educational needs assessment.

The first UIHC Advanced Management Institute was offered in January of 1990. The class was composed of 28 middle managers who were nominated and selected by a senior leadership selection committee. Selection was based upon performance and potential to lead the organization. One-third of the class was physicians. The weeklong program, comprising individual and team learning activities, was taught by on-campus, seasoned faculty and off-site faculty from the Wharton School of the University of Pennsylvania and from the University of North Carolina, Chapel Hill. The program content fostered team learning and covered health care finance, conflict management and negotiation, organizational development, human resources development, and other areas.

The program was an outstanding success, and the week of social and work interaction in a relaxed environment served as a catalyst for an enthusiastic, strong, and supportive network of individuals. The week provided a comprehensive perspective of work at University Hospitals and a greater understanding of the multiplicity of roles. For the physicians, this was particularly insightful, and they have served as some of the strongest supporters of the program. Because of the initial success, second and third Institute programs have been offered, bringing the total number of graduates to nearly 90. Using the strategy of task alignment (Beer et al, 1990), the organizational development plans for UIHC have called upon the graduates to serve in a variety of leadership roles, but particularly in the design and implementation of TQM.

TQM Steering Committee

In June of 1990, the Administrator appointed the TQM Steering Committee, which was charged with planning a customized approach to implementation of total quality management at the UIHC. The Steering Committee was composed of approximately 25 managers, who represented the areas of physical therapy, pharmacy, nursing, telecommunications, social service, dietary, material services, staff relations, patient and guest relations, and others. Physician involvement included representation from Pediatrics, Ophthalmology, Pathology, and Internal Medicine. Nearly 90 percent of the Steering Committee members were graduates of the UIHC Management Institute. The Steering Committee was able to build upon the camaraderie and candor that had developed in the Institutes to chart the complex design of TQM into the organizations infrastructure. Later in 1990, an Executive Quality Council, the policy group, composed of overlapping membership between the Steering Committee and senior leadership, was formed.

In order to accomplish the work in an efficient manner, the Steering Committee was divided into five working groups. Each working group was chaired by and included members from the Steering Committee, but additional institutional experts were added to increase involvement and drive the process into the organization. The Working Group on Communication was charged with designing a communication plan to begin the awareness process and keep the staff up to date on the plans and progress. One of its achievements was the initiation of a monthly column that appears in *The Compass,* the staff newsletter. This column has been authored by a variety of staff members and details the progress of TQM. Communication is one of the key components in tying the organization together and increasing the involvement of staff.

The Working Group on the Health Care Customer addressed the issue of identifying baseline expectations of UIHC customers. A customer is defined as any individual or group who has expectations or makes a quality judgment about our service. Customers are both internal and external. For the UIHC, external customers include patients, patient family members, visitors, referring physicians, and regulatory agencies. Internal customers are clinical and professional staff, students, and others. TQM involves using feedback about service expectations as the cornerstone of the quality improvement process. This group identified all sources of current customer feedback in the form of surveys. It developed a matrix of

---

Commitment to Quality

All members of the UIHC family are committed to continuous improvement in the quality of our services through an environment and performance which fosters excellence in patient care, teaching, and research. Respect and a caring attitude guide our daily actions toward patients, staff, trainees, students, and others we serve.

As an organization committed to the highest quality of patient care, our quest to SERVE is based upon:

*S*ervice	The patients and others we serve are our first priority.
*E*ducation . . .	We value education and research as our investment in the future.
*R*espect	Respect for each individual is the cornerstone of our services.
*V*ision	We share a vision that encourages all staff to exceed the expectations of those we serve.
*E*xcellence . .	We take pride in working together to continuously improve and excel in everything we do.

From the University of Iowa Hospitals and Clinics (UIHC)

---

chronic quality problems, which were identified as "Opportunities for Improvement." Later, this matrix would serve as the focus for the identification of the first Quality Improvement Teams.

Two other achievements of this group were the development of a centralized complaint mechanism, coordinated through patient representatives. Also, in view of the emphasis placed on interdepartmental relationships by the JCAHO Agenda for Change, the working group conducted focus groups in order to design a blueprint for an interdepartmental survey tool. This tool provides a consistent measurement device, throughout the UIHC, for identifying customer expectations between departments.

The third working group, Management's Commitment to Quality, developed the organizational value statement "Commitment to Quality" (see the box above). This statement was validated among nearly 400 staff members throughout the organization and has served as the cornerstone of the quality improvement process.

The Working Group on Education was charged with identifying the learning needs of staff in regard to TQM. This group developed and piloted the first training program to be offered. This initial program, "TQM for Managers," was targeted to an audience of about 500 managers at the level of first line and above. The purpose of this program, which included clinical staff, was to provide an overview of why the

UIHC was implementing TQM and how it would be accomplished.

At this point, it is crucial to note a number of key decisions that had been made by the Steering Committee and the Executive Quality Council. First, it was decided that training would not commence until substantial progress had been made in the groundwork for TQM and that implementation would begin in the near future. The intent was to avoid premature readiness of the organization. Therefore, TQM for managers did not begin until November of 1991, over a year into the planning process.

A second key decision regarding training was to avoid mass training. The approach was designed to eliminate any non-value-added efforts and to use existing staff in an efficient and effective manner. Teaching TQM techniques to a diverse audience, without a common frame of reference, would be difficult. Also the lack of application, or a delay in the application of techniques, would deter the retention of learning and increase staff frustration. Though TQM overviews would be integrated in hospitalwide orientation, mass training of staff would be avoided, at this time. For team training, just-in-time training techniques would be used where a project for improvement is defined, a team is formed to address the problem, and then trained in quality improvement techniques.

The final working group was the Working Group on Staff Involvement. This group was charged with integrating TQM into the grassroots level through the vehicle of a staff-suggestion program. This program would solicit quality improvement ideas from staff and would reward staff involvement. The underlying philosophy behind this approach was that those closest to the customers and processes would have a clearer understanding of expectations and how service-delivery processes might improve. This management strategy is also driven by the inherent assumption that the people involved in health care processes want to do their best to help the organization.

During the process of planning, the working groups, the Steering Committee, and the Executive Quality Council used quality improvement techniques and strategies to accomplish the work and facilitate group interaction. Each meeting was viewed as a learning opportunity and members learned and practiced brainstorming, affinity diagramming, force field analysis, rank ordering and multivoting, cause and effect diagramming, flowcharting, and other techniques. Because the Executive Quality Council also serves as the senior administrative team for the hospital, quality improvement tools and techniques are utilized, not only as learning opportunities, but as creative thinking and planning tools. An example of one such use is found in the Affinity Diagram (Fig. 17-1), which explores the issues that need to be addressed by university teaching hospitals in the year 2000.

Total quality management moves an organization from the "performance mode" to a "learning mode" (Fritz, 1991). The members of these groups worked to customize the process, foster creativity and innovation, and facilitate behavioral change through the use of these techniques.

IMPLEMENTATION APPROACH

Implementation of TQM can take a number of approaches. The University of Iowa Hospitals and Clinics determined that a centralized approach would be taken the first year, with decentralization occurring during the second year of implementation. The rationale for the centralized approach was to allow the leadership to acquire experience in the process and to test the UIHC training prototype.

To facilitate the centralized approach, eight core instructors received training from an external firm. Core instructors would serve not only as instructors, but as facilitators to the initial quality improvement teams. These core instructors were carefully selected; criteria included teaching experience, status as a leadership role model, and high interest in involvement. The core instructors included the hospital administrator, the director of nursing, the director of hospital information systems, the director of social service, the director of architectural, engineering and environmental services, the director of patient and guest relations, a professor, and chairman, of the Department of Ophthalmology, and the director of quality management. After core instructor training, the training materials were evaluated and the UIHC training prototype, Quality Improvement Team Training, was designed. The problem-solving approach developed for the UIHC was a composite of the work of the National Demonstration Project on Quality Improvement in Health Care, GOAL/QPC, Florida Power and Light, and other leaders in TQM (see the box on p. 185). This training included eight modules, with a programmed instruction module for self-paced learning designed for the team leaders.

SELECTION AND IMPLEMENTATION OF QUALITY IMPROVEMENT TEAMS

During the first year of implementation, it was determined that teams would be selected in three phases. A team application form and project selection checklist (see the box on p. 186) were developed, and ideas for teams were solicited from the TQM Steering Committee membership. Among the criteria for team formation were that the project must flow from one of the areas identified in the Matrix of Opportunities for Improvement (Fig. 17-2), the project must be of high priority to the health care customers, it must be supported by the appropriate affected managers, and it

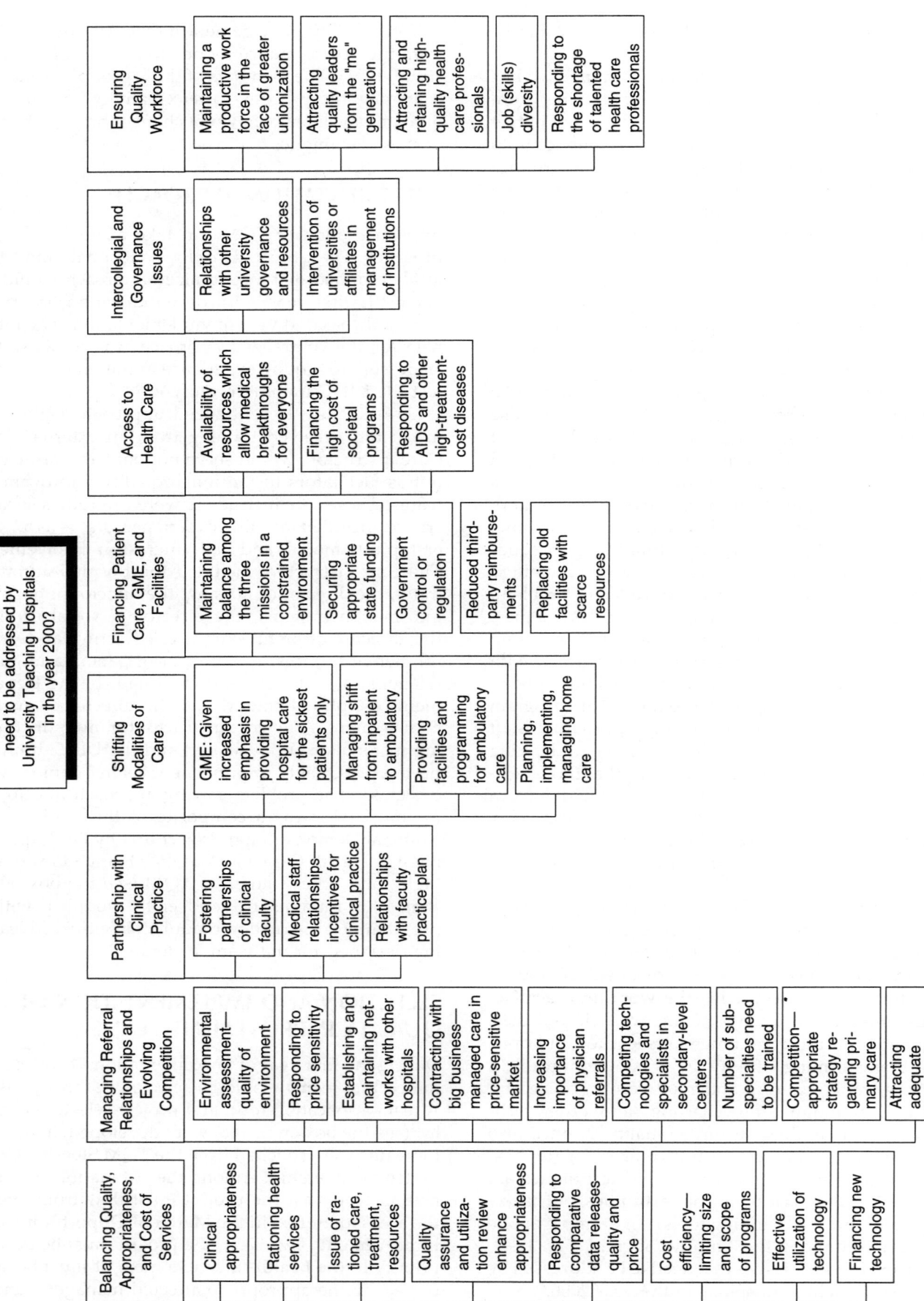

Fig. 17-1 Affinity diagram: issues that need to be addressed by university teaching hospitals.

Total Quality Management Quality Improvement Process		
1. Project Organization and Definition	**Quality Improvement Techniques***	
Goal: Develop a problem statement that describes the problem in terms of what it is specifically, where it occurs, when it happens, and its extent.		
Identify and list problems	Brainstorming Nominal group process Pareto Input-process-output-model	Flowchart Check Sheet
Determine customers	Brainstorming Input-process-output-model	Flowchart
Clarify customer expectations and establish quality indicators	Survey Focus group Brainstorming	Check sheet
Construct problem statement; identify gap between present and expected outcomes	Run chart Histogram Pie chart Stratification	Pareto chart Check sheet Flowchart
2. Diagnostic Journey		
Goal: Develop a complete picture of all the possible causes of the problem; then agree on the basic causes.		
Analyze symptoms of the problem	Brainstorming	
Formulate theories of causes	Nominal group technique Scatter diagram	
Test causes	Check sheet Pareto	
Identify root causes	Cause and effect diagram	
3. Remedial Journey		
Goal: Develop an effective and implementable solution and action plan.		
Consider alternative solutions	Brainstorming Force field analysis	
Design solutions and controls	Pie chart Bar graphs	
Address resistance to change	Flowchart Solution selection matrix	
4. Continuous Improvement Cycle		
Goal: Implement the solution and establish needed monitoring procedures and measures.		
Implement solutions	Pareto chart Histogram	
Check performance	Stratification Control chart	
Monitor control systems	Process capability	
From the University of Iowa Hospitals and Clinics **Note: Techniques are not all inclusive, nor need all be used in each step.**		

must have the potential for a 400 percent return on investment (ROI). The idea behind the 400 percent ROI was that teams should not be formed and trained, incurring institutional expense, if the problem to be addressed is not significant. And although most experts advise starting with functional teams, the UIHC determined that cross-functional teams would be where TQM could best impact change. It was also the intent of the Steering Committee and Executive Quality Council to form teams to address problems where traditional management methods had failed.

The first phase of team selection resulted in the submission of more than 30 ideas for teams. Using a rating tool and individual raters, the Executive Qual-

---

Total Quality Management: Project Selection Checklist

Instructions

If you have selected and defined an appropriate project for improvement, you should be able to check most, if not all, of the items listed below. If you cannot check all of these items, you may want to reevaluate your choice of project.

_____ 1. The process or project is directly related to the UIHC mission.

_____ 2. The process targeted for improvement has a direct impact on the UIHC's external/internal customers.

_____ 3. The process or work area has a lot of visibility.

_____ 4. All of the managers concerned with this process agree that it is important to study and improve this process.

_____ 5. Enough managers and staff involved in the project area will cooperate to make this project a success.

_____ 6. This process is not currently being changed in any way, nor is it scheduled to be overhauled in the near future.

_____ 7. The project is defined as one clearly defined process that has easily identified starting and ending points.

_____ 8. The process is not being studied by another group.

_____ 9. One cycle of the process is completed each day or two.

_____ 10. The problem statement for this team describes a problem to be studied, or an improvement opportunity, not a solution to be tried.

_____ 11. Data on the area is available or already collected.

From the University of Iowa Hospitals and Clinics

---

ity Council selected three projects. The first three teams were formed to address the problems of (1) lack of physician orders in the medical records, (2) cancellation of surgery because of incomplete preoperative work-ups, and (3) homegoing prescriptions for inpatients.

Three facilitators were identified from the core instructor group. Facilitators were then assigned to a problem area based on their lack of familiarity with the process under study. The rationale for this strategy was to eliminate any leadership bias and allow the facilitators to guide the team, composed of experts, in the process. Because the common and fatal flaw in many managers is "jumping to solutions," this approach was designed to decrease this possibility in the teams.

The facilitators met with the manager(s), who submitted the project ideas to select the appropriate team members. Members were selected on the basis of their expertise, interest, commitment and their knowledge of the process under study and availability. This time-consuming, careful process of team selection resulted in teams of about seven members. Each team included at least one physician and members representing at least five areas of the hospital. The team leaders were selected based upon their ability to work with group dynamics and knowledge of the process under study. The three team leaders were the director of medical records, a pharmacist, and a surgeon.

In order to accomplish training of the three teams together, team training was offered at 7 a.m. weekly

for 90 minutes. Training strategies included a small amount of didactic content but focused heavily on team learning either through assignments identified by the core instructor or led by the facilitators. Teams were able to progress at their own pace through the problem-solving process, and much of the team work was accomplished by individual and group "homework" accomplished away from the training sessions. Official team training ended after eight sessions, but the teams continued to meet with the facilitators to work through their problems.

The quality improvement team formed to address the problem of documentation of physician orders in the medical record was confronted with a hospital-wide challenge. Team members were selected on the basis of their knowledge, interest, availability, and clinical location. To provide this multidisciplinary coverage, the team included representatives from Medical Records, Medical Nursing, Pediatric Nursing, Laboratory, Respiratory Therapy, and Utilization Review, and a physician representative. Interested parties, identified as "sponsors," were kept appraised of team progress through minutes and regular team presentations.

The first order of business was to identify the customers affected by the process and their expectations. Following this, it was necessary to clearly identify the problem and its magnitude and the primary locations of the problem. A problem statement evolved after much discussion, as each team member had a different view of the problem. Only after looking carefully at the process was the team able to agree on a state-

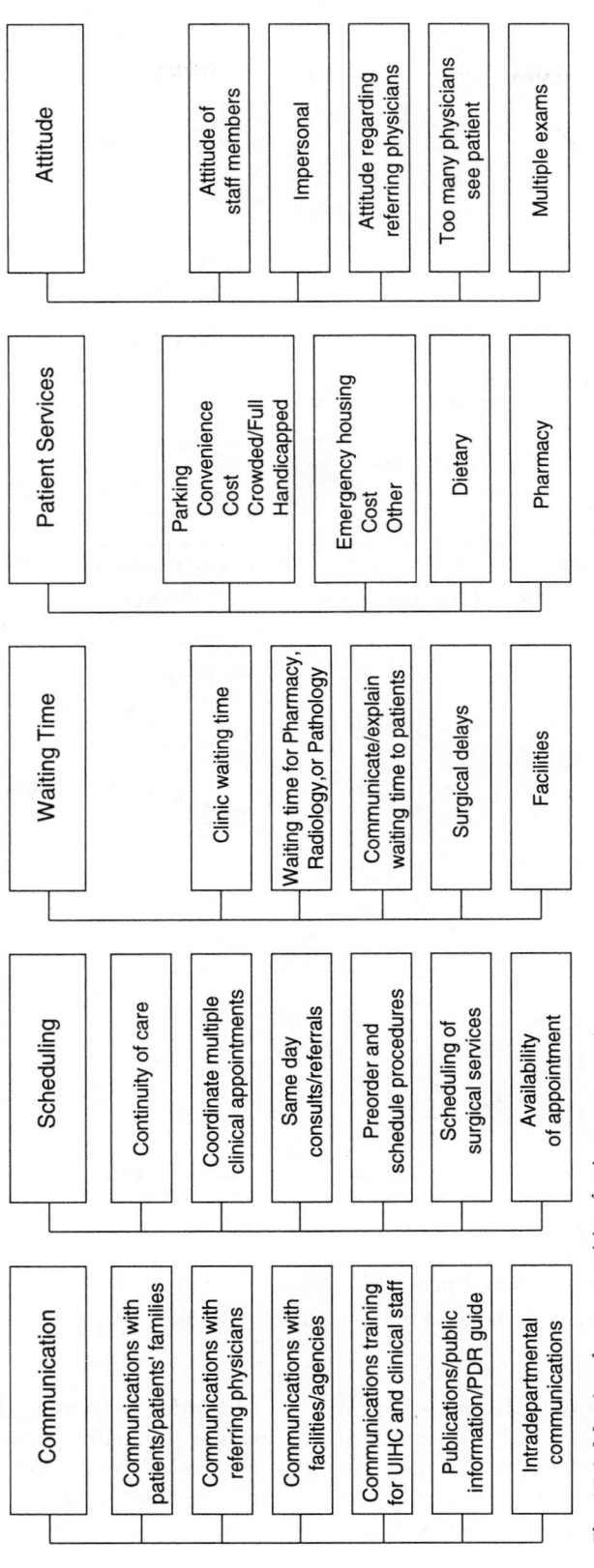

Fig. 17-2 Matrix of opportunities for improvement.

Communication

- Communications with patients/patients' families
- Communications with referring physicians
- Communications with facilities/agencies
- Communications training for UIHC and clinical staff
- Publications/public information/PDR guide
- Intradepartmental communications

Scheduling

- Continuity of care
- Coordinate multiple clinical appointments
- Same day consults/referrals
- Preorder and schedule procedures
- Scheduling of surgical services
- Availability of appointment

Waiting Time

- Clinic waiting time
- Waiting time for Pharmacy, Radiology, or Pathology
- Communicate/explain waiting time to patients
- Surgical delays
- Facilities

Patient Services

- Parking
  Convenience
  Cost
  Crowded/Full
  Handicapped
- Emergency housing
  Cost
  Other
- Dietary
- Pharmacy

Attitude

- Attitude of staff members
- Impersonal
- Attitude regarding referring physicians
- Too many physicians see patient
- Multiple exams

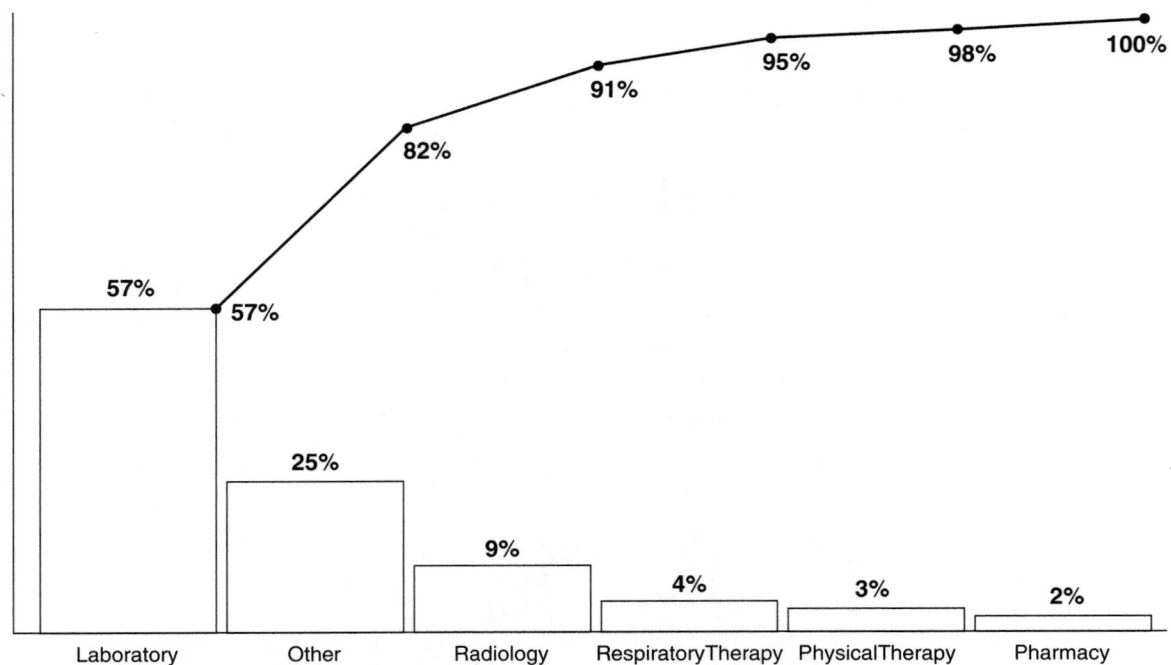

Fig. 17-3 Pareto chart: dollar amount lost per service category (7/01/91 to 3/31/92).

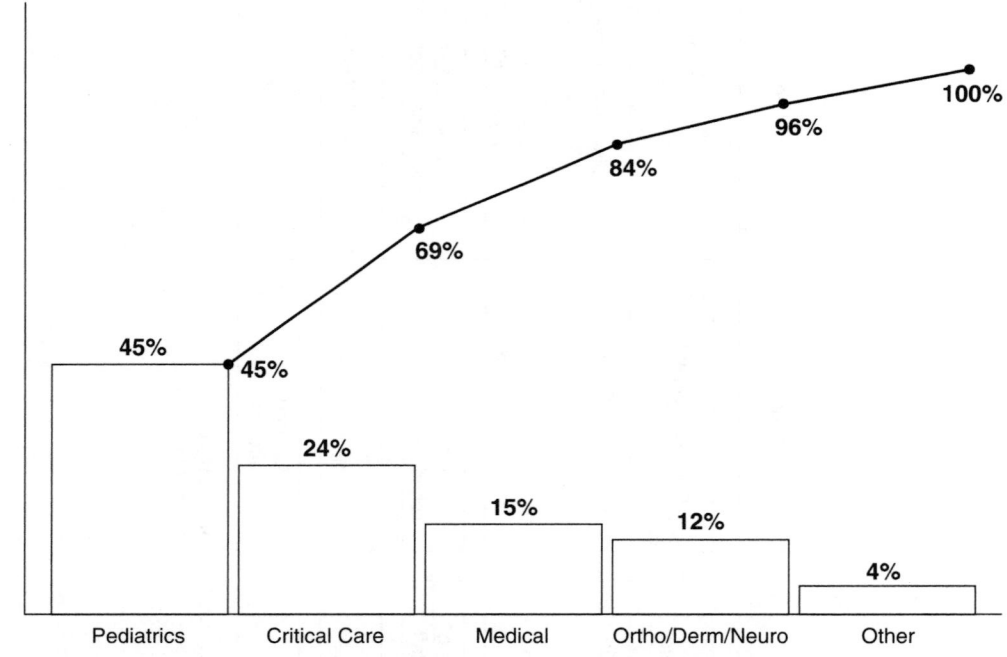

Fig. 17-4 Pareto chart: dollar amount lost per division fiscal year (7/01/91 to 3/31/92).

ment. The problem the team would address was that physician orders did not always get in the medical record. Though the treatment or laboratory test was actually performed on the patient, there was often no record of an order. Therefore, when a chart was audited by the Iowa Foundation for Medical Care for Medicare cost outlier payment, no order meant no reimbursement.

In order to localize the problem and determine its extent, the team audited 135 records during three quarters of the current fiscal year. The dollars or reimbursement denied, the service category involved (laboratory, pharmacy, radiology, respiratory therapy, etc.), and the specific clinical areas were identified. As noted in the Pareto charts (Figs. 17-3 and 17-4), 82 percent of the problem was with laboratory

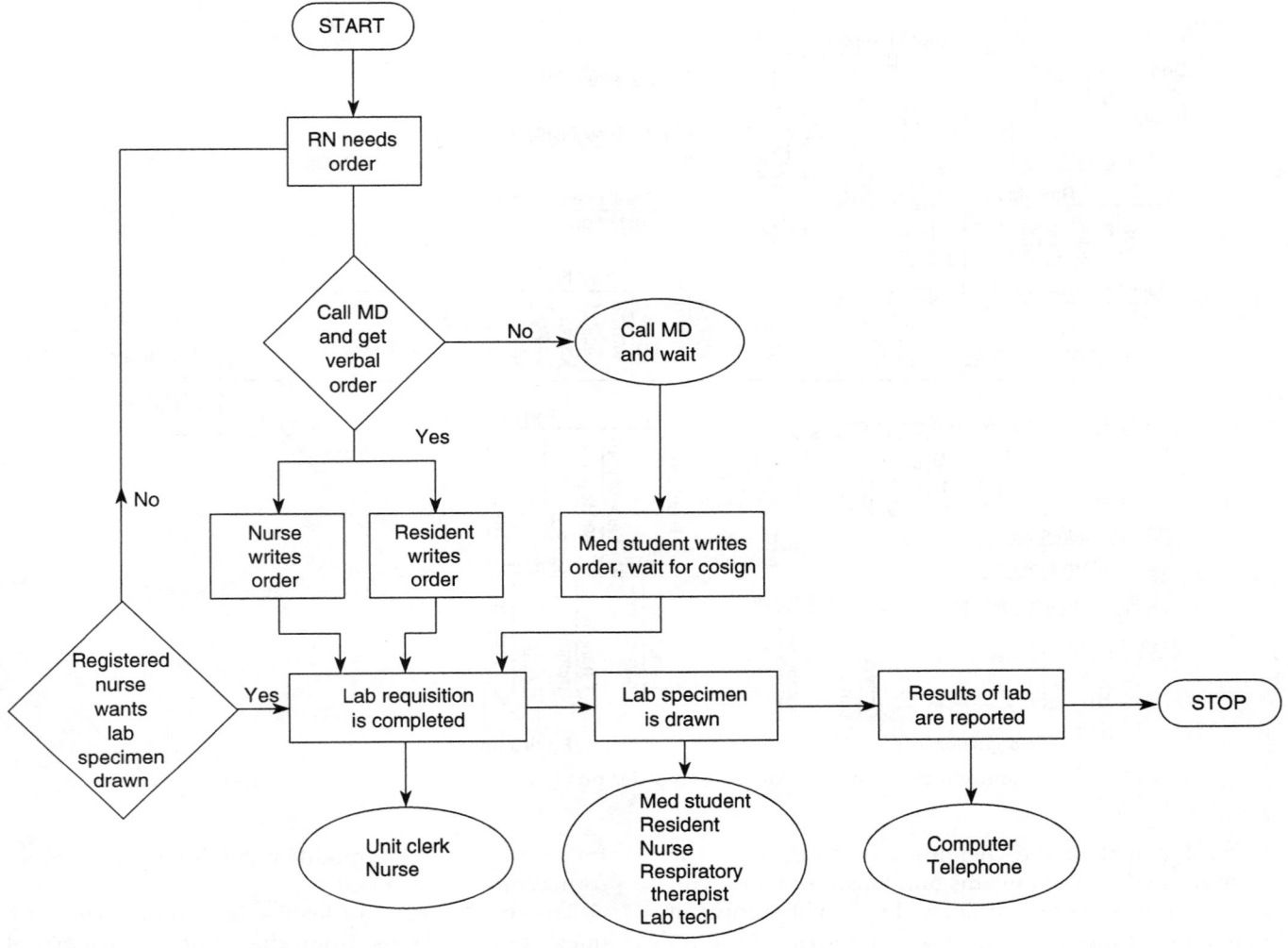

Fig. 17-5 Flowchart: registered nurse obtains order for a laboratory test.

and miscellaneous "other" orders. The "other" category was primarily composed of special care beds. The clinical areas where orders were not being written were Pediatrics and Critical Care. This, though logical because of the high acuity of the patients and the number of Medicare patients, was validated with data collection.

Because the primary problem area was identified as laboratory orders, the team's next step was to flowchart the process of how laboratory tests are ordered. Two of the team members visited all Pediatric and Medical Patient care units and interviewed staff on the units. From the information acquired, four flowcharts were generated; they illustrated how medical students, physicians, nurses, and respiratory therapists actually acquired lab tests. From Fig. 17-5, the reader will note that there are multiple pathways. One includes bypassing the medical record completely. The team members also discovered a tremendous variation from clinical unit to unit and among staff members. Addressing this variation and reduc-

ing it would be one of the goals of the team in identifying a new process.

Why was getting the order in the chart a problem? Identification of the underlying causes of the problem was a key component of team work. The team addressed this by developing a cause and effect (fishbone) diagram of the causes (Fig. 17-6). The team worked further to identify the root causes. The root causes are the primary or critical underlying causes. They were in the areas of role autonomy and diversity, the order form itself, lack of knowledge regarding the implications of not getting an order on the chart (lack of reimbursement, continuity of care, potential liability), and the process of taking verbal orders. Any solution the team would develop would need to address the root causes in order to be successful.

Finally the team was ready to begin formulating a solution selection matrix. The matrix would address the root causes and clarify what changes need to be made. But essential to the success of any new process

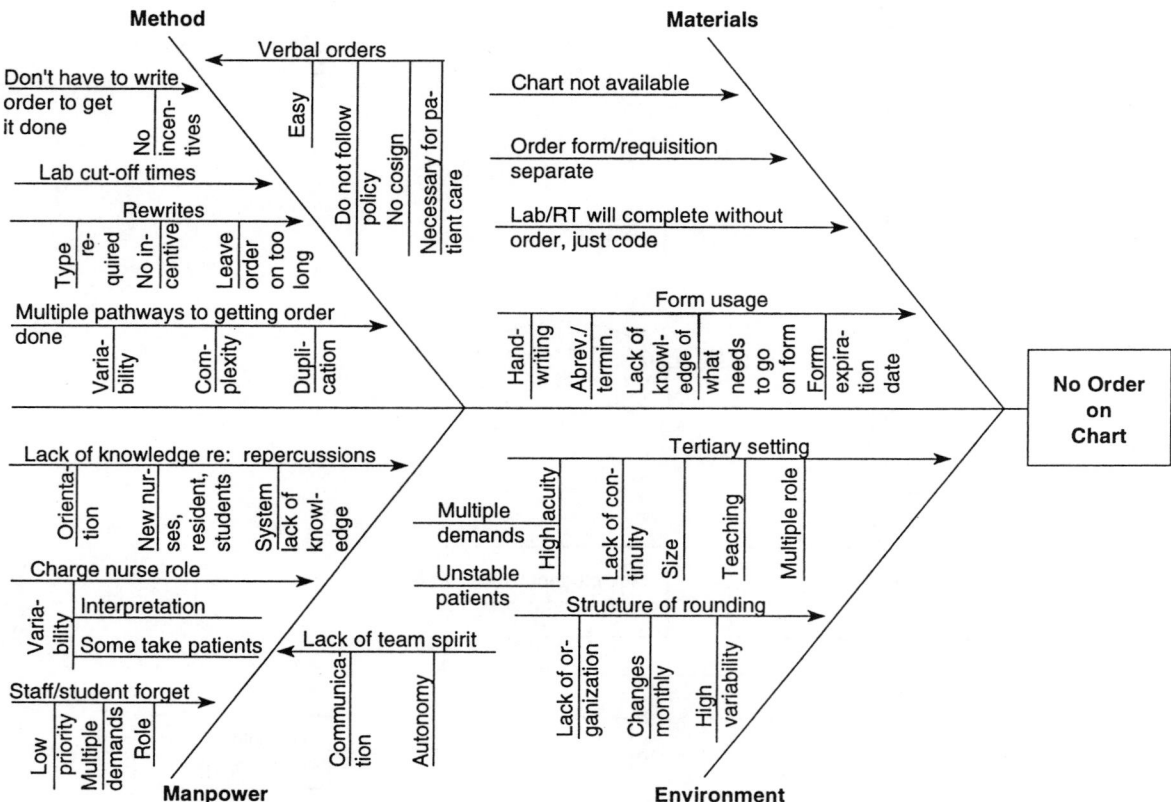

Fig. 17-6 Cause and effect (fishbone) diagram: no order on chart.

is involvement of the customers in its design. The team formed two miniteams and began to work with nurses on three clinical units to develop blueprints of new and simpler, yet effective, processes. These receptive clinical units would be the first to pilot the new system.

During the process, team enthusiasm has been very high. Team work required numerous small group or individual homework assignments, which were always addressed with a high degree of accountability. Team members were struck by the power of the process, and were kept on track by their facilitator, who assisted with group dynamics and helped with training the team in new tools and techniques. During team presentations, interest throughout the hospital was high, and team members sensed tremendous support and reward for their work. Though the process does have frustrating moments, and is not without political overtones, one team member summed it up by saying, "It works!"

The second phase of team selection took a different tack. In fact, some famous words of Ralph Waldo Emerson, "The voyage of the best ship is a zigzag line of a hundred tacks," generally served as the style of decision making. Each time, experience, learning, and the new perspective gained often led to a change in strategy. Instead of maintaining a direct approach—the traditional planning style—UIHC ef-

forts and plans were modified continually as new information was obtained.

The second phase of team selection involved a request for proposals from the entire management staff. Nearly 40 proposals were submitted. Three proposals that addressed highly different areas, and involved new clusters of staff, were selected. The teams formed to address two areas in the Department of Housekeeping focused on increasing customer awareness and instituting a self-directed work team approach. The third team would address increasing efficiency in the Department of Dietary.

As mentioned earlier, the first year of implementation at the UIHC took a centralized approach. During the second year, the process would need to be decentralized in order to allow greater involvement and encourage the departments to identify and prioritize opportunities for improvement.

Decentralization will involve identifying approximately 30 professional and clinical staff for core instructor training. Staff selected for training will need to meet the following criteria:

1. To have experience and great interest in teaching
2. To be viewed as a role model, exemplifying the management style and principles of TQM; participative; viewed as a leader and change agent
3. To be willing and able to commit to teaching and facilitating two teams per year

University of Iowa Hospitals & Clinics
Targeted Opportunities for Continuous Quality Improvement
Cost of Poor Quality (COPQ)   **Budget Form B-1**

_____ Budgetary Unit
1992-93

Due Dates
Dept to FM & C: 1/29/92
FM & C to Adm: 2/09/92
Adm to FM & C: 2/28/92

A | Opportunity for Improvement:

B | Service ("Customer") Requirements:

C | Costs of Poor Quality:

D | Improvement Goal:

PREPARED BY: _____ Date: _____
PREPARED BY: _____ Date: _____
Admin. Staff _____ Date: _____ ☐ APPROVED ☐ NOT APPROVED
Sr. Admin./Deputy Admin. _____ Date: _____ ☐ APPROVED ☐ NOT APPROVED
Administrator _____ Date: _____ ☐ APPROVED ☐ NOT APPROVED

COMMENTS:_____

Financial Management Use Only

Fig. 17-7 Targeted opportunities for CQI form.

4. Supported by one's department head and recommended by peer group

THE BUDGET CYCLE AND TQM

Although TQM focuses on improving processes, another facet is understanding the concept of the cost of poor quality and ways to decrease these costs throughout the organization. Because health care organizations are functioning under restrictive reimbursement regulations and federal and state cutbacks, and with health care costs approaching 14 percent of the gross national product, there is an increasing pressure to measure and control costs. Exploring the cost of poor quality in every area is a way to increase cost effectiveness and efficiency as well as free up dollars for new initiatives.

This concept, and the drive for continuous quality improvement, served as a catalyst for another organizational change. Previous to TQM, the budget cycle began with goals and objectives, requests for new initiatives, and general operating expenses. During the first year of implementation, the budget cycle was dramatically modified to produce an ideological change and further involve the various cost centers in quality improvement.

This ideological change was based on the following premises. Total quality management provides a fundamentally different view of the relationship between cost and quality. Quality health care does not cost more; in fact, it costs less. Over the years, many programs and systems have evolved that have not been efficient, effective, or targeted to meet the evolving expectations of those we serve, our customers. Health care delivery and its support systems that do not function at the highest level or are not targeted to meet valid and measurable service requirements generate something called the "cost of poor quality."

The cost of poor quality (COPQ) is the sum of all costs that would be eliminated if there were no quality problems. In industry, the COPQ has been estimated to be as much as 25 cents of every dollar of operating expenses. At the UIHC, managers were asked to reexamine work design and question whether existing systems and processes were meeting the expectations of those served and whether they functioned in a cost-effective and efficient manner. During this first cycle of change, managers were asked to focus on two areas within the COPQ: internal and external failure costs.

Internal failure costs are costs caused by system inefficiencies, inaccuracies, or dissatisfaction such as

TABLE 17-1 Targeted Opportunities for Continuous Quality Improvement at UIHC

Themes	Select Excellent Examples	Poor Examples
Work redesign Reducing overtime Reducing internal failure costs, such as medication errors, scheduling errors, infections, etc. Increasing patient access to services Reduction of waiting time Reduction of unnecessary lab tests and rework Reduction of discharge delays Improving the capture of patient charges Decreasing lost referrals	Development of a Care Map for cesarean-birth patients to decrease variation in LOS, tests, and procedures, and to increase efficiency and effectiveness of health care delivery A reduction of routine, often unnecessary, daily lab tests Reduction in repeat imaging of patients; cost of film and processing, wear on equipment, expense in additional treatment units, treatment delays, patient and physician dissatisfaction Projected reduction of overtime by $34,500 Reduction of lost referrals by establishing centralized scheduling function using existing staff Reduction of discharge delays and staff time, and improvement of the documentation process Reduction of inventory carrying costs, printing costs; and elimination of obsolete products	Requests for new technology that did not include a cost-benefit analysis Requests for equipment to increase efficiency that did not explore work redesign Plans for improvement that were not unit or departmentally focused Plans that blamed another area for their problems Remodeling requests

lapses, errors, product failure inside the hospital, mistakes in patient care, staff turnover, patient falls, nosocomial infections, excessive waiting times, litigation, poor surgical quality, and customer complaints. These costs can be in the areas of content and delivery quality. *Content* quality refers to the technical quality; *delivery* quality is the manner in which the services are delivered.

External failure costs are caused by defective or nonconforming products from outside the hospital reaching the customer. Examples include surgical packs not containing all components, lack of sterility in product, damaged products, and delay in receipt of products. These costs can also be incurred in the areas of content and delivery quality.

All cost centers, over three hundred, were asked to brainstorm with their staff, identify costs of poor quality, and select one for improvement in the coming fiscal year. The managers were then asked to submit their ideas on the form provided (see Fig. 17-7). The number of responses and their variety and creativity were outstanding. A description of some of the ideas submitted is depicted in Table 17-1.

It is important to note that requests for improvement opportunities did not require absolute quantification in dollars to demonstrate improvement. For example, it is difficult to determine the cost of individual complaints for a service area. What can be quantified is the number of complaints and how they decrease with process im-

provement. One of the dangers of TQM is to focus too much on cost at the expense of service and work environment improvement. It is one way to disenchant staff about the process.

CONCLUSION

TQM is a long-range strategy for an institution. Planning generally involves one year; implementation and roll-out require a three-to-five year process. TQM is not a program or a project, but a process of organizational change and human resource development. This highly dynamic process lends itself well to changing environmental demands and the increasingly sophisticated expectations of those served by the organization.

The focus is on meeting strategic targets for improvement identified by those we serve. TQM builds on existing strength yet allows for innovation at the grassroots level in order to design services and foster a work environment that better meets the needs of patients, families, students and staff.

REFERENCES

Beer M, R A Eisenstat, B Spector (1990, Nov/Dec): Why change programs don't produce change, *Harvard Business Review*, 151-166.

Fritz R (1991): *Creating*, New York, Fawcett-Columbine Book, Ballantine.

IMPROVING QUALITY AND PERFORMANCE: LESSONS LEARNED

Patricia Schroeder

Quality improvement remains a new science in its applications to health care. Early lessons can, however, guide future efforts. Much has been learned from the work of those organizations that have already attempted QI implementation. The chapters in this book have described efforts that were viewed as successful, that made tangible and intangible advances for quality within the organization.

Despite these positive results, many health care organizations are failing in their attempts to implement QI. Some experts predict that fewer than 20 percent of all hospitals will succeed in QI efforts (Sahney, 1992, James, 1992). While such a grim outlook may be premature, or even extreme, this prediction suggests that there is much more to QI implementation than what may appear at first glance. True success changes the organization down to its core, and such change does not come easily or quickly.

How can one ensure at the outset that one's efforts will result in the organization's successful transformation to QI? The answers may be found in looking at early efforts and defining key strategies that worked, as well as hazards or obstacles that thwarted quality initiatives.

KEY STRATEGIES FOR SUCCESS

The preceding examples of successful QI efforts share a number of common features. Obviously, all were from hospitals, all projects cited were led by nurses, and all were part of a larger, organizationwide, long-range commitment to quality. A closer look, however, clarifies several other common attributes that were central to success.

Project Selection

The selection of early quality improvement projects is critical. Groups selected projects dealing with high-priority issues: those that addressed long-term, irritating problems or projects that carried the potential of great benefit. Projects were also highly visible and meaningful, with progress toward resolution being apparent and of benefit to many within the organization.

Collaboration

All the projects reported here required both intradepartmental and interdepartmental collaboration. Re-

ports spoke to a growing team spirit, greater awareness of the roles of others, and greater willingness to identify shared solutions. Quality improvement projects broadened perspectives of all involved and increased sensitivities to the work of others.

Empowerment

Work on quality improvement initiatives helped staff members live the concepts of empowerment. That is, rather than talking about empowerment, or learning about it, groups were confronted with the pain and pleasure of accountability. Decisions took longer to reach, and outcomes were not always what each group member had originally hoped for, but there was widespread agreement that a sound rationale underpinned the decisions.

Innovation/Creativity

Quality improvement requires innovation and creativity. Group members were required to look beyond stale, Band-Aid solutions. Greater awareness of root causes of problems and multidimensional processes spurred new ideas and approaches. Progress toward improvements also required multiple strategies and actions on the part of all involved.

Time and Support

Improving quality requires time and support. In all instances of QI project success, staff members were required to spend time on the project. Some spoke of "sacred time" regarding project meetings. Freeing up time for this work required support from managers and colleagues alike. In today's busy health care organizations, "extra" time is an unavailable commodity. Yet, in these instances, improvement in quality was considered of primary importance—a means to an end in providing better care and service.

PITFALLS OF QUALITY IMPROVEMENT EFFORTS

Even the most successful QI initiatives encounter pitfalls along the way. Some pitfalls are minor and, while throwing the group a bit off course, are easily rectified. In fact, they help groups to refocus, recommit, and learn more about the QI process for future work. Other pitfalls are major, resulting in a long-term standstill or, worse, regression. Frustration and cynicism peak, and quality improvement appears to be a passing fad that has lost support.

Organizations early to implement QI initiatives have taught many lessons about common pitfalls to avoid.

QI is a science and an art, but it is not a religion.

It is not uncommon to hear QI concepts presented with religious zeal, emphasizing the importance of "true believers," "moments of truth," and "total commitment" (Zemke, 1992, p. 8). Theorists become prophets, whose concepts must be followed without question. Followers exchange critical thinking for blind obedience.

We are learning, however, that even the strongest of beliefs will not change an organization. Effectiveness requires strategy and actions.

Actions do not always equal progress.

In many organizations, early QI efforts create much activity. Many organizations talk about quality. Education in quality is prevalent. Many become involved. But the knowledge that QI implementation takes years makes us too complacent with a lack of real progress. We mistake activity for forward movement, and we fail to recognize that little progress is made toward change, little benefit is obtained for the effort and money expended, and little or no application of QI concepts occurs beyond the committee meetings and project teams.

We are learning that creating a busy quality agenda does not ensure progress toward culture change. Strategic planning and leadership are required to move the quality initiative forward, to change the status quo, and to imprint the quality-oriented mission on the minds, attitudes, and behaviors of all employees.

Quality improvement creates a power shift.

Empowerment has been a buzzword in health care for many years. Its use goes beyond quality improvement initiatives. The concept of empowerment sounds appealing, painting a picture of employees who are more self-directed, accountable, and effective. Yet, too often there is a lack of recognition that as decision making shifts hands, so does power. In some organizations, leaders would promote empowerment but would not choose to support, or would even undermine, the power shift.

Placing greater decision-making responsibility in the hands of the front line produces consequences. These results need to be supported, even nurtured, by leaders if the employee is to continue making decisions and taking actions.

It is critical that the organization help employees receive the knowledge and skills necessary for critical decision making. Education will also be needed for managers and other leaders if they are to thrive in the realities of an empowered environment.

Quality improvement creates stress for middle managers.

Quality improvement literature speaks frequently of the new roles for senior management, as well as the new roles for the front-line employees, but there is little that directly describes the resulting new role for middle managers. Much about the role can, however, be inferred. For example, business literature speaks frequently about the benefit of flatter organizations, those with fewer layers of managers between the top and the bottom. Examples of specific projects support this premise, reporting dramatic improvements in service and substantial cost savings, created by eliminating management layers.

Quality improvement in today's environment requires new skills for managers. Shared decision making, greater collaboration, a focus on customer-defined quality, and greater cost efficiency are some of today's challenges. At a time when managers may feel more vulnerable than ever, they need to learn new skills for leadership. These expectations create a time of great stress and confusion. To compound the dilemma, while senior managers often speak about new QI approaches to leadership, the norms of the organization may continue to expect and reward old behaviors.

Great attention must be focused on the role of middle managers, and the expectations of them in a QI-oriented organization. Education and support must be provided to smooth the transition of these times.

Quality improvement can create a shift from clinical quality to systems perspectives.

Traditional quality assurance programs were primarily clinical in focus. This outlook reflected accrediting expectations, mandating providers of clinical services to monitor and evaluate quality. Few nonclinical (or nonmandated) departments carried out quality assurance efforts. Given QI's roots in manufacturing and systems applications, early QI efforts have frequently focused on service aspects of health care organizations. For example, waiting time, access to equipment, and availability of services are common systems applications of QI techniques. Such issues are important for internal and external customers alike, but are less likely to improve clinical outcomes than they are to increase satisfaction of patients and employees.

It is essential that quality efforts seek some balance in the effect on clinical and service outcomes in addressing processes. Improvement in care and service, as well as in processes and outcomes is necessary to better meet the needs of health care consumers.

Data access is essential for QI effectiveness.

Understanding of and belief in QI concepts was initially considered the most vital part of making quality happen. Experience has taught that data access and information systems are equally critical. Quality will not improve without measurement and data to reflect current status and ongoing progress. Most health care agencies collect tremendous amounts of data and have some available computer assistance. Yet these same agencies too often realize that they have collected data that are meaningless in today's customer-focused perspectives.

Much work will be needed to develop meaningful measurement tools and methods, and to establish integrated automated systems useful in improving quality.

Quality improvement requires ongoing commitment and visibility.

Initial QI implementation is an exciting and creative time. The early enthusiasm is contagious and often generates early gains. Senior managers are visible and vocal in their support of QI. Communications about early efforts typically pervade the organization.

Enthusiasm can easily wane after the first few years. Senior managers may begin to devote time to other pressing issues, believing that QI is self-perpetuating once initiated. Frustration can ensue when "easy" problems have not been solved or when unrealistic expectations for QI have not been met.

Times of waning enthusiasm require a refocusing of efforts and recommitment to the process. Organizations must again find creative ways to communicate their commitment to QI and to make achievements more visible. Strategic plans must reflect continued expectations for progress. Communication channels must be flooded with reports of successful and enthusiastic efforts to improve quality.

Quality must be rewarded.

It is well understood that to reinforce widespread change, one must support and reward the new behaviors or the performance desired. This is easier to say than it has been to effect in the name of quality improvement.

Attempts at establishing new reward systems have received mixed reviews. For example, some quality-specific reward systems are based on the use of token rewards, such as recognition certificates, gift certificates, and pins or coins. Anecdotally, in a practice setting they have been described by different members of the same staff as anywhere from "the most positive thing I've seen in a long time" to "a professionally offensive token." Responses to other types of reward systems have been equally mixed.

We must return to very basic questions in order to create effective approaches to rewarding quality. These questions include:

What aspect of quality will be rewarded?
How and when will this aspect of quality be measured?
What do employees see as rewarding?

COMPONENTS OF EFFECTIVE QUALITY SYSTEMS

Experience in applications of QI to health care has taught us that, irrespective of strategies or pitfalls, certain components will always be necessary to create an effective quality system. These include:

- Standards and guidelines specifying processes of care and service within the organization
- Individual performance feedback/appraisal mechanisms
- Intradisciplinary quality assessment and improvement approaches
- Interdisciplinary quality assessment and improvement approaches
- A focus on quality by the organizational culture
- Interorganizational benchmarking approaches.

Early lessons regarding the implementation of QI and the relationships between these components will provide great help to the organizations that follow. But there is much yet to learn if we are to increase beyond 20 percent the number of health care organizations successfully implementing QI.

Many deep questions about quality improvement remain.

- How can we most effectively adapt QI concepts and methods to the nuances and demands of today's health care settings?
- How can we most efficiently reorganize health care organizations to better meet consumer needs, when current regulations and reimbursement structures function in contradiction to QI methods?
- Is successful implementation of QI related to the societal culture in which the organization functions, and if so, how does one deal with organizations and employees who bring ethnically diverse backgrounds to the workplace?
- Are QI concepts and methods the magical answer for creating the new organization, or can improvements of equal magnitude be possible through the presence of consumer-oriented values, creative and committed "key players," and sophisticated data systems?

These questions and many others will continue to pervade our thoughts, research, literature, and experiences. Perhaps this book succeeds in raising more questions about QI than answers. American health care organizations have embarked on an attempt to create change of a magnitude that has never been seen before. We seek to change the focus, functions, and culture of our settings for health care delivery. The extent to which we will succeed remains to be seen.

The extent to which we have the opportunity for QI also remains to be seen. While many from the manufacturing sector claim widespread support for QI, some are now saying that tough economic times require organizations to cut costs first, and worry about quality later. Stratton (1992) draws the contrasts between Ford Motor Company's slow steady approach to improvement and General Motors' approach, in an effort to catch up to others in the industry, of cutting the work force first, then improving quality. He asks, "Has the time for new quality improvement efforts passed? If a company isn't 5 to 10 years into a well-developed quality improvement process, should it give up?" (Stratton 1992, p. 5)

CONCLUSION

Many changes are on the horizon for health care. Quality improvement can be a guiding force during these times of transitions. QI must never be considered merely a new label, task, or a defined program. Quality improvement is a mindset and an expectation that must pervade all people, plans, and processes within an organization. To the extent it is less it undermines its capacity to succeed.

REFERENCES

James B (1992, May 28): Presentation, Annual meeting of grant recipients, Robert Wood Johnson Foundation "Improving the Quality of Hospital Care" grant, Salt Lake City, Utah.

Sahney V (1992, May 14): Presentation, Implementation, observed barriers, and management of continuous quality improvement, National Quality of Care Forum, Morristown, NJ.

Stratton B (1992, February): Has time run out for a better idea? *Quality Progress*, p. 5.

Zemke R (1992, February): Faith, hope, and TQM, *Training*, p. 8.

GLOSSARY

affinity diagram A tool used to identify patterns and categories in broad or complex issues.

benchmarking The process of using industry leaders and the best demonstrated levels of excellence as the unit of comparison for one's own agency, with an ongoing effort to achieve and surpass that performance.

brainstorming A creative approach to engage all group members in sharing suggestions, options, and ideas in an open, nonjudgmental environment.

cause and effect diagram A tool used to help identify the multiple causes of any final result, outcome, or problem. Also called a *fishbone diagram* because of its appearance.

common cause variation The spectrum of outputs or results of a process that are related to the process itself.

control chart A tool used to demonstrate trends in output data over time, within the context of pre-established, statistically determined upper and lower control limits.

data Facts, or a collection of facts, used to make a judgment.

deploy To strategically disseminate, as in allocating responsibility for aspects of the quality plan to many people.

deployment chart A tool used to link the steps of a process with the persons responsible for them.

fishbone diagram See *cause and effect diagram.*

flowchart A tool used to create a picture or step-by-step description of a process.

focus group An assembly of individuals meeting to provide feedback on a predetermined topic with which they have some experience.

histogram A tool (graph) used to demonstrate frequency distribution.

indicator A measurement tool or statement used to assess a characteristic of quality.

Ishikawa diagram See *cause and effect diagram.*

key processes Sets of activities that are particularly important to an organization because of their impact, cost, or relevance to the consumer.

monitoring The process of data collection over time.

multivoting A selection process used by a group to reduce a long list of options to a reasonable number.

nominal group process An activity used to generate ideas within a group that is less "free flowing" than, for instance, brainstorming.

paradigm The collection of fundamental beliefs that underlie the way things are done; a model or approach.

Pareto chart A tool (bar graph) used to prioritize action, by visually highlighting and separating the "vital few from the trivial many."

PDCA cycle A model for planning and problem solving, consisting of the steps Plan, Do, Check, Act. Also called the *Shewhart cycle.*

performance assessment and improvement The label coined by the JCAHO that uses an organized problem-solving approach to enhance the impact of structure, process, and outcome to improve achievement of patients, practitioners, and organizations (customers).

processes Series or set of activities carried out to achieve a certain end result.

process variation The spectrum of end results (output) of a set of activities. Consists of common cause variation and special cause variation.

run chart Tool (graph) that depicts data over time, and allows reader to identify trends

scatter diagram Tool (graph) used to identify relationships between two factors or variables. Also called a *scattergram.*

Shewhart cycle See PDCA Cycle.

special cause variation Variation in process output that is caused by unusual circumstances.

197

statistical process control The use of mathematics and measurement to study and strategically direct the way work is carried out.

tree diagram A tool used to break down a goal, problem, or idea into manageable tasks or action steps.

trend A pattern in data that points to its meaning, or to the need for other data collection, analysis, and/or action.

trend chart See *run chart.*

INDEX

A

Accountability
    at Johns Hopkins Hospital, 172-173
    at Medical University of South Carolina Medical
        Center, 151
    for quality, 15
Action plan development
    at Johns Hopkins Hospital, 176-177, 178f
    at St. Vincent Medical Center, 100
Affinity diagram, 42-43, 44f
American Nurses Association (ANA), 62
Automation needs, in quality improvement, 13

B

Baldrige, Malcolm, National Quality Award, 16-17
Bellin Hospital (Green Bay, Wisconsin), 116, 117f
    improvement team at, 116-118
    steps in process
        act: hold gain; repeat cycle, 126-127f, 128f
        assembling team, 118
        check: determining if intended need met, 124-126
        do: implementing change on pilot basis, 123-124,
            125f, 126f
        establishing real causes of problem, 122, 123ft
        locating and isolating problem, 118-120f, 119f
        plan: change, 122-123, 124f
        recognizing and celebrating, 127-128f
        understanding cause of variation, 120, 121f, 122
        verifying problem exists, 118
Benchmarking
    application of, at Lakeland (Florida) Regional Medical
        Center, 83
    interorganizational, in quality improvement, 10
Beth Israel Hospital (Boston), quality initiative at,
    137-140f, 139f, 141f, 142-145, 142f, 143f, 144f
Bon Secours Hospital (Grosse Pointe, Michigan)
    merging of quality assurance and quality
        improvement at, 85-86
        data collection, 87
        decubitus protocol, 91
        documentation, 89, 90f, 91
        education, 93
        nosocomial decubiti as indicator, 86-87
        nursing department involvement, 86
        quality improvement tools used, 88-89
        skin integrity task force, 91, 92f, 93f
        unit-based quality assurance council
        involvement, 89
    quality assurance structure at, 85
Boss, as hero in traditional organizations, 54
Bottom line fixation, in traditional organizations, 54
Boundaries, collaboration across, 13
Brainstorming, 29-30
    application of, at Medical University of South
        Carolina Medical Center, 152f
Bureaucratic mindsets, in traditional organizations, 54

C

Cause and effect diagram, 36, 37f, 38
    applications of
        at Beth Israel Hospital (Boston), 140, 141f
        at Froedtert Memorial Lutheran Hospital, 166f,
        167, 167f
        at Johns Hopkins Hospital, 174
        at Medical University of South Carolina Medical
        Center, 152f
        at University of Iowa Hospitals and Clinics, 189,
        190f
Change
    creating through quality initiative, 137-140f, 139f,
        141f, 142f, 142-145, 143f, 144f
    evaluating process, at New York Hospital, 134, 135f
    need for, at New York Hospital, 131-132
    precipitating, in organizational conduct, 18-19t
    process of, at New York Hospital, 133-134
Check sheets, 24-25, 27f
Cleveland Clinic Foundation, 102, 103f, 104t
    patient satisfaction as indicator of quality at, 105-107,
        108f, 109t, 111-115, 112t, 113t
    quality improvement and 10-step process at, 104-105
Collaboration, in quality improvement, 7, 13, 147, 193
Commitment, in quality improvement, 13, 14, 57
Communication
    in quality improvement, 59, 147
    in traditional organizations, 55-56
Continuous quality improvement, 5-6
    incident reporting within framework of, 130-134,
        133f, 135f, 136
Control, new definitions of, in quality improvement,
    58-59
Control charts, 31-32, 33f, 38f
    application of, at Bon Secours Hospital (Grosse
        Pointe, Michigan), 88f
Crosby, Philip, 4, 6, 170
Customer orientation, in quality improvement, 6
Customer requirements, establishing, at Johns Hopkins
    Hospital, 175-176t
Customer satisfaction, at Froedtert Memorial Lutheran
    Hospital, 158
Customer/supplier relationship, at Johns Hopkins
    Hospital, 175t

D

Data
    for quality initiative, 142-143f, 144f
    in quality improvement, 8-9, 13, 22-23
    using, 23
Data collection, 23
    at Bon Secours Hospital (Grosse Pointe, Michigan),
        87
Decubitus protocol, at Bon Secours Hospital (Grosse
    Pointe, Michigan), 91
Deming, W. Edwards, 4, 6, 8, 16, 48, 85, 130, 170